PROTEIN SCIENCE AND ENGINEERING

ANGIOTENSIN: NEW RESEARCH

Protein Science and Engineering

Additional books in this series can be found on Nova's website
under the Series tab.

Additional E-books in this series can be found on Nova's website
under the E-book tab.

Endocrinology Research and Clinical Developments

Additional books in this series can be found on Nova's website
under the Series tab.

Additional E-books in this series can be found on Nova's website
under the E-book tab.

PROTEIN SCIENCE AND ENGINEERING

ANGIOTENSIN: NEW RESEARCH

SŌTA HARADA
AND
ITSUKI MOI
EDITORS

Nova Science Publishers, Inc.
New York

For permission to use material from this book please contact us:
Telephone 631-231-7269; Fax 631-231-8175
Web Site: http://www.novapublishers.com

Library of Congress Cataloging-in-Publication Data

Angiotensin : new research / editors, Sota Harada and Itsuki Moi.
p. ; cm.
Includes bibliographical references and index.
ISBN 978-1-62100-773-9 (hardcover)
I. Harada, Sota. II. Moi, Itsuki.
[DNLM: 1. Angiotensins. QU 68]
572'.65--dc23
2011038153

Published by Nova Science Publishers, Inc. † New York

CONTENTS

PREFACE

The renin angiotensin system (RAS) maintains the cardiovascular homeostasis and is involved in the pathogenesis of several disorders related to heart and kidney. There are several peptides under RAS in which angiotensin (Ang) II is the major contributor. In this book, the authors present topical research on angiotensin. Some of the topics discussed include the influence of renin-angiotensin-aldosteron system genes on hypertrophy development in hypertrophic caradiomyopathy; cardiac renin angiotensin system and exercise training; the role of the counter-regulatory renin angiotensin system in the heart and new roles for the neuropeptide angiotensin II.

Chapter 1 - Left ventricular hypertrophy (LVH) is a harbinger of morbidity and mortality, while its regression is associated with improved clinical prognosis. It is therefore imperative to understand the mechanisms that influence the development of hypertrophy and identify markers indicative of the risk of developing extensive hypertrophy, before its occurrence. The renin-angiotensin-aldostererone system (RAAS) is involved in LVH indirectly, through the key roles it plays in blood pressure regulation, and also directly, as some of its components also have direct hypertrophic effects; thus, this system has been the focus of numerous studies seeking genetic modifiers of LVH. Hypertrophic cardiomyopathy (HCM), an inherited condition, characterised by highly variable extent and distribution of LVH, which is caused primarily by defective sarcomeric proteins, is a disorder in which RAAS variants appear to modulate the extent of hypertrophy development. Early investigations of the role of this pathway in hypertrophy development, in the context of HCM, were largely centred on the genes encoding angiotensin converting enzyme and angiotensin II type 1 receptor, while downstream RAAS genes remained largely neglected. Recent association studies have, however, identified variants in additional RAAS genes that individually and collectively influence the penetrance and extent of LVH in HCM. Other investigations have provided evidence for local Angiotensin II generation, alternatively named tissue RAAS, which may also influence hypertrophy development. Furthermore, pharmacological inhibition of RAAS in anti-hypertrophic therapy has recently gained renewed interest with the development of a direct renin inhibitor. Taken together, these studies justify a renewed look at the individual and compounded effects of RAAS components on hypertrophy within the context of HCM. In this review the authors discuss the involvement of specific RAAS components in hypertrophy development and further highlight their hypertrophy modifying role in HCM with special emphasis on knowledge gained from association studies. To illustrate the value and possible caveats of the candidate gene association approach, the authors discuss results from the authors' research on family cohorts in which HCM-causing founder mutations segregate. The authors also discuss the need for studies that comprehensively cover genes comprising the RAAS to describe a subset of functional RAAS variants that work together to confer an increased risk for hypertrophy development in HCM patients.

Chapter 2 - Cardiac hypertrophy is a central feature in both pathological and physiological remodeling. In cardiovascular disease, pathological remodeling with hypertrophy or dilatation leads to heart dysfunction and failure, and is at least partly caused by altered cardiac gene expression and molecular phenotype. Although the response compensates for reduced contractility in the short term, the long term effect is progressive dysfunction. In contrast, physiological hypertrophy and remodeling induced by exercise training (also known as athletes' heart) is considered beneficial, as it supports the increased O_2 demand. Exercise induces functional and structural changes in the cardiovascular system and the type of training (endurance vs. strength training) is of special importance as shown in the meta-analysis by Pluim et al. which confirmed the hypothesis of two different forms: the endurance trained and the strength trained heart. Endurance-trained hearts show an eccentric hypertrophy, whereas a concentric hypertrophy develops in strength-trained hearts. Within a few weeks of training such structural changes may occur but in both cases there is no sign of loss of ventricular function as observed in decompensated cardiac hypertrophy. As a result of these structural adaptations cardiac output rises significantly when compared with that of untrained individuals. The structural cardiac remodeling induced by exercise training can be dependent of local or systemic factors.

Chapter 3 - The counter-regulatory renin angiotensin system (RAS) is centred around the angiotensin converting enzyme (ACE) homologue ACE2. ACE2 metabolizes angiotensin (Ang) II to Ang-(1-7), decreasing AngII and increasing Ang-(1-7) levels. ACE2 also converts AngI to Ang-(1-9), which can be further converted to Ang-(1-7) via ACE-mediated metabolism. Ang-(1-7) has been shown to counteract AngII actions mainly via stimulating the protooncogene Mas receptor. Thus the ACE2/Ang-(1-7)/Mas axis has received much recent focus as a potential therapeutic target in cardiovascular disease. In experimental models the heart has been a major focus of this research in pathophysiologies such as cardiac remodelling following experimental myocardial infarction, ischaemia reperfusion injury, cardiac hypertrophy in aortic banding and AngII infusion models and heart failure. In these settings administration of the peptide Ang-(1-7), or over-expression of ACE2 via somatic gene transfer or transgenic strategies mediates clear therapeutic benefit in reversing many of the phenotypes in these models. This experimental evidence is supported by clinical research which has shown that in patients on ACE inhibitors or angiotensin type 1 receptor antagonists ACE2 and Ang-(1-7) levels are upregulated, suggesting they may contribute to the therapeutic benefit of these drugs in patients following myocardial infarction and in heart failure. While these studies have provided clear evidence for ACE2 and Ang-(1-7) as potential therapeutic targets there still remains much to be understood about the counter-regulatory RAS in the heart. Certain studies using transgenic or somatic overexpression of ACE2 in the heart have demonstrated a severe effect on cardiac conduction and promotion of cardiac fibrosis. Furthermore, recent new discoveries in the RAS may also play a role in the counter-regulatory RAS. For example, Ang-(1-9) may inhibit ACE-mediated generation of AngII by binding the same catalytic site as AngI. Furthermore, Ang-(1-9) reduces cardiac hypertrophy in rat myocardial infarction and has also been demonstrated to inhibit cardiomyocyte hypertrophy directly via the angiotensin type 2 receptor. Ang-(1-9) is produced at enhanced levels in cardiac lysates from heart failure patients. The role of the AngI metabolite Ang-(1-12) in cardiac pathophysiology is still unknown, however it has been shown to be a substrate for the production of AngII and Ang-(1-7) from cardiomyocytes. In this article the authors will review the current status of knowledge regarding the role of the counter-regulatory RAS in the heart and focus on the future of exciting research in this field which may further our understanding of cardiovascular disease and identify new targets for the development of novel therapies.

Chapter 4 - Angiotensin II (Ang II) is known as a peripheral hormone involved in the control of blood pressure and fluid homeostasis. The study and characterization of Ang II and its receptors in the brain has opened a new vision of its physiological role and also offers a variety of research fields. Ang II is involved in the response to stress, which stimulates the brain and the peripheral (hormonal) Ang II systems. Activation of brain angiotensin II AT_1 receptors is required for stress-induced hormone secretion, including CRH, ACTH, corticoids and vasopressin, and for stimulation of central sympathetic activity. The blockade of peripheral but also brain AT_1 receptors prevents the hormonal and sympathoadrenal response to isolation stress and prevents the formation of stress-induced gastric ulcers, through ischemia and inflammation. The AT_1 receptor antagonists prevent inflammation (neutrophil infiltration and increase in ICAM-1 and TNF-α) in the gastric mucosa and partially inhibit sympathoadrenal stimulation, without affecting the protective effect of glucocorticoid release during stress. The coordination of behavioral and autonomic responses to stress is partially under the control of extrahypothalamic, including cortical, CRF neurons expressing CRF_1 receptors. AT_1 receptor activation is thus also involved in the cortical decrease of CRF_1 binding induced by stress. A large number of studies have been conducted on the effect of drugs of abuse on hypothalamic and extrahypothalamic CRF systems in the brain and on the role of CRF in mediating the behavioral and physiological effects of drugs of abuse. It is also known that dopaminergic neurotransmission in the nucleus accumbens and caudate-putamen plays a critical role in the locomotor and stereotypic effects of psychostimulant drugs. Ang II receptors are found on the soma and terminals of dopaminergic neurons and it has been shown that Ang II, acting through its AT_1 receptors, facilitates the release of dopamine in the rat striatum in vitro and in vivo. Repeated exposure to amphetamine, as with most addictive drugs, results in progressive and lasting enhancement of their psychomotor and positive reinforcing effects. Neuroadaptive changes in mesotelencephalic dopaminergic projections play a key role in the induction and expression of amphetamine sensitization. Recently, the authors found evidence showing that brain AT_1 receptor activation is involved in the neuroadaptive changes induced by amphetamine. The results of studies on the physiological role of brain Ang II offer new pharmacological tools for the treatment of some stress-related disorders such as drug abuse.

Chapter 5 - Protein concentrates from ungerminated and germinated lima bean *Phaseolus lunatus* seed flours were hydrolyzed with alcalase 2.4L or pepsin-pancreatin sequential hydrolysis, and ACE inhibitory activity measured in the different hydrolysis treatments. A 2^3 factorial design with four replicates of the central trial was used. Evaluated factors were protein concentrate source (ungerminated seeds, PC_1; germinated seeds, PC_2), enzyme/substrate ratio E/S (1/50 or 1/10) and hydrolysis time (0.5 or 2.0 h for alcalase; 1 or 3 h for pepsin-pancreatin). Degree of hydrolysis (DH) was high for the alcalase hydrolysates (24.12 - 58.94%), but the pepsin-pancreatin hydrolysates exhibited the highest ACE inhibitory activity (IC_{50} = 0.250 - 0.692 mg/mL). Under the tested conditions, the hydrolysates with the highest ACE inhibitory activity were produced with sequential pepsin-pancreatin using either PC_1 at 1 h hydrolysis time and a 1/10 E/S ratio or PC_2 at 1 h hydrolysis time and a 1/50 E/S ratio. Lima bean protein hydrolysates prepared with alcalase or pepsin-pancreatin are a potential ingredient in the production of physiologically functional foods with antihypertensive activity.

Chapter 6 - Angiotensin I-converting enzyme (ACE, EC 3.4.15.1) is a zinc metallopeptidase involved in release of angiotensin II (Ang II) and inactivation of bradykinin (BK), two peptide hormones which play key roles in regulation of blood pressure, renal and cardiovascular functions. Ang II is an end-product of the highly regulated renin-angiotensin-aldosterone system (RAAS) while bradykinin is an end-product of the kallikrein-kinin system (KKS). Ang II is produced by the RAAS system from the precursor angiotensinogen, cleaved by the enzyme renin to angiotensin I (Ang I), and then cleaved by ACE to Ang II. Ang II is considered the most active agonist of this system, and its physiological actions are implemented through stimulation of specific receptors distributed widely throughout the body. Ang II is known to bind to the AT1 and AT2 binding site subtypes. Stimulation of the AT1 receptor results in a signaling pathway cascade in several cell types, leading to processes such as vasoconstriction, inflammation and cell proliferation. These are extremely important in many cardiovascular diseases, including hypertension, atherosclerosis and ventricular hypertrophy. The AT2 receptor is mainly expressed during the fetal stage and is only minimally expressed in adults under normal circumstances. Its role in the adult cardiovascular system remains unclear, but it apparently produces oppositional effects to the AT1 receptor. The existence of two active sites for ACE has generated speculation about their functional significance. *In vitro* these two domains display relatively broad substrate specificity, including cleavage of Ang I and BK. However, some biochemical features differentiate these active sites. ACE- specific inhibitors are one of the most widely prescribed drug classes in cardiology and are used for treatment of hypertension and heart failure. This overview discusses the pathophysiological role of ACE and its enzymatic products, principally Ang II.

Chapter 7 - Cardiovascular diseases are leading cause of morbidity and mortality in developed countries. Renin-angiotensin system (RAS) and its effector molecule, angiotensin (Ang) II, play an important role in the pathophysiology of cardiovascular and kidney diseases. Most of the known pathophysiological effects of Ang II are mediated by Ang type 1 receptors (AT_1Rs), and up-regulation of AT_1Rs is an important event involves in undesired cardiovascular-renal crosstalk. Many lines of evidences have shown that reactive oxygen species (ROS) and reactive nitrogen species (RNS) play significant roles in regulation of AT_1R signaling. In the authors' study, the authors reveal that AT_1R-stimulated ROS production mediates activation of mitogen-activated protein kinases (MAPKs), leading to hypertrophic growth of cardiomyocytes and excessive cytokine production by cardiac fibroblasts. These findings indicate that ROS work as a crucial second messenger in Ang II-induced signaling. Endogenous ROS apparently increase AT_1R expression level, while RNS down-regulates the expression of AT_1R. The differences in the effects of ROS and RNS on AT_1R expression can be explained by the local covalent modification of cysteine thiols that are found at active or allosteric sites of effector proteins. This review introduces the recent findings on molecular mechanisms underlying reduction/oxidation (redox)-dependent post-translational regulation of AT_1R signaling in the cardiovascular system. These findings will provide a new understanding on the importance of cross talk between Ang II signaling and ROS/RNS in the development of heart failure.

Chapter 8 - Cardiac remodeling is characterized by excessive production of extracellular matrix (ECM) proteins by specialized cells referred to as cardiac myofibroblasts. Cardiac myofibroblasts function both as autocrine and paracrine cell types secreting pro-fibrotic factors, which accelerates production of ECM proteins. Among these pro-fibrotic factors, Angiotensin II (Ang II) plays a predominant role by influencing multiple pathways that promote ECM production and adverse remodeling. Agents that block Ang II and its receptors reduce ECM synthesis and improve cardiac function. These effects are similar to those obtained by peroxisome proliferators activated receptor–γ (PPAR-γ) agonists. Both Ang II receptor inhibitors and PPAR-γ agonists appear to have similar beneficial effects on cardiovascular diseases, diabetes and metabolic syndromes. These similar effects suggest cross-regulatory interactions between Ang II and PPAR-γ pathways. The significance of these interactions regulating cardiac remodeling is discussed in this chapter.

Chapter 9 - The regulation of cell volume is fundamental to cell survival. Here I discuss the factors involved in the regulation of cell volume in cardiac cells of the failing heart and the influence of cell swelling on the activation of ionic channels, particularly of the swelling-activated chloride channels. Emphasis is given to the novel finding that angiotensin II causes cell swelling in cardiac cells. Finally, the role of cell swelling on gap junction permeability and its consequence for impulse propagation and generation of cardiac arrhythmias is discussed.

Chapter 10 - The renin angiotensin system (RAS) maintains the cardiovascular (CV) homeostasis and is involved in the pathogenesis of several disorders majorly related to heart and kidney. There are several peptides under RAS in which angiotensin (Ang) II is the major contributor. It was reported about the role of Ang II and its receptor Ang II type 1 (AT1) in mediating the CV remodeling during heart failure. Another receptor AT2 acts primarily opposite to that of AT1. Ang (1-7) is a peptide which can prevent the ventricular remodeling during cardiac complications acting via Mas receptor. Diabetes mellitus is characterized by multiple organ damage and also increases the prevalence and severity of CV diseases. Hyperglycemia activates the local RAS, resulting in the formation of Ang II and stimulation of the endogenous cell death pathway. Cardiac remodeling, including fibrosis and left ventricular hypertrophy, is found in the diabetic heart as a result of the activation of the RAS. Blockade of the AT1 receptor by Ang receptor blocker (ARB) can be effectively used to prevent the cardiac remodeling in the form of hypertrophy and fibrosis during diabetic conditions. By blocking the actions of Ang II on AT1 receptors, ARBs facilitate its action on AT2 receptors and also improves the conversion of Ang II to Ang (1-7), which upon acting on Mas receptor to counteract the activated RAS in diabetic cardiomyopathy.

Chapter 11 - The goal of this chapter is to review the most relevant scientific evidence supporting the role of Angiotensin II (Ang II), the major hormone associated with hypertension, in the pathogenesis of dry age-related macular degeneration (AMD), a leading cause of blindness among the elderly and to highlight the importance of hypertension treatment to reduce the risk for developing AMD. AMD is a late onset (after age 50), progressive degeneration of the retina associated with vision loss coupled with a spectrum of specific clinical, physiological and histopathological features. The early or dry stage of AMD is characterized by the accumulation of drusen, specific lipid rich deposits under the retina whereas the late or wet stage is characterized by growth of abnormal new vessels under the retinal pigment epithelium (RPE) from the subjacent choroid, termed choroidal neovascularization (CNV). Extracellular matrix turnover (ECM) and inflammation are key cellular processes that play a central role in the pathogenesis of AMD. The scientific evidence to support the proposed role of Ang II-mediated RPE effects on subretinal deposits formation and inflammation is reviewed in depth.

Chapter 12 - Angiotensin II (Ang II), the active peptide of the renin–angiotensin system, binds and activates two major receptor subtypes, namely AT_1 and AT_2. The classical effects of Ang II in the control of blood pressure and fluid homeostasis are mediated by AT_1 receptors. The AT_2 receptor is involved in vasodilatation, inhibition of the cell proliferation, induction of programmed cell death and cellular differentiation. Ang II AT_2 receptor expression is highly modulated during development. In the fetus, AT_2 receptors predominate in all tissues and decline shortly after birth, being restricted to a few organs including brain. Interpretation of the function of Ang II in cerebellum necessitates a thorough understanding about the localization and signal transduction of Ang II receptors. A clear complementary pattern of AT_1 and AT_2 binding labeled by [^{125}I] Ang II was observed on adjacent layers in young rats within the cerebellar cortex. By using specific markers of the Purkinje cells (PCs) (Zebrin II and calbindin28K), the authors demonstrated that Ang II AT_2 receptors co-localized with the PCs as a monolayer, in correspondence with the well-defined layer observed by binding autoradiography at differential developmental stages (P0 to P60). Blockade of AT_2 receptors with PD123319 during late pregnancy caused a lost of AT_2 binding in the external granular layer (EGL) in P0 pups. A detailed histological analysis evidenced an enlarged EGL in the cerebellar cortex. It is well known that PCs migrate early during fetal stage (E14) toward the cerebellar cortex. Aiming to elucidate the non-classical signaling pathway of Ang II AT_2 receptors in rat hindbrain the authors selected P15, a critical developmental stage. Following Ang II stimulation, SHP-1 associates to AT_2 receptors but not to AT_1 subtype. Immunocomplexes obtained with anti-AT_2 or anti-SHP-1 exhibited PTPase activity, blocked by PD123319 (AT_2 antagonist) or PP2. SHP-1 activation was correlated with tyr-phosphorylation level of SHP-1 in immunocomplexes. Both immunocomplexes contained c-Src and PP2 blocked SHP-1 tyr-phosphorylation as well as activation and association SHP-1 to c-Src. Taken together, the localization of AT_2 receptors in the Purkinje cells, the effect of blockade during late pregnancy on the development of the cerebellar cortex and the signal transduction mechanisms, a potential role for AT_2 receptors can be assigned on neuronal migration and cerebellar cortex organization.

Chapter 13 - The Renin Angiotensin System (RAS) has been shown to be involved in the progression of several diseases. The association of RAS and disease is the mechanistic basis behind medications that block its components, such as Angiotensin II (ANGII) Type 1 Receptor (AT_1R) blockers (ARBs) or Angiotensin Converting Enzyme (ACE) inhibitors (ACEi). Disorders such as hypertension, heart disease, chronic renal disease and diabetic nephropathy are treated with these medications; however, blocking the RAS is not effective in all patients. The exact role the RAS plays in the progression of disease is not completely understood. *In vivo* imaging techniques to investigate RAS alterations would be of great value to further understand RAS contribution to disease states. Characterization experiments and initial testing in animal disease models of AT_1R and ACE specific radiotracers are ongoing, with several potential candidate tracers having been identified which would allow for non-invasive *in vivo* imaging modalities such as Single Photon Emission Tomography (SPECT) and Positron Emission Tomography (PET). This chapter will summarize RAS alterations in diseased tissue, the relevance of *in vivo* imaging, and novel tracer development and evaluation.

In: Angiotensin: New Research
Editors: S. Harada, I. Moi, pp. 1-57

ISBN: 978-1-62100-773-9

Chapter 1

THE INFLUENCE OF RENIN-ANGIOTENSIN-ALDOSTERONE SYSTEM (RAAS) GENES ON HYPERTROPHY DEVELOPMENT IN HYPERTROPHIC CARDIOMYOPATHY

Nadia Carstens[1], Lize Van der Merwe[2,3] and Johanna C. Moolman-Smook[1*]

[1] MRC Centre for Molecular and Cellular Biology,
Dept Biomedical Sciences, University of Stellenbosch Health Sciences Faculty
Tygerberg, South Africa.
[2] Biostatistics Unit, Medical Research Council of South Africa,
Tygerberg, South Africa.
[3] Dept Statistics, University of Western Cape, Bellville, South Africa.

ABSTRACT

Left ventricular hypertrophy (LVH) is a harbinger of morbidity and mortality, while its regression is associated with improved clinical prognosis. It is therefore imperative to understand the mechanisms that influence the development of hypertrophy and identify markers indicative of the risk of developing extensive hypertrophy, before its occurrence. The renin-angiotensin-aldostererone system (RAAS) is involved in LVH indirectly, through the key roles it plays in blood pressure regulation, and also directly, as some of its components also have direct hypertrophic effects; thus, this system has been the focus of numerous studies seeking genetic modifiers of LVH.

Hypertrophic cardiomyopathy (HCM), an inherited condition, characterised by highly variable extent and distribution of LVH, which is caused primarily by defective sarcomeric proteins, is a disorder in which RAAS variants appear to modulate the extent of hypertrophy development.

---

* Address for Correspondence: J. C. Moolman-Smook MRC Centre for Molecular and Cellular Biology, Room 4036, Teaching Block, University of Stellenbosch Health Sciences Faculty, PO Box 19063, Francie van Zijl Drive, Tygerberg 7505, South Africa , Tel: +27-21-9389693; Fax: +27-21-9389476 Email: hm@sun.ac.za

Early investigations of the role of this pathway in hypertrophy development, in the context of HCM, were largely centred on the genes encoding angiotensin converting enzyme and angiotensin II type 1 receptor, while downstream RAAS genes remained largely neglected. Recent association studies have, however, identified variants in additional RAAS genes that individually and collectively influence the penetrance and extent of LVH in HCM. Other investigations have provided evidence for local Angiotensin II generation, alternatively named tissue RAAS, which may also influence hypertrophy development. Furthermore, pharmacological inhibition of RAAS in anti-hypertrophic therapy has recently gained renewed interest with the development of a direct renin inhibitor.

Taken together, these studies justify a renewed look at the individual and compounded effects of RAAS components on hypertrophy within the context of HCM. In this review we discuss the involvement of specific RAAS components in hypertrophy development and further highlight their hypertrophy modifying role in HCM with special emphasis on knowledge gained from association studies. To illustrate the valuc and possible caveats of the candidate gene association approach, we discuss results from our research on family cohorts in which HCM-causing founder mutations segregate. We also discuss the need for studies that comprehensively cover genes comprising the RAAS to describe a subset of functional RAAS variants that work together to confer an increased risk for hypertrophy development in HCM patients.

1. Left Ventricular Hypertrophy (LVH)

Left ventricular hypertrophy (LVH) is acknowledged as a major risk factor for cardiovascular morbidity and mortality [1;2]. More specifically, increased LVH has been shown to predict the development of congestive heart failure [3], coronary heart disease [4], stroke [5], cardiac arrhythmias [6] and sudden cardiac death (SCD) [7]. Regression of LVH, on the other hand, is associated with a higher life expectancy [8] and improved clinical prognosis [9;10]. It is therefore vital to understand the underlying determinants of LVH to eventually facilitate more effective therapeutic intervention; in the meantime, the identification of molecular markers associated with LVH would enable improved risk stratification for cardiac morbidity in susceptible individuals.

Previous studies have shown that LVH is the most common cardiac complication of hypertension [11]. The effect of hypertension-control has been evident from studies such as the Heart Outcomes Prevention Evaluation (HOPE) and Losartan Intervention for Endpoint reduction (LIFE) clinical trials that investigated the effect of renin-angiotensin-aldosterone system (RAAS) inhibitors on cardiac hypertrophy in hypertensive cohorts. In the HOPE trial, cardiovascular morbidity and mortality was significantly reduced by regression of LVH with the angiotensin-converting enzyme (ACE) inhibitor ramipril [3]. Similarly, the LIFE study reported that the angiotensin receptor-blocker losartan was able to reduce left ventricular mass (LVM), an indicator of LVH, which, in turn, reduced the risk for SCD, myocardial infarction and stroke, independent of systolic blood pressure or other treatment administered [12;13]. However, antihypertensive treatment has not reduced morbidity and mortality from cardiovascular disease associated with LVH as would be expected by the degree of blood pressure reduction [14]; furthermore, LVH has also been observed in normotensive subjects [11;15]. Consequently, LVH is not only attributable to pressure overload, but also to other, non-hemodynamic effects, some of which pertain to direct effects of RAAS components [16;17].

Various RAAS components have been shown to individually and collectively influence hypertrophy development [18;19]. For instance, the main effector molecule of the RAAS, Angiotensin (Ang) II, is known to exert hypertrophic effects on neonatal [20;21] and adult [22-24] cardiomyocytes and has been implicated in numerous pro-hypertrophic cardiac networks [25]. Schunkert et al. found that Ang I to Ang II is involved in rat hearts with adaptive LVH, indicating increased RAAS components to hypertrophy [26]. In addition, Dostal and Baker demonstrated that Ang II-induced cardiac hypertrophy was prevented when an Ang II type 1 receptor (AT_1R)-antagonist was administered, an effect that was not achieved with a reduction in blood pressure, leading the authors to conclude that this effect was blood pressure-independent [27]. This was later confirmed in double transgenic rats harbouring human renin and human angiotensinogen genes [28;29].

However, Ang II is involved in complex pathways that influence LVH in a manner that is not yet completely understood, and the full contribution of the different RAAS components to hypertrophy development remains to be elucidated. This is not an easy analysis to perform in complex conditions in which hypertrophy is but one of the features of the disease, such as hypertension, and is more easily achieved in more simple conditions.

One such condition is hypertrophic cardiomyopathy (HCM), an inherited condition that is caused primarily by defective sarcomeric proteins, and which is characterised by highly variable extent and distribution of LVH. In this disorder, RAAS gene variants, possibly amongst others, appear to modulate the extent of hypertrophy development [30-33]. This disease has proven to be a valuable model to investigate the molecular mechanisms involved in hypertrophy development as its strong familial nature makes it amenable to the use of powerful molecular genetic techniques, while its autosomal dominant inheritance pattern ensures at least larger cohorts of study subjects than some of the other, rarer, genetic disorders which feature cardiac hypertrophy [34].

2. Hypertrophic Cardiomyopathy (HCM)

HCM is a primary cardiac disorder characterized clinically by LVH occurring in the absence of increased external loading conditions [35], as well as by diastolic dysfunction, arrhythmias and sudden death [36;37]. The prevalence of HCM has been shown to be approximately 1 in 500 in young adults through population-based clinical studies [38], although a much higher prevalence is expected in older individuals, based on the fact that HCM penetrance is age dependant [39].

In HCM, cardiac mass is increased due to left ventricular wall thickening that is frequently asymmetric and most often involves thickening of the interventricular septum [36]. Clinical diagnosis of HCM is established most easily with two-dimensional (2D) echocardiography by imaging the hypertrophied, but non-dilated, left ventricular chamber [40]. However, clinical presentation in patients with HCM varies greatly, some patients present with minimal or no symptoms and have a benign, asymptomatic course, while others develop more serious complications, such as cardiac arrhythmias and heart failure, with one of the most severe endpoints being sudden cardiac death [36;41]. This clinical variability is further observed in the extent and distribution of hypertrophy, which ranges from extensive and diffuse to mild and segmental, with no particular pattern considered typical [42].

HCM is classically described as a disease of the sarcomere [43]. Primary HCM is inherited as an autosomal dominant trait, and to date more than a thousand different causal mutations have been identified within 13 sarcomere- and myofilament-related genes, which contribute in part to the heterogeneity of the disease [44;45].

It has been suggested that the prognostic significance of a given causal mutation is related to its influence on the magnitude of hypertrophy [46;47]: some mutations are associated with severe hypertrophy, an early onset of disease and higher susceptibility to SCD, while others are associated with a relatively benign outcome [48;49]. Furthermore, the dose of these mutant proteins in an individual has been shown to have a strong impact on the clinical course of HCM: individuals with homozygous or compound heterozygous mutations in sarcomere protein genes exhibit more severe clinical phenotypes [50;51]. Even so, the clinical presentation varies even between individuals from the same family with identical causal mutations [52], as well as between different families, with intrafamilial and interfamilial variability reaching similar levels [53-55]. Thus, sarcomeric mutations account for but a fraction of the diversity of hypertrophic phenotypes seen in HCM [35], suggesting that the clinical heterogeneity of HCM can be viewed as a product of the causal sarcomeric mutation as well as additional genetic and environmental factors.

The case for genetic modifiers of HCM is predicated on the fact that a discrepancy exists between sarcomere-related mutations and the resulting cardiac phenotype. For instance, Fananapazir and Epstein [54] provided evidence for modifier genes in HCM when they described a Caucasian as well as a Korean kindred with an identical disease causing mutation (R403Q) in the *MYH7* gene. The R403Q mutation was associated with 100% disease penetrance and a high incidence of SCD in the Caucasian kindred, while no SCD was observed in the Korean kindred; because of the significantly different clinical presentation of HCM between the two families, the authors concluded that the genetic background of the individuals along with environmental factors are responsible for the phenotypic diversity. This was later corroborated by other studies [53;56-58].

Transgenic animal models have also proven valuable in confirming a role for genetic modifiers on the cardiac phenotype in HCM, aided by the ability to control environmental influences and the genetic background of inbred strains of animals [59]. Semsarian and co-workers [60] studied a mouse model of HCM, α-MHC$^{403/+}$; the α-MHC$^{403/+}$ missense mutation in mice is equivalent to the human *MYH7* R403Q mutation. By breeding the α-MHC$^{403/+}$ mice into different genetic backgrounds of two distinct inbred mouse strains, they were able to identify a range of phenotypic differences in terms of hypertrophy, histopathology and exercise capacity. Given that the mice strains were housed under the same environmental conditions, the study provided confirmation for the role of genetic modifiers in HCM.

Interestingly, founding mutations have been reported in populations from Europe, the United States of America and South Africa [44;61]. Such populations, in which apparently unrelated families share causal mutations, are particularly valuable for genetic studies, as they offer a more homogeneous population in which to assess the role of additional genes in a clinical phenotype, which, as modifiers, are neither necessary nor sufficient to cause the condition. Thus, although HCM is regarded as a monogenic disease due to the necessity for a causative mutation to trigger the development of the phenotype, it can also be regarded as a complex trait due to the variability introduced by the involvement of additional genetic loci and environmental factors, each probably contributing to the phenotype to varying extents.

Various genetic mapping approaches have been employed to identify quantitative trait loci (QTLs) that alter the hypertrophic phenotype of HCM, the most common being candidate gene association analysis. Components of the RAAS are particularly plausible candidate modifiers of LVH in HCM, not only due to their effect on blood pressure, and thus indirect effect on LVM, but also due to their direct hypertrophic effect on cardiomyocytes [31;33;62].

3. Renin-Angiotensin-Aldosterone System (RAAS)

The RAAS exerts its main effect through Ang II, which has the ability to act as a systemic hormone (circulating RAAS) and as a local factor (tissue RAAS) [63]. A schematic overview of the RAAS is given in Figure 1. Briefly, the biologically inert decapeptide Ang I is cleaved from angiotensinogen by the aspartyl-protease, renin, and subsequently hydrolyzed to the active octapeptide Ang II by ACE1 within the circulation, or by ACE1-independent mechanisms, involving, for instance, chymase. A second ACE, ACE2, has also been discovered, which converts Ang I to Ang-(1-7), which has been shown to counteract the vasoconstrictive effects of ACE.

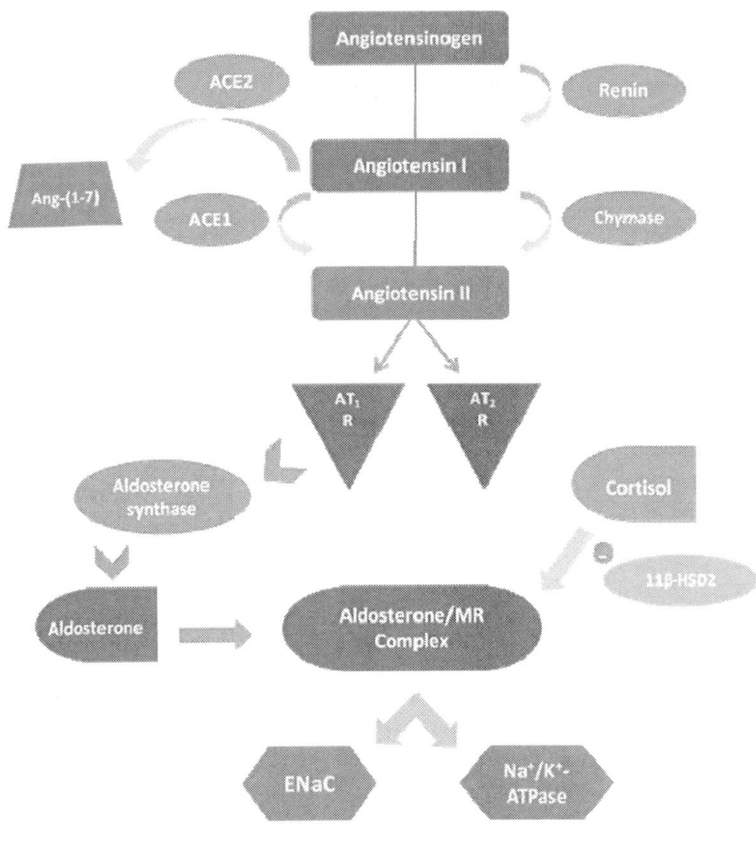

Figure 1. A schematic representation of the renin-angiotensin-aldosterone system (RAAS).

Ang II exerts its main biological effects by binding to highly specific Ang II receptors. To date, two main receptors have been characterized in humans: the Ang II type I (AT_1R) and Ang II type II (AT_2R), each with their own signalling cascade and physiological function [64;65]. Binding of Ang II to the AT_1R, triggers the synthesis of aldosterone via aldosterone synthase (*CYP11B2*). Aldosterone is a mineralocorticoid that exerts its function by, in turn, binding to the mineralocorticoid receptor (MR), which increases the transcription of MR-responsive genes [66]. The MR binds both aldosterone and glucocorticoids, such as cortisol, with equal affinity. However, the enzyme 11 β-hydroxysteroid-dehydrogenase type 2 (11β-HSD2) increases the MR specificity for aldosterone by inactivating the glucocorticoids [67]. The MR/aldosterone complex then exerts its Na^+-regulating effects in three phases [68;69]. The first is a latent period that lasts for about an hour, during which aldosterone-induced transcription and translation takes place. The second is an "early response" phase, lasting up to three hours, during which Na^+ transport is increased, mainly by increasing the open probability and number of active epithelial Na^+ channels (ENaC). A further increase in Na^+ transport is observed during the "late response", that lasts for about 24 hours, and during which expression of ENaC as well as Na^+/K^+-ATPase subunits are increased [70;71].

Early investigations of the role of the RAAS pathway in hypertrophy development, in the context of HCM, were largely centred on the genes encoding ACE and the AT_1R, while downstream RAAS genes remained largely neglected. Recent association studies have, however, have identified variants in additional RAAS genes that individually and collectively influence the penetrance and extent of LVH in HCM. Other investigations have provided evidence that local Ang II generation in the myocardium, alternatively named tissue RAAS, is closely linked to the development of cardiac hypertrophy [72]. Recent studies have identified additional RAAS proteins that impact on hypertrophy development in a blood pressure-dependent as well as Ang II-independent manner. This calls for an expansion of the "classical" RAAS to include these newly identified RAAS components as well as a re-evaluation of our current knowledge of the role of RAAS components in the hypertrophic phenotype of HCM. Furthermore, pharmacological inhibition of RAAS in HCM as anti-hypertrophic therapy has recently gained renewed interest with the development of a direct renin inhibitor [73;74]. Taken together, these studies justify a renewed look at the individual and compound effects of RAAS components on hypertrophy within the context of HCM.

In this chapter we will discuss the involvement of specific RAAS components in hypertrophy development and further highlight their hypertrophy-modifying role in HCM, with special emphasis on knowledge gained from association studies.

To illustrate the value and possible caveats of the candidate gene association approach, we discuss results from our research on family cohorts in which HCM-causing founder mutations segregate. Finally, we discuss the need for studies that comprehensively cover genes comprising the full RAAS in order to identify a comprehensive subset of functional RAAS variants that work together to confer an increased risk for hypertrophy development in HCM patients.

3.1. Angiotensinogen (*AGT*)

Angiotensinogen, which is the first component of the RAAS, is encoded by the *AGT* gene. This gene consists of five exons and four introns and spans 12 kb on chromosome

1q42-43. Angiotensinogen remains a popular candidate modifier for essential hypertension and -associated end-organ damage, as there exists a significant correlation between plasma *AGT* concentration and blood pressure in humans [75]. Additionally, mice overexpressing the *AGT* gene exhibit elevated blood pressure in a dose-dependent manner [76;77], while *AGT* gene-knockout mice show reduced blood pressure levels [78].

Xu et al. [79] reported that transgenic mice overexpressing the rat angiotensinogen gene developed severe chronic hypertension coupled with cardiac hypertrophy and impaired cardiac function. Single nucleotide polymorphisms (SNPs) and related haplotypes in this gene have additionally been associated with essential hypertension and elevated blood pressure in some populations [80-83], but not all [84]. However, two SNPs in *AGT*, T174M and M235T, were related to blood pressure-independent LVM-reductions in hypertensive patients with echocardiographically-diagnosed LVH who were treated with the AT_1R-antagonist irbesartan, but not in such patients treated with the beta-1 adrenergic receptor-blocker atenolol (data from the Swedish Irbesartan Left Ventricular Hypertrophy Investigation versus Atenolol (SILVHIA) trial [85].

The involvement of *AGT* polymorphisms in LVH development remains controversial, as some studies report significant associations between *AGT* variants and LVH, while other studies fail to replicate these results [86-89]. One explanation for this discrepancy is the fact that *AGT* polymorphism frequencies vary greatly according to ethnic origin [90], which makes association studies on these polymorphisms sensitive to false-positive results due to population stratification. In such studies, false-negative results often occur in populations where one allele is largely predominant due to the limited statistical power of the resultant association studies [82]. For instance, in a meta-analysis of 69 studies with a combined sample size of 27 906, the overall prevalence of the M235-T allele was 52.1%. The prevalence of the M235-T allele was however significantly dependent on race, being 78.0 % in Asians, 77% in blacks and only 42.2 % in Caucasians [91].

Kuznetsova et al. [92] studied the European Project On Genes in Hypertension (EPOGH) cohort, which consisted of 221 nuclear families from three Caucasian populations, respectively from Poland, Russia and Italy, to investigate to what extent LVM was associated with the M235T and -6 G/A polymorphisms in the *AGT* gene. They reported that the significant association that they observed between these polymorphisms and LVM were dependent on age, gender, ecogenetic context and appeared to be modulated by the trophic effects of salt intake on LVM. These observations point towards the importance of adjusting for relevant confounders in *AGT* association studies to avoid spurious significance of results.

These factors were taken into consideration when Tang et al. investigated the effect of the above polymorphisms in a cohort of 605 predominantly Caucasian patients obtained from the Hypertension Genetic Epidemiology Network (HyperGEN) [93]. The authors reported that LVM as well as LVM_{index} and the M235-T allele were negatively associated in hypertensive patients, but positively associated in normotensive patients, in a model adjusted for the potential confounding effect of weight, height, age, sex, systolic blood pressure, diastolic blood pressure, presence of diabetes, and antihypertensive medication use. The link between hypertrophy and *AGT* therefore extends beyond the known impact of angiotensinogen on blood pressure. This concept is also borne out biologically, as angiotensinogen has been shown to be expressed in myocardial tissue, where it is able to induce cardiac hypertrophy, independent of systemic blood pressure [94-96]. Moreover, mice expressing *AGT* exclusively in the liver and brain, showed reduced cardiac hypertrophy when compared to mice expressing *AGT* in the liver, brain and heart with a similar blood pressure [97].

Three *AGT* SNPs have been investigated for their role in hypertrophy development in HCM, in particular. These include a threonine to methionine substitution in exon 2 at position 174 of mature Angiotensinogen (T174M), a 704 T>C substitution, which results in a methionine to threonine substitution at position 235 (M235T) in the same exon, as well as a promoter variant 6 bp upstream from the transcription initiation site (-6 G/A). Most of the HCM studies focussed on the M235T variant.

Just as in hypertension studies, the involvement of the M235T variant in HCM is controversial, as some studies report a correlation between this polymorphism and HCM [98-101], whereas other studies do not [33;102;103]. Ishanov et al. [99] revealed that the M235-T allele frequency was higher in Japanese patients with sporadic HCM, than in their unaffected siblings and offspring. These findings were replicated in a study on 96 Japanese HCM patients (43 with familial HCM and 53 with sporadic HCM) and 105 of their unaffected siblings and children [100]. Another study [101] reported similar results from an investigation of 150 South Indian HCM (90 sporadic HCM and 60 familial HCM) patients and 165 age- and sex-matched healthy controls, without known hypertension or LVH. Significant differences were detected in genotypic distribution as well as the allelic frequencies of the M235T polymorphism between patients with sporadic HCM and controls, although these findings were not replicated in patients with familial HCM [101].

In contrast, Yamada et al. found no significant association between this variant and non-familial HCM in a Japanese cohort [103]. No significant association was found between M235T and cardiac hypertrophy indices in a cohort of 389 unrelated patients with HCM [33]. Similarly, Coto et al. reported no significant association between the M235T variant and cardiac hypertrophy in a study on 245 echocardiographically-diagnosed HCM-patients and 300 healthy controls [104]. Furthermore, none of the most commonly studied *AGT* SNPs (M235T, T174M, and -6 G/A) had a significant influence on a composite LVH score or LVM in a cohort of 108 genetically independent HCM patients [105].

In addition to relatively small sample sizes, none on these studies accounted for the confounding effects of the primary HCM causal mutation or any other known hypertrophy covariates in their analyses.

Furthermore, the question of the functionality of the M235T SNP remains. This polymorphism was associated with a stepwise-increase in angiotensinogen levels in Caucasian subjects, as well as a corresponding moderate increase in risk of hypertension in both Caucasian and Asian subjects in a meta-analysis of 127 publications [106]. The M235-T genotype did, however, not predict plasma angiotensinogen levels in Asian and black subjects, or blood pressure, risk of ischemic heart disease, or myocardial infarction in either of these ethnic groups [106].

The M235T variant is in tight linkage disequilibrium (LD) with the -6G/A variant in the proximal promoter of the *AGT* gene [93;107]. This substitution affects specific interactions between at least one trans-acting nuclear factor and the promoter of *AGT*, thereby influencing the basal rate of transcription of the gene, which initially explained why T235-homozygotes have plasma angiotensinogen levels that are 10–20% higher than M235-homozygotes [108].

However, later analyses of transgenic mice expressing either the -6G/235M or the -6A/235T haplotype in the 13.5-kb human *AGT* gene showed that both transgenes exhibited the same transcriptional activity and produce similar plasma levels of human Angiotensinogen [109]. These results suggest that variation at the -6-position may only be a marker, and may not in itself be functional. However, mice carrying the -6G/235M haplotype showed a slight but significant increase in blood pressure and relative heart weight, as well as compensatory downregulation of endogenous renin expression, which led the authors to speculate that these haplotypes might affect the cardiovascular system and the regulation of blood pressure differently [109].

Jain et al. found that -6G/A can act as a marker for three other promoter SNPs, as well as for 3 additional intragenic SNPs, where the -6G and -6A variants each tag a different haplotype of these polymorphisms. To inspect the physiological effect of these haplotypes, they generated double transgenic mice containing either the -6A or -6G haplotype of the human *AGT* gene, and also the human renin gene (*REN*). Transgenic mice containing -6A haplotype had increased plasma *AGT* levels and increased blood pressure, compared with those with the -6G haplotype [110].

Grobe et al. developed triple-transgenic mice carrying a null mutation in the endogenous murine angiotensinogen gene, while expressing either the -6G/235M or -6A/235T haplotype of the human *AGT* gene, and either an overexpressed and poorly regulated, or a tightly regulated human *REN* gene. Mice expressing the -6G/235M haplotype on the well-controlled renin background exhibited increased blood pressure and cardiac hypertrophy. In contrast, mice with the -6A/235T haplotype in a poorly regulated renin background exhibited increased cardiac and renal growth and increased blood pressure sensitivity to a high-salt diet, leading the authors to conclude that the differential effects of these haplotypes on cardiovascular end-points are context dependent and sensitive to genetic background and environmental influences [111].

There is, however, a lack of studies that explore the *physiological* effects of *AGT* variants on hypertrophy development specifically in HCM.

3.2. Renin and Renin-Associated Genes

Renin is a rate-limiting component of the RAAS, as it controls the initial conversion of angiotensinogen to Ang I. While there is a paucity of research on the role of renin and its associated proteins in hypertrophy development in HCM, it remains an exciting and promising field of research, which is currently offering promising prospects for hypertrophy research that might be transferable to hypertrophy in HCM. In addition, the recent development of a direct renin inhibitor, aliskiren, renewed interest in renin as a potential therapeutic target in cardiac hypertrophy management [74;112]. As this direct renin inhibitor controls the rate-limiting step of the RAAS and decreases plasma renin activity (PRA), it is thought to offer superior benefits to ACE- and AT_1R blockers in treating cardiovascular disorders, as these latter blockers interfere with the negative feedback loop exerted by Ang II on renin formation that elicits a rise in plasma renin concentration [113].

Aliskiren ameliorated cardiac hypertrophy in rats expressing both human renin and angiotensinogen [114] and was proven to be at least as effective as ACE inhibition and Ang receptor blockade in LVH reduction in spontaneously hypertensive rats [115]. Aliskiren was also shown to ameliorate cardiac remodelling and hypertrophy after myocardial infarction with doses that did not affect blood pressure in mice [116]. The recent Aliskiren in Left

Ventricular Hypertrophy (ALLAY) study reported that aliskiren was as effective as the Ang-receptor blocker losartan in LVM regression, making aliskiren a potential treatment option in patients with LVH [73].

Renin is generated from preprorenin in a number of steps: Prorenin is generated from preprorenin in the juxtaglomerular cells of the kidney by the removal of 23 amino acids, and is later converted into mature renin. Recent research has identified three additional proteins that associate with renin and prorenin *in vivo*. This includes a protein that is able to inhibit renin upon binding to it, namely the renin-binding protein (RnBP), as well as two receptors for renin. The mannose-6-phosphate/insulin-like growth factor II receptor (M6PR/IGFII) has been suggested as a clearance receptor in cardiomyocytes, as it only binds glycosylated forms of prorenin and facilitates its subsequent internalisation and degradation [117]. The (pro)renin receptor (PRR), on the other hand, is a promising candidate for tissue uptake of renin, as it binds both renin and prorenin and activates prorenin non-proteolytically [118].

The presence of renin in the heart is a matter of great controversy, as evidence for local renin synthesis has not been conclusive. It is now widely accepted that cardiac renin is taken up from the circulation, either due to diffusion into the interstitium [119;120], or through specific functional binding sites and renin receptors [121;122]. In addition, the heart can generate renin locally from circulating prorenin by proteolytic cleavage and non-proteolytic activation through the PRRs in myocardial tissues [123-125]. Interestingly, the plasma concentration of prorenin is ten times greater than that of renin [126] and circulating prorenin levels may reach as high as 100 times the level of renin under conditions of renal damage and cardiac hypertrophy [127].

Veniant and colleagues developed a transgenic rat line that expresses prorenin exclusively in the liver. These rats demonstrated a 400-fold increase in plasma prorenin, but exhibited normal plasma renin levels and blood pressure. However, these animals developed severe liver fibrosis as well as cardiac and aortic hypertrophy [128]. This study gained more attention with the cloning of the PRR [123]. When renin and prorenin are bound to this receptor, a five-fold increase in angiotensinogen to Ang I conversion is noted, and these physiological effects are exerted in a manner completely independent of Ang II generation [129;130]. In a study on neonatal rat cardiomyocytes, Saris et al. [131] demonstrated that prorenin bound to the PRR activated the p38 MAPK/HSP27 pathway; they postulated that this activation is responsible for the severe hypertrophy observed by Veniant et al. Similarly, renin and prorenin have been proven to induce DNA synthesis and activate the p42/p44 MAPK intracellular pathways and stimulate the release of plasminogen activator inhibitor (PAI)-1, as well as transforming growth factor-β1 (TGF-β1), through binding with the PRR [132]. These are profibrotic, inflammatory and hypertrophic signalling pathways that function independent of Ang II generation [118;133-135]. These pro-hypertrophic signalling cascades are not inhibited by ACE inhibitors, aliskiren or AT_1R blockers [113]. This and other studies [136-138] supports growing evidence that renin and prorenin *per se* exerts hypertrophic cellular effects, independent of Ang II generation, at least some of which involve the PRR.

A protein that corresponds to the "handle" region of prorenin, which inhibits the binding of prorenin to the PRR [139], has been shown to reduce cardiac hypertrophy and improve left ventricular function in spontaneously hypertensive rats on a high salt diet [127]. This effect was however not replicated in high renin conditions [140].

The PRR is identical to ATPase-associated protein 2 (encoded by the *ATP6AP2* gene), an accessory protein to a vacuolar proton-transporting ATPase (v-H^+-ATPase). In a study in

Xenopus embryos and in human cultured cells, Cruciat et al. showed that ATP6AP2 functions in a renin-independent manner as an adaptor between Wnt receptors and the v-H^+-ATPase complex [141]. Aberrant Wnt signalling has previously been linked to cardiovascular hypertrophy [142].

Recently, Connelly et al. corroborated the co-localization of PRR with v-H^+-ATPase in the heart and reported an increased expression of PRR in the hearts of transgenic animals with diabetic cardiomyopathy [143]. This increased expression of PRR was associated with diastolic dysfunction, interstitial fibrosis as well as cardiomyocyte hypertrophy. Direct renin inhibition then reduced cardiac PRR expression in these animals, in association with improved cardiac structure and function [143].

The PRR is therefore able to influence hypertrophy development through local RAAS activation as well as through Wnt signalling, making it an attractive target for antihypertrophic treatment [144]. More research is however needed to fully elucidate the contribution of the PRR to cardiac hypertrophy in general, as well as to the role of PRR in HCM [145].

Furthermore, previous studies have shown that M6PR/IGFII is also able to bind prorenin and renin on cardiomyocytes [146;147], and to generate renin from prorenin through proteolytic cleavage [148]. This binding and activation did not result in Ang II generation in cardiomyocytes [149].

Takahashi et al. reported another protein that was capable of forming a complex with renin, which they named RnBP [150]. Further *in vitro* studies showed that this protein is able to form a heterodimer with renin and subsequently to inhibit its activity [151]. This protein was later found to be identical to the enzyme N-acetyl-D-glucosamine 2-epimerase (NAGE) [152]. In a study of RnBP-knockout mice, Schmitz et al. were unable to detect any effect of RnBP-deficiency on renal and circulating RAAS or on blood pressure, leading the authors to speculate that RnBP does not play a role in the regulation of plasma renin and RAAS activity [153]. However, Bohlmeyer and colleagues investigated the expression of RnBP in failing human hearts, with end-stage idiopathic dilated cardiomyopathy. They found that RnBP expression was restricted to endothelial cells in non-failing hearts, while RnBP gene and protein expression was selectively activated in the ventricular cardiomyocytes of failing hearts [154]. Interestingly, they reported that the highest RnBP mRNA levels were detected in a subject with significant LVH. Additionally, RnBP was redistributed from a cytosolic to a sarcolemmal/sarcomeric fraction, which led the authors to conclude that RnBP may be involved in the modification of cardiac cytoskeletal proteins.

Knoll et al. investigated the effect of a RnBP gene (*RENBP*) T61C variant on several cardiovascular parameters in 505 randomly selected Caucasian individuals [155]. Males ($n = 293$) and females ($n = 212$) were analysed separately, as the RnBP gene is X-linked, and individuals on antihypertensive medication were excluded. The authors reported an association between this variant and plasma prorenin, as well as the renin/prorenin ratio, but found no significant association with circulating renin, blood pressure, heart rate or LVM in men. These findings were not replicated in females [155]. In contrast, Gu et al. reported a strong association between markers rs1557501 and rs2269372 in *RENBP* and systolic blood pressure responses to low-sodium diets in a cohort of 1906 individuals from Han Chinese families who took part in the Genetic Epidemiology Network of Salt Sensitivity (GenSalt) [156].

Research on renin and renin-related proteins largely focussed on identifying these proteins in different *in vivo* settings, to pinpoint their physiological function. While association has been detected between *REN* [157], *RENBP* [156] and the PRR gene, *ATP6AP2*, [140] variants and blood pressure regulation, no study has detected an effect of polymorphisms in these genes on hypertrophy *per se* or within the context of HCM to date.

3.3. Angiotensin Converting Enzyme (ACE)

ACE, encoded by the *ACE1* gene, is a transmembrane-ectopeptidase that is responsible for the conversion of Ang I to the active Ang II and the inactivation of bradykinin. This gene remains the most commonly studied candidate modifier gene for HCM, as Ang II and bradykinin exert strong cardiovascular effects in opposing directions. While Ang II promotes hypertension and cardiac hypertrophy, bradykinin exerts cardioprotective effects.

ACE1 expression is increased in many forms of cardiovascular hypertrophy [26;158], while serum ACE activity is significantly related to LVM, independent of systemic blood pressure [159]. ACE inhibitors, together with AT_1R blockers, are currently the gold standard for antihypertensive therapy [139]. Furthermore, inhibition of ACE with ramipril is associated with LVH regression, independent of its effect on blood pressure [3], while ACE inhibition improved left ventricular function in patients with hypertrophic obstructive cardiomyopathy [160]. These data are complemented by meta-analyses of clinical trials that suggest that ACE inhibitors are effective in causing LVH regression, even after adjustment for treatment duration and change in blood pressure [161-163].

An insertion/deletion (I/D) polymorphism, involving the presence (I) or absence (D) of 287 bp Alu repeats in intron 16 of *ACE1*, accounts for 47% of the total variability in serum ACE levels [164]. Circulating ACE levels in plasma were nearly 60% higher in DD-homozygotes, compared with II-homozygotes [164]. This polymorphism is consequently thought to be functional as it exerts and incremental effect on plasma and tissue ACE levels, where II-homozygotes exhibit the lowest levels of plasma and tissue ACE, heterozygotes the intermediate and DD-homozygotes the highest [35;165].

However, in a meta-analysis of 49 959 individuals [166], the prevalence of the D-allele was significantly influenced by ethnicity, as the D-allele prevalence was 56.2% in Caucasians, 60.3 % in blacks and 39.1% in Asians. This group added to these findings in a more recent meta-analysis on echocardiographic phenotypes across 38 studies [167] by reporting that both DD-homozygotes and ID-heterozygotes had elevated LVM and an increased mean wall thickness when compared to II-homozygotes. The authors did, however, mention that these results should be interpreted with caution as adjustments for environmental and lifestyle confounders of LVM were inconsistent across studies and they observed a significant publication bias for studies reporting an association between LVM and the I/D polymorphism, which may have lead to an overestimation of the pooled association [167]. In contrast, a study on 2439 subjects from the Framingham Heart study did not find a significant association between ACE DD-genotypes and echocardiographically-determined LVM [168].

In the first study of this polymorphism in HCM, Marian et al. reported a significant association between the DD-genotype and an increased risk of sudden cardiac death in HCM patients [169]. Later, other studies reported a significant association between the D-allele and increased LVH indices, but this association was not replicated in all studies (Table 1).

One explanation for this discrepancy could be that association between the I/D polymorphism and hypertrophy indices is context-dependent and sensitive to hypertrophy- and environmental confounders in HCM [180].

Table 1. Summary of association studies on the influence of ACE I/D polymorphism on HCM phenotypes

Study Cohort	Results
389 unrelated HCM patients	DD-genotype associated with increased left ventricular wall thickness in MYBPC3 carriers, but not MYH7 carriers [33]
100 HCM patients and 106 of their unaffected siblings and offspring	DD-genotype associated with increased risk of SCD in HCM [169]
114 genetically affected HCM patients	Significant association between D-allele and hypertrophy, which is influenced by HCM-causal mutation [170]
118 Indian HCM Patients and 164 ethnically, age- and gender-matched controls	Prevalence of DD-genotype significantly higher in patients compared to controls and was associated with increased risk of HCM, after adjustment for age, sex, body mass and smoking [171]
62 Australian HCM patients	DD-genotype associated with greater progression of LVH, independent of age, body mass and blood pressure [172]
183 Caucasian HCM patients	DD-genotype significantly associated with LVH, independent of age, sex, weight and body surface area [173]
50 unrelated HCM patients and 50 healthy controls	DD-genotype more prevalent in HCM patients [174]
80 Japanese HCM patients and 88 of their unaffected children and siblings	DD-genotype more prevalent in HCM patients [175]
71 Japanese patients with nonfamilial HCM and 122 healthy controls	No association between DD-genotype and indices of hypertrophy [103]
136 Brazilian HCM patients	Serum ACE activity, but not I/D polymorphism affected LVH in HCM [176]
104 unrelated Caucasian HCM patients	No association between D-allele and LVM, but variant affected plasma ACE levels [177]
126 genetically diagnosed Japanese HCM patients	D-allele associated with decreased posterior wall thickness, decreased ejection fraction and increased left ventricular end-systolic dimension; no association with septal thickness or maximal left ventricular wall thickness [178]
63 HCM patients and 20 healthy controls, all Caucasian	Increased QT dispersion in HCM patients with DD-genotype [179]
245 unrelated HCM patients and 300 healthy controls, all Spanish Caucasians	No association between I/D polymorphism and risk of cardiac hypertrophy [104]

Tesson et al. assessed the effect of the I/D polymorphism in families that harbour HCM causal genes in the cardiac myosin binding protein C (*MYBPC*) or β-myosin heavy chain

(*MYH7*) genes and found that the association between this polymorphism and LVH was dependent on the specific HCM mutation [170]. When all genetically-affected individuals were analysed together, they found no significant association. A significant association was, however, reported between the ACE D-allele and interventricular septal thickness in individuals with the R403Q mutation in *MYH7* [170]. Different HCM mutations show definite variability in phenotypic expression, as some are associated with severe cardiac hypertrophy, while others offer more benign outcomes [48;49]. It is therefore conceivable that the effect of primary HCM causal mutation cannot be discounted in HCM association studies. Most of the studies in Table 1 did, however, not account for this effect.

Another general difficulty for HCM association studies is shown by the study of Lechin et al. [173]. This group used regression analysis to show that ACE I/D genotypes only accounted for 3.7% of the variability in LVM index and 6.5% of a LVH score used to quantify the extent of hypertrophy in unrelated HCM patients [173]. This allows for the possibility that ACE variants only make a modest contribution towards hypertrophy in HCM and speaks to the possibility that there might be a number of modifying variants and genes that affect the HCM phenotype.

Buck et al. reported that ACE activity, rather than ACE polymorphisms, affected LVH in HCM, although this study is somewhat hampered by the small sample size [176]. However ACE activity is obviously determined by genetic variation within the ACE1 gene. Thus, it remains puzzling that the I/D variant is not located in a coding region and does not exert any clear effect on gene transcription, which points to a very real possibility that it might only be a marker for a functional variant in close proximity [181;182]. The precise location of this proposed functional variant is still uncertain, although it is thought to be most likely located between intron 18 and the 3' UTR [180;183]. On the other hand, Kammerer and co-workers recently suggested a QTL on chromosome 4 that impacts on ACE activity [184], and a yet another possibility for a functional variant exists in the 5' gene region [185;186].

3.4. Angiotensin Converting Enzyme 2 (ACE2)

A second ACE, ACE2, which is thought to be an essential regulator of cardiovascular function [187] was recently reported. This homologue of *ACE1* removes the C-terminal phenylalanine from Ang II, to form Ang-(1-7), which is a ligand of the G-protein-coupled receptor Mas. ACE2-null mice develop progressive Ang II-mediated age-dependent cardiomyopathy, which is associated with increased oxidative stress as well as pathological hypertrophy [188]. ACE2-deficiency also exacerbated adverse cardiovascular remodelling in mice with Ang II-induced hypertrophy, whereas recombinant human ACE2 reduced Ang II-induced hypertrophy in wild type mice and partially prevented the development of dilated cardiomyopathy in pressure-overloaded mice [189]. The beneficial effect of ACE2 on adverse cardiac remodelling is furthermore evident from a number of animal models [190-192]. In addition, Ang-(1-7) has been shown to attenuate cardiac hypertrophy and dysfunction through a direct local effect in transgenic animal models [144].

Lieb et al. previously reported that the minor alleles of four SNPs in the X-linked *ACE2* gene were associated with LVM_{index} as well as interventricular septal thickness in males (but not females) from the general population in the MONICA (MONitoring trends and determinants in CArdiovascular disease) Augsburg survey [193]. These four SNPs (rs4646156, rs879922, rs4240157 and rs233575) showed high pairwise LD and a common haplotype, consisting of the minor alleles of these SNPs, was associated with an increased odds-ratio (OR) for LVH (OR 3.10, p=0.006) in a model adjusted for age, body mass, antihypertensive medications and systolic blood pressure. Males carrying this haplotype displayed modestly increased LVM_{index} and interventricular septal thickness [193].

Subsequently, Wang and co-workers investigated the effect of two other SNPS on HCM in a Chinese population, as the minor alleles of rs879922 and rs4240157 were present at too low frequency, and rs4646156 and rs233575 were not polymorphic, in the Chinese population [194]. They reported that the T-allele of rs2106809 and C-allele of rs6632677 conferred an increased risk for HCM in males, from a study of 261 HCM patients and 600 healthy controls [194]. These SNPs were in strong LD with each other, and the TC haplotype was associated with an increased risk for HCM and modestly increased interventricular septal thickness, independent of age, body mass and blood pressure. The primary disease-causing HCM mutations of these patients were, however, unidentified and were therefore not adjusted for in the analyses. These findings could also not be replicated in females.

The G-allele of rs879922 was recently reported to be significantly associated with cardiac hypertrophy in a South African HCM family cohort, independent of the primary HCM causal mutation and known hypertrophy covariates, viz. blood pressure, age, sex, body surface area (BSA), heart rate and hypertension diagnosis [32]. After adjustment for known hypertrophy covariates, the G-allele significantly increased LVM by 18.7 g, maximum interventricular septal thickness by 1.9 mm and maximum posterior wall thickness by 0.7 mm [32].

Although ACE2 is clearly a plausible hypertrophy modifier in HCM, more studies are needed to fully elucidate the contribution of *ACE2* variants to hypertrophy in HCM as none of these variants have any obvious functional roles.

3.5. Cardiac Chymase (CMA)

Ang II production in the heart can also be attributed to a serine protease named cardiac chymase (CMA). Indeed, Urata et al. showed that CMA accounts for 80% of the Ang II generated in the human ventricle [195]. Chymase is produced from mast cells in the heart and is not inhibited by ACE inhibitors [196]. Transgenic mice expressing human CMA showed elevated blood pressure and increased LVM [197], while cardiac chymase activity was increased in the hearts of naturally-occurring cardiomyopathic hamsters [198;199]. Hoshino et al. showed that a CMA-inhibitor significantly increased survival rate, while attenuating cardiac hypertrophy and end-diastolic left ventricular pressure, in a hamster model of myocardial infarction [200].

Two biallelic markers of the cardiac chymase A gene (*CMA*) on chromosome 14q11 have been studied in hypertrophy association studies: a 1625 G/A transition in intron 2, termed CMA/A, and a -1903 G/A transition in the 5' untranslated region, termed CMA/B [174;201]. He et al. investigated the antihypertrophic properties of the ACE I/D and the CMA/B polymorphisms in a clinical trial on the effect of the ACE inhibitor benazepril on 157 Chinese patients with essential hypertension [201]. Benazepril significantly reduced blood pressure and LVH in these patients. Patients treated with benazepril that harboured the ACE DD genotype showed a significantly higher reduction in echocardiographically determined LVM and LVM_{index} when compared to II and ID genotypes. No association was, however, found between the CMA polymorphism and regression of LVH in these patients [201].

Conversely, Gumprecht et al. reported that the CMA/B polymorphism, together with the ACE I/D polymorphism, conferred a genetic predisposition to increased risk of the development of LVH in Caucasian type-2 diabetics [202].

The CMA/B was not associated with the extent of LVH in one study of a cohort of 50 unrelated HCM patients and 50 healthy controls [174]. In a later study, the same group reported that CMA polymorphisms did not affect blood pressure, posterior- or interventricular septal thickness in patients with acute myocardial infarction [203]. In a family-based association study, the CMA/B polymorphism showed a significant association with LVM in an unadjusted analysis, but the same SNP did not show a significant association with LVM or interventricular septal thickness in a multivariate analysis in which age, sex and the presence of hypertension were adjusted for ($p = 0.06$) [31].

3.6. Angiotensin II Type 1 Receptor (AT_1R)

The main effector molecule of the RAAS, Ang II, when bound to the AT_1 and AT_2 receptors, influences cardiac hypertrophy, remodelling and contraction in multiple blood pressure independent ways. Binding of Ang II to the AT_1R activates multiple intracellular pathways that involve phospholipids, calcium, reactive oxygen species (ROS) and kinases [204]. These AT_1R-mediated pathways elicit cardiovascular hypertrophic effects that are well documented, which includes vasoconstriction, aldosterone release and growth stimulation [27;205].

Moreover, overexpression of the AT_1R leads to increased cardiac mass and cardiomyocyte hypertrophy in mice [206]. It was recently shown that increased cardiac expression of the AT_1R gene (*AGTR1*) in cardiomyocytes of adult transgenic mice caused blood pressure-independent hypertrophy by promoting cardiomyocyte growth, which progressed to pathological remodelling upon further stimulation [207]. Moreover, large clinical trials have concluded that AT_1R antagonists reduce LVH and other cardiac morbidities in humans [208;209].

AT_1R-antagonists are currently being explored as potential therapeutic options for hypertrophy and associated morbidities in HCM [210]. Four small pilot studies in patients with non-obstructive HCM showed slight improvements in cardiovascular morphology and function [211-214]. The most recent of these studies reported that the long-term administration of the AT_1R-antagonist candesartan in HCM patients was associated with significant regression of LVH, improvement of left ventricular function, and exercise tolerance. This effect was dependent on the specific HCM causal mutation [213]. These studies are however still too small to allow definitive conclusions to be drawn and more research is needed in this regard.

Castellano et al. studied the effects of an A/C transversion at position 1166 in the 3' untranslated region of *AGTR1* (rs5186) on the regulation of blood pressure and cardiovascular structure in 212 subjects randomly selected from a general population in northern Italy [215]. They reported that blood pressure levels were significantly lower in CC-homozygotes, but no association was found with echocardiographically -determined LVM after adjustment for potentially confounding variables (age, sex, height, weight, blood pressure and smoking)

[215]. Similarly, a study on 141 Caucasian patients with normal coronary arteries did not find association between the A1166C, or the ACE I/D polymorphism, and left ventricular function or LVM [216].

Wang et al. studied the effects of *AGTR1* C-512T, A1166C and L191L polymorphisms on the progression of blood pressure and LVM in a longitudinal study involving 581 European American and African American youths [217]. When analysed as a single variant, the L191L polymorphism showed a significant systolic blood pressure-lowering effect in youths with a high socioeconomic status, and a diastolic blood pressure-lowering effect in African American youths. However, haplotype analysis identified a protective haplotype (C-521, 191L and A1166) for LVM in the entire cohort. Individuals homozygous for this haplotype showed a significant decrease of 12.9g in LVM when compared to the most common reference haplotype (–521T, 191L and A1166) [217].

Ishahov et al. reported that this polymorphism did not contribute significantly to hypertrophy development in hypertensive (n = 53) or HCM (n = 96) patients [218]. However, subjects with a family history of HCM, but who did not manifest the disease clinically, had a four-fold increase in C-allele carrier status compared to patients without a family history of HCM [218]. Conversely, the 1166C-allele was associated with increased LVM in 104 unrelated HCM patients, independent of age, gender, peak left ventricular outflow gradient, plasma renin, and the ACE I/D polymorphism [177]. Coto et al. reported a significantly higher frequency of 1166C-allele carriers among echocardiographically-diagnosed HCM patients compared to controls (OR = 1.56; 95%CI = 1.09-2.23) [104]. This allele was also associated with higher left ventricular wall thickness in HCM patients [104].

In contrast to these studies, in which only echocardiographic criteria were used to diagnose HCM, Funada et al. studied the effect of this polymorphism in 126 genotype-identified HCM patients from 49 Japanese families [178]. These patients were diagnosed with HCM through standard echocardiographic criteria and the diagnosis was confirmed with genetic testing for sarcomeric gene mutations. While this resulted in an improved diagnosis, the authors did unfortunately not adjust the subsequent association analyses for these sarcomeric mutations, which may have yielded more informative results. They reported that the A1166C alone did not influence LVH, but when analysed in combination with the ACE I/D polymorphism, the two SNPs significantly affected adverse cardiac remodelling [178]. This SNP was additionally found to associate with LVH in a study on 26 individuals from a single family with HCM caused by a previously identified myosin binding protein C mutation [31]. A recent study [219] proposed a biochemical mechanism of action for the A1166C polymorphism. This SNP is located in the 3' untranslated region in a target site for the hsa-miR-155 micro-RNA, which is able to bind to 3' untranslated regions through complementary base-pairing and thus to repress mRNA expression post-transcriptionally. Using reporter silencing assays, Sethupathy et al. showed that hsa-miR-155 downregulates the expression of only the 1166A, and not the 1166C-allele, which results in increased translation of *AGTR1* in C-allele carriers [219]. It is however unsure at this stage whether *AGTR1* and hsa-miR-155 is concomitantly expressed in the heart and more studies are therefore needed to fully explore the functionality of this SNP, while the possibility still exist that it might be in LD with a truly functional mutation. However, this highlights a mechanism by which apparently non-functional polymorphisms can have effects on expression of genes, and thereby may affect biochemical pathways and physiological systems.

3.7. Angiotensin II Type 2 Receptor (AT_2 R)

Cardiac expression of the AT_2R is upregulated in heart failure, myocardial infarction and cardiac remodelling [220-222]. Previous studies in adult rat hearts have suggested that AT_2Rs have antihypertrophic effects on the heart that counterbalance the hypertrophic effects of the AT_1Rs [223;224]. In a study on adult rat hearts, Bartunek et al. demonstrated that AT_2R inhibition amplifies LVH in response to Ang II. They perfused normal and hypertrophied hearts either with only Ang II or Ang II together with an AT_2R blocker and measured new protein synthesis within the left ventricles of these hearts. AT_2R blockade in Ang II-treated rats resulted in an amplified left ventricular growth response to Ang II, which was coupled with reduced left ventricular cGMP content, and enhanced membrane protein kinase C translocation [225].

The AT_2R gene (*AGTR2*) is located on the X-chromosome and consists of three exons and two introns; the entire open reading frame of the gene is situated in the third exon. Zhang et al. reported that an rs5193/rs5194 haplotype in *AGTR2* is associated with a cardioprotective role in Cantonese patients with essential hypertension [226].

A commonly occurring AT_2R polymorphism, rs1403543, designated as either -1332 G/A or +1675 G/A [227;228] is, however, the most frequently studied SNP in hypertrophy association studies. This polymorphism is located at a lariat branch-point in the first intron, 29 bp before exon 2, in a region that is important for transcriptional activity [228;229]. Nishimura et al. postulated that this polymorphism is functional and may affect pre-mRNA splicing [230], although a later study provided evidence that it modulates AT_2R protein expression, but not mRNA splicing [229]. Warnecke et al. concluded that +1675 G/A is associated with increased AT_2R protein levels, which may be protective in LVH development [229].

In a study of 60 normotensive and 60 untreated, mildly hypertensive students at a Bavarian university, Schmieder and colleagues found that the +1675 A-allele is significantly associated with an increase in echocardiographically determined LVM and relative left ventricular wall thickness in young, mildly hypertensive males [231]. The +1675 A-allele was additionally associated with LVH in males aged 55–74 from the Glasgow Heart Scan Old (GLAEOLD) cohort [232]. These findings were, however, not replicated in the similar, but larger Glasgow Heart Scan (GLAECO) cohort, and the authors subsequently concluded that further research into the role of *AGTR2* in LVH was needed [232].

In contrast, Alfakih et al. reported an association between +1675 G-allele and LVM_{index} as determined with magnetic resonance imaging (MRI) in patients with systemic hypertension [227]. MRI is credited with being a more reliable measure of cardiac hypertrophy than M-mode and 2D-echocardiography, even though echocardiography is still widely used to estimate LVM as it is more readily available as a clinical tool [233].

Deinum et al. investigated the effect of an *AGTR2* +3123 A/C polymorphism (rs11091046) on LVH in 103 unrelated HCM patients [234]. Multiple regression analysis showed that the *AGTR2* +3123 C-allele decreased LVM_{index} in female subjects, independent of plasma renin, the +1166 A/C *AGTR1* variant or the I/D *ACE* variant. However, this study of ungenotyped cases did not account for differences in the primary HCM causal mutation, which may have had confounding effects on the association. A later study reported a significant association between the +1675 A-allele and decreased LVH in a HCM family cohort, independent of the primary HCM causal mutation, blood pressure, age, sex, BSA, heart rate and hypertension diagnosis [30].

3.8. Aldosterone Synthase (*CYP11B2*)

Recent studies in perfused hearts and cultured cells reported increased cardiomyocyte contractile force and cardiomyocyte hypertrophy in response to aldosterone administration [235-237]. Serum aldosterone was, furthermore, significantly related to LVM as well as septal and posterior wall thickness in a population based sample of 615 middle-age subjects [159]. Tsybouleva and co-workers showed that myocardial aldosterone levels were increased by 4.5-fold in HCM hearts, when compared to healthy donor hearts, and that mRNA levels from the aldosterone synthase-encoding gene, *CYP11B2,* increased 7-fold in HCM [238].

The -344T/C polymorphism in the 5' promoter region of the *CYP11B2* was significantly associated with levels of plasma aldosterone in a cohort of 216 patients with essential hypertension, after adjustment for age and 24h urine Na^+-excretion [239]. This polymorphism also predicted statistically significant variations in left ventricular diameter and LVM, independent of sex, body size, blood pressure, physical activity, smoking, and ethanol consumption in 84 healthy Caucasians [240]. The -344T/C polymorphism resides in a putative binding site for steroidogenic transcription factor-1 (SF-1); the -344 C-allele is associated with a four-fold increase in SF-1 binding and could therefore possibly influence gene expression [241]. Bassett et al. confirmed that the C-allele binds SF-1 more strongly that the T-allele, but added that SF-1 failed to stimulate CYP11B2 expression *in vivo* [242].

A study on two larger cohorts from the MONICA study did, however, not replicate these associations [243]. A later meta-analysis (that included data from these as well as a number of subsequent studies) investigated the effect of this polymorphism on left ventricular structure-related phenotypes [244]. The -344T/C variant was not significantly associated with LVM or interventricular septal wall thickness in a pooled sample of 2157 unrelated subjects, although hypertensive subjects ($n = 332$) homozygous for the T-allele showed a 6.9% increase in LVM, compared to CC-homozygous subjects [244]. Posterior wall thickness was 2.4 % lower in homozygous CC individuals in a subject pool of 1994 from 10 homogeneous studies; this effect was increased to 11% when only hypertensive individuals were analysed [244].

While this meta-analysis only included data from unrelated people in case-control study designs, another study investigated the effect of this promoter variant as well as five other *CYP11B2* polymorphisms (singularly and in combined haplotypes) on heart size, in 955 members from 229 British families [245]. The additional five variants included an intron 2 conversion (I2C) polymorphism, in which intron 2 of the neighbouring 11 beta-hydroxylase gene (*CYP11B1*) gene has been transferred to *CYP11B2,* as well as four other SNPs in the coding region (A2713G, A4550C, T4986C and G5937C). While the authors found no association with the -344T/C SNP, they reported a significant association between G5937C and interventricular septal thickness, whereas the I2C and A4550C polymorphisms associated with left ventricular cavity size. Measured haplotype analyses confirmed the association of I2C and G5937C polymorphisms with interventricular septal thickness, and alleles at the I2C polymorphism with left ventricular cavity size. These *CYP11B2* polymorphisms contributed to 2.4 and 2.0–3.4% of the variability in septal wall thickness and left ventricular cavity size, respectively [245].

Two independent studies later reported strong LD between *CYP11B2* polymorphisms and variants in the neighbouring *CYP11B1* gene [246;247]. The enzyme encoded by the latter gene catalyses the final step in cortisol biosynthesis. Studies later showed that aldosterone synthesis is highly heritable and is affected by genotypes at *CYP11B2* as well as *CYP11B1* [248;249]. The association found between *CYP11B2* polymorphisms and cardiovascular phenotypes could therefore perhaps be explained (or influenced) by LD across the CYP11B1/B2 locus, but more studies are needed to fully explore this notion.

Patel et al. reported that *CYP11B2* −344T/C genotypes did not influence LVM or interventricular septal thickness in 142 genetically-independent echocardiographically-diagnosed HCM patients [250]. However, Ortlepp et al. later found that this polymorphism significantly associated with both of these hypertrophy phenotypes after age, sex and the presence of hypertension was controlled for, in a single family with HCM caused by a previously identified myosin binding protein C (MyBPC) mutation [31]. In contrast to the study by Tsybouleva et al., Chai et al. reported that plasma and left ventricular tissue levels of aldosterone in 79 genetically-independent subjects with HCM were not significantly different from those in age-matched controls [251]. They reported a significant association between the *CYP11B2* −344T-allele and LVM_{index} as well as interventricular septal thickness in men, but not in women. Multiple regression analysis showed that the effect of the −344T-allele on interventricular septal thickness occurred independently of renin or the *ACE* I/D, *AGTR1* +1166 A/C or *AGTR2* +3123 A/C polymorphisms [251].

These studies did, however, not investigate the effect of the entire CYP11B1/B2 locus on hypertrophy indices in HCM and more research is thus needed to fully elucidate the contribution of CYP11B1/B2 variants to hypertrophy development in general, an in HCM in particular.

3.9. Mineralocorticoid Receptor (MR)

The MR, encoded by *NR3C2*, is responsible for the downstream RAAS functions, as it binds to aldosterone to form an MR/aldosterone complex, which, in turn, activates aldosterone-induced early and late response gene transcription and signalling cascades to mediate cellular Na^+ homeostasis via its downstream effectors. The MR is a member of the steroid/thyroid/retinoid/orphan receptor family of transcription factors and has been identified in cardiac tissue in previous studies [252]. Functional polymorphisms in *NR3C2* have been shown to result in a rare condition called pseudohypoaldosteronism type I, which is characterized by unresponsiveness to aldosterone, severe salt wasting, extreme hyperkalaemia and elevated PRA [253;254].

Interestingly, through its binding to the MR, aldosterone is able to directly induce cardiomyocyte hypertrophy [255;256]. Nagata et al. investigated the effect of MR-blockade on cardiac hypertrophy in rats with salt-sensitive hypertension and concluded that MR-blockade attenuates LVH, in the absence of an antihypertensive effect [257]. Correspondingly, the MR antagonist spironolactone attenuated LVH in uremic rats without a significant reduction in blood pressure [258]. Several further animal studies, including some using HCM model animals, illustrated beneficial cardiovascular effects with cardiomyocyte-specific MR blockade [259;260].

Overexpression of the human MR in mice resulted in mild dilated cardiomyopathy in conjunction with a significant increase in heart rate, while blood pressure levels remained unchanged [261]. Tsybouleva and colleagues investigated the effect of MR blockade in a transgenic mouse model of human HCM (cTnT-Q92). They were able to demonstrate that MR blockade with spironolactone reduced myocyte disarray and interstitial fibrosis, and also improved diastolic function; they concluded that aldosterone, throught the MR, significantly affects the relationship between sarcomeric dysfunction and the cardiac phenotype of HCM [238]. Similar approaches were, however, not as effective in feline HCM models [210;262]. One study speculated that this might be due to inadequate dosage of RAAS inhibitors as more research is needed on the dosage required to adequately disrupt the RAAS in feline models [262].

In another transgenic mouse model of cardiac hypertrophy, Zhang et al. show that conditional and cardiomyocyte-restricted overexpression of the human MR promoted LVH and diastolic, but not systolic, dysfunction through redox-dependent, blood pressure–independent effects in response to Ang II infusion [263]. MR blockade with canrenoate was shown to decrease the expression of TGF-β and significantly reduced LVH and cardiac fibrosis in these mice, which is consistent with earlier studies where MR blockade reduced hypertrophy indices determined with MRI in transgenic rats [264].

In humans, MR antagonists were shown to reduce ventricular remodelling, sudden cardiac death and myocardial fibrosis in the randomized aldactone evaluation study (RALES) and in the eplerenone post-acute myocardial infarction efficacy and survival study (EPHESUS) clinical trials. These effects were also independent of the antagonist's effect on blood pressure, providing evidence that MR blockade offers cardioprotective effects in patients with heart failure and systolic left ventricular dysfunction [265;266]. The MR blocker spironolactone is currently still being investigated as an experimental therapy option in HCM, as small preliminary studies showed beneficial cardiovascular effects, but more research is essential in this regard [267].

Previous reports show a significant association between *NR3C2* polymorphisms and blood pressure control in hypertensive populations [268-270], but there is currently a lack of information on the involvement of *NR3C2* variants in both overload-induced and blood pressure-independent hypertrophy. One possible explanation for the lack of knowledge in this regard is the size of the MR gene, as it spans about 360 kb and contains 10 exons. A minimum of about 20 SNPs is needed to at least capture the main haplotypes for a given population in this gene through linkage disequilibrium unit (LDU)-based density as well as tag SNP selection.

3.10. 11β-HSD2

The MR is able to bind both aldosterone and cortisol, but under normal circumstances it is protected from cortisol occupancy by the short-chain dehydrogenase/reductase 11β-HSD2, which degrades cortisol to corticosterone, which is then unable to bind to the MR [271]. Null mutations in this gene causes apparent mineralocorticoid excess (AME), a rare form of congenital hypertension, characterised by severe hypertension, hypokalemia and low aldosterone levels, as well as associated end-organ complications such as renal or cardiovascular damage [272].

Transgenic mice overexpressing 11β-HSD2 in cardiomyocytes were normotensive, but spontaneously developed cardiac hypertrophy, fibrosis, and heart failure and died prematurely on a normal salt diet [273]. In addition, the MR blocker spironolactone improved adverse left ventricular remodelling in rats by modulating MR and 11β-HSD2 expression levels [274]. Recently, Bailey et al. showed that *HSD11B2-null* heterozygote mice, which express only 50% of normal enzyme levels, develop salt-sensitive hypertension [275]. These mice exhibited a salt-induced increase in heart:body weight ratio, which was partially reduced by spironolactone [275].

11β-HSD2 is consequently an attractive candidate gene for hypertension in humans and polymorphisms in this gene have been associated with blood pressure regulation in several populations [276]. However, little is known about the role of this gene in hypertrophy development, although one study reported a correlation between urinary 11β-HSD2 activity and LVM in essential hypertension [277].

3.11. Downstream RAAS Effectors

Various studies have implicated altered intracellular Na^+ in cardiac hypertrophy [278;279]. Thus far we have discussed the indirect (blood pressure-dependent) as well as the direct hypertrophic effect of certain RAAS components on hypertrophy in HCM. Another potential mechanism whereby RAAS genes can alter the HCM hypertrophic phenotype is by altering the balance of intracellular Na^+, which plays a crucial role in the structural, mechanical, and electrical properties of the myocardium. The MR/aldosterone complex exerts its effects on Na^+ homeostasis via the ENaCs, as well as via Na^+/K^+-ATPase.

3.11.1. Na^+/K^+-ATPase

The Na^+/K^+-ATPases catalyze the exchange of Na^+ and K^+ ions across plasma membranes and are essential downstream effectors of the MR/aldosterone complex. The Na^+/K^+-ATPase is a heteromeric protein that consists of α- and β-subunits [280]. The α-subunit is a polytopic membrane protein that confers the catalytic activity of the enzyme and contains binding sites for Na^+, K^+ and ATP [281]. The β-subunit modulates the pump function and is important for the efficient translation of the α-subunit on the endoplasmic reticulum, membrane insertion and correct folding of the α-subunit as well as the expression of the enzyme on the plasma membrane [282].

To date, four isoforms of the α-subunit (α1, α2, α3 and α4) and three isoforms of the β-subunit (β1, β2 and β3) have been described in mammals, which exhibit tissue-specific expression [283]. Previous studies have confirmed the expression of the α1, α2, α3, β1, β2 and β3-subunits in human hearts [284-286]. Studies in animal hypertrophy models have additionally demonstrated that the expression of Na^+/K^+-ATPase α- and β-subunit isoforms are altered in hypertrophied ventricles [287-290].

In the first report on Na^+/K^+-ATPase isoform expression in the myocardium of normal and failing human hearts, Allen et al. reported that none of the three α-subunits showed altered expression in the left ventricles of failing hearts [291]. Later, Shamraj et al. reported that Na^+/K^+-ATPase isoform expression is indeed altered in failing compared to nonfailing human hearts [292]; this finding was subsequently corroborated by other groups [285;293].

The Na^+/K^+-ATPase also serves as a receptor for ouabain and other related cardiac glycosides. Previous investigations have established that the positive inotropic effects of cardiac glycosides on the myocardium is due to partial inhibition of the cardiac Na^+/K^+-ATPase, which causes a small increase in intracellular Na^+ and, in turn, affects the Na^+/Ca^{2+} exchanger, ultimately leading to increased intracellular Ca^{2+} and force of contraction [294;295]. Fedorova et al. reported that the development of LVH and subsequent transition to heart failure in Dahl salt-sensitive rats on a high Na^+ diet was associated with shifts in left ventricular Na^+/K^+-ATPase isoform composition and sensitivity to ouabain [296].

Huang et al. demonstrated that partial inhibition of the Na^+/K^+-ATPase by ouabain in cultured neonatal rat cardiomyocytes induced hypertrophic growth, which was coupled with increased expression of TGF-β and other late response markers indicative of cardiac hypertrophy [295]. Subsequent studies by the same group revealed that the hypertrophic response that follows Na^+/K^+-ATPase inhibition was also associated with p42/44 MAPK and ROS-dependent pathways [288;297].

Animal knockout-models suggest differential roles for α- and β-subunits in the heart. The hearts of heterozygous Na^+/K^+-ATPase α1-knockout mice were hypocontractile, while the hearts of heterozygous α2-knockout mice were hypercontractile as a result of increased Ca^{2+} transients during the contractile cycle [298]. In contrast, homozygous Na^+/K^+-ATPase β2-knockout mice exhibited ventricular hypertrophy without any diminution of Na^+/K^+-ATPase enzymatic activity [299]. Homozygous knockout mice in which the Na^+/K^+-ATPase β1 gene was inactivated exclusively in the ventricular cardiomyocytes exhibited mild hypertrophy, coupled with reduced contractility and ventricular function in aging mice [300].

Polymorphisms in the α1-subunit gene (*ATP1A1*) [301;302], as well as in the β1-subunit gene (*ATP1B1*) gene [303;304], were previously associated with essential hypertension. *ATP1B1* variants have also been associated with QT-intervals in long-QT patients [305]. However, the effect of genetic variation in the Na^+/K^+-ATPase subunit isoforms on cardiovascular hypertrophy remains unclear.

3.11.2. Amiloride-Sensitive Epithelial Sodium Channels (ENaCs)

The amiloride-sensitive epithelial sodium channels (ENaCs) are also important regulators of intracellular Na^+, as they are responsible for the electrodiffusion of Na^+ through epithelial cells. Each ENaC consists of three homologous subunits, i.e. an α-, β-, and a γ-subunit [306], encoded by the *SCNN1A, SCNN1B,* and *SCNN1G* genes, respectively.

Gain-of-function mutations in ENaC subunit genes can cause a rare condition called Liddle syndrome. These mutations prevent the degradation of ENaCs, resulting in excessive Na^+-absorption, K^+-wasting, systemic hypertension, as well as an elevated incidence of early cardiovascular disease and LVH [307-309].

The association of the ubiquitin ligase Nedd4-2 with an ENaC leads to ubiquitination of the ENaC and its subsequent removal from the plasma membrane. Nedd4-2 is therefore vital to the activity and regulation of ENaCs. In a study on Nedd4-2-knockout mice, Shi and colleagues demonstrated that these mice had elevated blood pressure and impaired ENaC activity, which was aggravated by a high salt diet [310]. Ultimately, these animals developed cardiac hypertrophy and systolic dysfunction [310].

The role of ENaC mutations in hypertension is well documented and the antihypertensive properties of the ENaC inhibitor, amiloride, have long been known [311;312]. However, studies in animal models of hypertension have shown that low doses of amiloride can reduce

LVH and other cardiovascular pathologies, despite the fact that blood pressure remained high [313;314]. These effects occurred independently of changes on serum K^+. These and other studies highlight the potential cardiovascular benefit of ENaC inhibition [315].

Interestingly, heterozygous αENaC-knockout mice appear to have an intact capacity to maintain blood pressure and Na^+ balance despite varying salt diets [316]. This ability to maintain normal blood pressure margins appears to be caused by increased RAAS activity through a compensatory upregulation of AT_1Rs [316]. In a study of rats on a salt-restricted diet, the AT_1R antagonist candesartan markedly decreased the quantity of ENaC α-subunits, which have been shown to be rate-limiting for assembly of mature ENaC complexes [317]. Candesartan administration was also found to increase the abundance of ENaC β- and γ-subunits in these rats [317].

These studies point towards a definite interplay between the ENaCs and RAAS components. Further studies are, however, needed to fully explore the nature of this interaction in pathological hypertrophy *per se* as well as within the context of HCM. Studies are additionally needed to investigate the effect of genetic variation in ENaC subunit genes on hypertrophy development.

4. RAAS Variants in HCM

It is then evident that almost all RAAS components have a plausible impact on hypertrophy development, whether due to hemodynamic changes, or completely independent from systemic blood pressure. The cardiac phenotype of HCM is complex in nature as a multitude of factors influences its phenotypic expression, whereas the contribution of genetic variation in the RAAS to the HCM phenotype is by no means resolved. A better knowledge of the underlying factors that influence this complex hypertrophic phenotype of HCM will ultimately contribute to better risk stratification of HCM patients, and, more immediately useful, may pinpoint hypertrophy-contributing pathways that may be more amenable to modulation than the primary sarcomeric gene mutation.

It is imperative to consider confounding issues when embarking on a new HCM association study. The most commonly addressed issue in association studies is understandably cohort size as it impacts directly on the power of that particular study, but HCM prevalence is estimated to be 1 in 500 in young adults [38], which makes the practicality of extremely large cohorts a challenge.

There are furthermore study parameters that pertain specifically to HCM association studies, which can significantly improve the interpretability of these studies. In the next section we discuss the family-based association approach to identify hypertrophy modulators in HCM using data generated from a South African HCM founder family cohort to highlight some of these issues.

4.1. An Investigation into the Influence of RAAS Genes on Hypertrophy in an HCM Founder Family Cohort

This study aimed to test for association between variants within RAAS genes and hypertrophy in HCM with adjustment for known hypertrophy confounders, and to quantify the effect of these variants on hypertrophy indices, using a family based association approach. To this end we selected polymorphisms to cover genes that represent the different steps in the RAAS.

4.2. Materials and Methods

4.2.1. Study Subjects

This study was approved by the University of Stellenbosch Health Science Faculty's Institutional Review Board (N04/03/062) and all subjects entered into the study gave written informed consent. During routine mutation screening for HCM-causing mutations, 27 consecutively referred probands carrying one of three mutations that occur as founder mutations in South Africa, i.e. R92W$_{TNNT2}$, R403W$_{MYH7}$, and A797T$_{MYH7}$ were identified [318]. Pedigree tracing was performed for these index individuals and their family members were invited to participate in this modifier gene study. Genomic DNA for all genotypic analyses was extracted from peripheral blood lymphocytes as described previously [55].Thus, a panel of 388 individuals that included genetically and clinically affected and unaffected family members was identified; these individuals were all screened for the presence or absence of all three founder mutations.

4.2.2. Clinical Evaluation

The subjects were clinically characterised by 2D-echocardiography performed by a single cardiologist who was unaware of the mutation status of each subject. Analyses included echocardiographic recordings in M-mode, 2D and Doppler blood-flow imaging using a 2.5Hz transducer in standard parasternal long-axis and short-axis, using apical four- and two-chamber views with a GE Healthcare Vivid7 cardiovascular ultrasound system. A total of 16 2D-echocardiographic measurements were taken according to the recommendations of the American Society of Echocardiography [319], as described previously [320]. This included six segments of the left ventricular wall at both the mitral valve and papillary muscle levels and four segments at the smaller supra-apex level.

LVM was calculated using the formula for the estimation of LVM from 2D left ventricular linear dimensions as recommended by the American Society of Echocardiography [319]:

$$LVM = 0.8 \times \left(1.04\left[(LVIDd + PWTd + SWTd)^3 - (LVIDd)^3\ \right]\right) + 0.6g\ ,$$

where LVIDd is the left ventricular internal diameter during diastole, PWTd is the posterior wall thickness during diastole, and SWTd is the interventricular septal wall thickness during diastole.

Due to the non-homogenous distribution of hypertrophy in individuals with HCM, echocardiographically-derived LVM is not considered to be the most accurate measure of LVH. In addition, a single measurement of hypertrophy such as maximum interventricular septal thickness or even maximum left ventricular wall thickness (mLVWT) does not reflect the full extent of hypertrophy in all individuals. We therefore calculated a cumulative wall thickness (CWT) score, which is the sum of all 16 wall thickness measurements. As the distribution of hypertrophy is variable in HCM, we also derived the first principal component (PC1) from these 16 measurements. PC1 best explained the variability in wall thickness for this particular cohort and is essentially a linear combination (weighted sum) of the 16 wall thickness values, which explains the largest proportion of the variation in all 16 measurements combined, as described previously [30].

Blood pressure measurements were taken twice in the sitting position and after 5 minutes of rest and the second measurement was used.

Subjects were identified as hypertensive if they had a systolic blood pressure ≥ 140 mm Hg or diastolic blood pressure ≥ 90 mm Hg, or if they were on anti-hypertensive medication. Medical history and covariates of cardiac structure (age, sex, BSA and heart rate) were noted for each participant.

4.2.3. RAAS Variant Genotyping

Polymorphisms with high reported heterozygosity values in dbSNP (http://www.ncbi.nlm.nih.gov/snp/) in *AGT*, *ACE1*, *ACE2*, *AGTR1*, *AGTR2*, *NR3C2* and *SCNN1B*, including variants previously investigated for association with LVH in other studies, were chosen for investigation.

AGT, *ACE1* and *AGTR1* variants were genotyped as summarized in Table 2, while *NR3C2* and *SCNN1B* SNPs were genotyped using ABI TaqMan Validated SNP Genotyping Assays. *ACE2* and *AGTR2* variants were genotyped in a smaller subset of the HCM founder cohort as described previously [30;32].

4.2.4. Statistical Analysis

Validation of input files and Mendelian inheritance within families were verified with Pedstats v. 6.11 [321], using X-chromosome settings where appropriate, and genotyping inconsistencies were resolved by re-genotyping. Pedstats was also used to asses Hardy-Weinberg equilibrium on unrelated individuals within the cohort. Quantitative transmission disequilibrium testing (QTDT) [322] was used to assess the (broad sense) heritability of all four hypertrophy traits (LVM, mLVWT, CWT, PC1) after adjustment for hypertrophy confounders. Each trait was transformed to approximate normality using quantile normalization [323] prior to all analyses.

The association between the various *AGT*, *ACE1*, *AGTR1*, *NR3C2* and *SCNN1B* variants and the four hypertrophy traits was assessed with specialised mixed-effects models using per-individual random effects, which are correlated according to kinship coefficients (R package kinship, function lmekin, www.r-project.org).

These models include environmental and polygenic variance components. All analyses were adjusted for covariates that are known to modulate cardiac hypertrophy, namely whether the individual carries a mutation or not, the identity of the primary HCM-causing mutation ($R92W_{TNNT2}$, $R403W_{MYH7}$, or $A797T_{MYH7}$), hypertension diagnosis, mean arterial pressure, sex, age at clinical assessment, BSA and heart rate (as a proxy measure for tachycardia). Such modelling results in the effect of the candidate gene variants being estimated after the effects of the covariates have been removed from the phenotype.

The association between variants in the X-linked *ACE2* and *AGTR2* genes and the four quantile normalised traits were analysed similarly as part of previous studies and are included here for discussion purposes [30;32].

The untransformed dataset was used to estimate informative covariate-adjusted effect sizes, as effect sizes calculated from the quantile normalised data cannot be interpreted in the context of the original measurements.

Table 2. Summary of methods used for genotyping of *AGT*, *ACE1* and *AGTR1* variants. All primer sequences are given in 5'-3' direction

Gene	Variant	Primer sequences	Genotyping method	Alleles: Restriction enzyme fragments (bp)
AGT	rs5051	F: catctgtccttctggccagc	SNaPshot	C/T
		R: ccgggctgaatgctaaagg	agaacaacggcagcttcttcccc	
	rs4762	F: ttccatggagctttgaatcc	SNaPshot	C/T
		R: ttgccttaccttggaagtgg	ccagctgctgctgtcca	
	rs699	F: ttccatggagctttgaatcc	SNaPshot	C/T
		R: ttgccttaccttggaagtgg	gacaggatggaagactggctgct ccctga	
ACE1	rs4340	F: gactctgtaagccactgctgg	1.5% AGE	I-allele: 737 D-allele: 450
		R: ccaacaccacattacctgcc		
	rs4365	F: cagccttgggtcttaacc	ASREA/12% PAGE	A-allele: 332, 316, 261, 129, 120, 40
		R: tggcagtgttagaatggc	*Alu*I	G-Allele: 332, 316, 175, 129, 120, 86, 40
	rs4303	F: ctcaccaacatcctggcttcc	SNaPshot	G/T
		R: gcctgcttcttcatgcatcg	acctccatgccttcgtccgccgc	
AGTR 1	rs5182	F: ttgtagccaaagtcacctgc	ASREA/12% PAGE	T-allele: 422, 309, 127, 68
		R: aatgtgcagtaccaggtgc	*Mnl*I	C-allele: 325, 309, 127, 97, 68
	rs2640539	F: tcctagacacgggacatcg	ASREA/1.5% AGE	G-allele: 992
		R: tggagggaaccttatggg	*Mspa*1	C-allele: 609, 383
	rs3772627	F: aatacagtgcagacctgg	ASREA	A-allele: 697, 423
		R: attgctgaggaagattgc	*Bsah*1	G-allele: 496, 423, 201
	rs11122575	F: caccttcaatgcagccaacc	SNaPshot	T/C
		R: tccttgcagcaccagttgg	tcttctatgtccctcacatagtattg caaatgaca	
	rs1926723	F: caccttcaatgcagccaacc	SNaPshot	A/G
		R: tccttgcagcaccagttgg		

4.3. Results and Discussion of Family-Based Association Study

All genotype frequencies, in a random sample of unrelated individuals, were in agreement with Hardy-Weinberg equilibrium. All four of the investigated hypertrophy traits, viz. LVM, mLVWT, CWT and PC1, were significantly heritable (Table 3).

The heritability value reported here for the CWT score and mLVWT is in accordance with earlier values reported for cardiac wall thickness [324;325].

However, previously published heritability estimates for echocardiographically determined LVM ranged from 0.17 to 0.69 in different populations, with the lowest values reported in healthy adults and the highest in monozygotic twins [324-330].

Table 3. Heritability (H^2) of the hypertrophy traits investigated in this study, after adjustment for hypertrophy covariates

	H^2	p-value
LVM	0.55	< 0.001
mLVWT	0.45	0.001
CWT	0.42	0.010
PC1	0.47	0.006

LVM= echocardiographically-derived left ventricular mass, mLVWT= maximum left ventricular wall thickness, CWT = cumulative wall thickness score, PC1 = first principal component.

Table 4. P-values for association of RAAS gene variants with hypertrophy measurements

		LVM	mLVWT	CWT	PC1
AGT	rs1926723	0.6798	0.4377	0.6734	0.7618
	rs11122575	0.3582	0.0623	0.1572	0.1450
	rs699	0.4604	0.9606	0.6836	0.5675
	rs4762	0.4520	0.4834	0.0918	0.0823
	rs5051	0.6944	0.9771	0.9482	0.7649
ACE1	rs4340 (I/D)	0.2542	0.2272	0.2008	0.2453
	rs4298	0.6998	0.6824	0.6290	0.3536
	rs4303	0.4418	0.4835	0.5716	0.4820
	rs4356	0.0795	0.0977	0.0645	0.0874
ACE2	rs1978124	0.2349	0.7125	0.3756	0.2821
[32]	rs2285666	0.7142	0.9594	0.7508	0.8158
	rs879922	0.0412	0.0185	0.0958	0.1113
	rs4646179	0.3408	0.1987	0.2563	0.4294
AGTR1	rs2640539	0.1666	0.0102	0.1021	0.1228
	rs3772627	0.8999	0.4134	0.5705	0.7406
	rs5182	0.3771	0.2243	0.2817	0.2005

		LVM	mLVWT	CWT	PC1
AGTR2	rs1403543	0.2260	0.0761	0.0850	0.0179
[30]	rs5194	0.9174	0.8168	0.7269	0.8398
	rs11091046	0.9627	0.6929	0.5641	0.5920
NR3C2	rs906124	0.4176	0.7432	0.8626	0.6621
	rs11933380	0.0766	0.9926	0.2834	0.2381
	rs745019	0.0347	0.5271	0.1771	0.1372
	rs1403142	0.3314	0.7610	0.2920	0.1881
	rs13150372	0.3795	0.6759	0.3839	0.3091
	rs7694706	0.0594	0.5933	0.4515	0.2802
	rs6535584	0.3629	0.6883	0.6742	0.4941
		LVM	mLVWT	CWT	PC1
	rs6535594	0.0813	0.8407	0.2321	0.1691
	rs7699349	0.3132	0.9693	0.7104	0.5424
	rs2883930	0.0963	0.1610	0.0587	0.0777
	rs4835508	0.7945	0.6930	0.1600	0.1176
	rs11945778	0.7464	0.9546	0.9556	0.9939
	rs3910047	0.8542	0.8323	0.5922	0.6149
	rs3846329	0.7874	0.8676	0.6242	0.6725
	rs2137334	0.6097	0.1428	0.1086	0.0709
	rs13118022	0.2148	0.7165	0.8758	0.9656
	rs4635799	0.6669	0.7220	0.6399	0.6704
SCNN1B	rs11074555	0.3634	0.3590	0.2676	0.1939
	rs9930640	0.1490	0.5519	0.6283	0.5972
	rs239345	0.6191	0.4640	0.2565	0.3369
	rs238547	0.4596	0.7492	0.5141	0.3343
	rs8044970	0.0694	0.0290	0.0996	0.0918
	rs152740	0.3194	0.4014	0.5912	0.5706
	rs250563	0.9596	0.5520	0.2524	0.2691
	rs2303153	0.4410	0.5723	0.8381	0.7350

LVM= echocardiographically-derived left ventricular mass, mLVWT= maximum left ventricular wall thickness, CWT = cumulative wall thickness score, PC1 = first principal component.

Despite the range of LVM heritability values reported in these studies, all of them agreed that adjustment for known hypertrophy confounders such as age, sex and blood pressure significantly affected these values. In the Northern Manhattan Family Study for instance, the heritability of LVM was estimated at 0.65 in a model adjusted for age and gender, while this value dropped to 0.49 in a model adjusted for age, sex, weight, height, systolic blood pressure, diabetes, and antihypertensive medication [328]. Furthermore, the heritability of LVM as determined by cardiac MRI was estimated at 0.84 after adjustment for age and sex in a recent study on twins [331]. The heritability estimates reported in this multigenerational

HCM founder family cohort then offers a relevant appraisal of the heritability of these four traits as it is independent of the known confounding effects of the primary HCM causal mutation, as well as other known hypertrophy covariates.

The results from the association analyses are shown in Table 4. We do not find association between the well studied *AGT* M235T (rs699) polymorphism and any of the investigated hypertrophy indices, which is in accordance with Brugada et al., who reported that none of the commonly studied *AGT* SNPs, viz. M235T, T174M (rs4762), and -6 G/A (rs5051), had a significant influence on a composite LVH score or LVM in a cohort of 108 genetically independent HCM patients [105], as well as with a number of previous studies [33;102;103]. However, our results are in contrast to other hypertrophy studies [98-101].

Similarly, we failed to find significant evidence for association with the *ACE* I/D polymorphism, which is in agreement with some previous studies [103;104;168;177], but in contrast to others [171-173]. A possible explanation for the inconsistent results on the association of these two genes and hypertrophy could be that the effect of genetic variation in these genes on hypertrophy is context dependent as mentioned previously [92;180] and that both the I/D polymorphism as well as the M235T show variable distribution across different ethnic groups and populations [90;91;166].

For instance, previous studies reported that the effect of the I/D polymorphism [33;170] is reliant on the primary HCM causal mutation of an individual. While we did not analyse the three different HCM mutation groups separately, as such stratification would result in lower statistical power due to smaller sample groups, we nevertheless generated association p-values that were adjusted for the confounding effect of the individual primary HCM-causal mutations.

In *ACE2*, in a previous study from our group [32], we found that an intronic polymorphism associated significantly with both LVM and mLVWT. The G-allele of rs879922 was associated with a significant increase of 13.71 g in LVM as well as a 1.68 mm increase in mLVWT. This is consistent with a previous report that this G-allele, singly as well as within a four-marker haplotype, modestly increased LVM and interventricular septal thickness in the general male population in Augsburg, Germany [193].

Furthermore, a significant association was found between the T-allele of an *AGTR1* intronic SNP (rs2640539) and a 1.22 mm increase in mLVWT. Our study did, unfortunately, not include the A1166C (rs5186) variant that is most frequently studied in HCM. The 1166C-allele was previously associated with increased LVM in 104 unrelated HCM patients, independent of age, gender, peak left ventricular outflow gradient, plasma renin, and the ACE I/D polymorphism [177]. Similarly, Coto et al. reported that this variant was significantly associated with left ventricular wall thickness in HCM patients [104].

Another previous study by our group reported a significant association between the *AGTR2* +1675 G/A SNP (rs1403543) and a composite hypertrophy score that best explained the variability in wall thickness in that particular cohort, PC1 [30]. A clear, although not significant, trend towards association was also seen between this polymorphism and mLVWT and CWT in this cohort. This is consistent with a previous study that reported an association between this +1675 G-allele and LVM_{index} as determined with MRI in a hypertensive cohort [227]. Unlike Deinum et al., we do not find association between the +3123 A/C polymorphism (rs11091046) and LVH [234]. This discrepancy could be due to the fact that, unlike the previous study [234], our study adjusted all analyses for the primary HCM causal mutation.

Interestingly, this is the first report of a significant association between SNPs in *NR3C2* as well as *SCNN1B* and hypertrophy traits in HCM. The G-allele of rs745019 in *NR3C2* associated with a significant increase of 10.75 g in LVM, while the G-allele of rs8044970 in *SCNN1B* caused a significant decrease of 1.28 mm in mLVWT.

The lack of reproducibility of past results is a great concern and also hampers the interpretability of RAAS association results in HCM cohorts [332]. For instance, we did not find association with either the *ACE* I/D or *AGT* M235T variants in our analysis, which is consistent with some studies [103;104;177], but in contrast to others [31;99;172;174]. One explanation for this discrepancy could be lack of adjustment for relevant confounders as discussed earlier, which further underscores the need for consistency in HCM association study designs.

Taken together, our results highlight a number of key concerns and limitations for association studies in HCM. The first concern is that of statistical power, which refers to the probability that a test statistic reflects a true association (or lack thereof) between a genomic variant and a specific disease trait [333]. Traditionally, the power of a modifier study relies on the marker allele frequency, cohort as well as true effect size, and the number of confounders adjusted for [334;335]. In addition, errors in phenotypic classification and genotype errors contribute significantly to the power of an association study [333]. Presently, no comprehensive method exists for calculating the power of an association study in extended families, while very few case-control HCM studies report power calculations. Although our cohort size can be considered modest by current standards, it is simply the reality that HCM cohorts will typically be relatively small, as seen in Table 1. The impact of cohort size on the statistical power of an association study can, however, not be ignored and results from smaller studies should consequently be interpreted with caution.

The power of a particular study is further hampered by the use of genetic markers that have a low minor allele frequency (MAF), especially when one considers the small effect sizes that seem to be the norm in HCM hypertrophy modifier studies [173;245], and the profound impact that these two parameters have on the statistical power to avoid spurious results [335]. The possibility exists that a polymorphism that serves as a marker for hypertrophy in one population might have a very low MAF in a different population, as seen in the study reported by Wang et al. [194]. Moreover, functional polymorphisms typically have low heterozygosity values, as these polymorphisms have direct impacts on disease phenotypes. It is therefore necessary to prioritise markers with a fairly high MAF in HCM association studies.

The use of a family-based association approach in this study provided certain benefits over case-control designs, as it offers additional quality control measures to ensure genotyping accuracy and the opportunity to circumvent the confounding effect of undetected population stratification. Moreover, populations carrying founder mutations provide added control over the genetic variability introduced by different HCM causal mutations, which is an extremely important confounding factor in HCM association studies, as HCM causal mutations show variable phenotypic expression in different genetic backgrounds [48;49].

Another area for concern is multiple testing, where an increased probability of obtaining a false positive result exists. A popular solution for this is to use a Bonferroni adjustment. This method assumes that all the performed tests are independent and each p-value is consequently multiplied by the number of tests performed. However, Bonferroni corrections can be overly stringent in any genetic association study, especially when the phenotypes investigated are correlated, such as using a number of hypertrophy traits [336], or when using a number of SNPs that are in some measure of LD with each other. Alternatively, Bayesian methods could be used for correction, but require prior knowledge of the probability of involvement, which is presently unknown for most genetic variants [337].

Most studies attempt to circumvent the multiple testing issue by only investigating one or two phenotypes. The most commonly studied phenotype in HCM is LVM as determined by echocardiography, as it is readily available as a clinical tool [233] and it provides a more comprehensive measure of the extent of hypertrophy than a single wall thickness measurement could. The extent and distribution of LVH in HCM is, however, extremely variable and asymmetric, as discussed earlier, while LVM is derived from geometric assumptions; hence echocardiographically determined LVM may be an inaccurate measure of total LVH in the context of HCM. Cardiac MRI is credited with being a more precise and reproducible measure of LVM than M-mode and 2D-echocardiography, although the substantial costs involved in the infrastructure prohibits many investigations from using this technique. Moreover, the heritability of echocardiographically-determined LVM is estimated between 0.17 and 0.69 as discussed earlier, while ECG and MRI measures are reported to be more heritable [324;331]. These estimates are however heavily cohort-specific and sensitive to hypertrophy confounders. Thus, a great need exists for a clear consensus on the most appropriate measure of hypertrophy across HCM association studies.

On the other hand, single measurements are difficult to interpret clinically as cardiac hypertrophy in HCM is mostly asymmetrical and no single measurement could give the most accurate representation of the degree of hypertrophy in all affected individuals. If one considers the association p-values in Table 3, it becomes apparent that information may be lost if one only considers mLVWT, for instance. One way to address this issue is to use composite scores that encompass a number of hypertrophy measurements to describe the extent of hypertrophy. A number of such scores, such as the Wigle score and the Maron-Spirito score, exist [47]; however, it is still uncertain which composite score offers the best estimate of the extent of hypertrophy.

In the absence of a consensus measurement that accurately reflects the degree and distribution of hypertrophy in HCM, we circumvented this difficulty by using a composite hypertrophy score derived by principal component analysis, PC1, which best described the variability in the 16 echocardiographically determined wall thickness measurements in our cohort. Thus, we analysed a single weighted average that takes the extent and distribution of hypertrophy into account without resorting to a geometrically inaccurate estimate of overall hypertrophy.

Cardiac hypertrophy is a classic complex phenotype as it is influenced by a multitude of factors such as blood pressure, age, sex etc. Failure to adjust for these factors might result in spurious association, which is a known artefact of association studies. In the present study we adjusted all analyses for the identity of the primary HCM-causing mutation (R92W$_{TNNT2}$, R403W$_{MYH7}$, or A797T$_{MYH7}$), hypertension diagnosis, mean arterial pressure, sex, BSA, heart rate and age at clinical assessment. We did however not adjust for circulating Ang II or other measures of plasma RAAS activity, which has the potential to mask or exaggerate the contribution of individual RAAS component to hypertrophy development.

The effect sizes reported here are modest, although comparable to those reported by previous studies [173;217;244;245]. For instance, in our study the T-allele of rs2640539 in *AGTR1* was associated significantly associated with an increase of 1.22 mm in mLVWT, whereas the G-allele of rs8044970 in *SCNN1B* was associated with a decrease of 1.28 mm in mLVWT, which is comparatively modest and therefore difficult to interpret clinically. The clinical relevance might, however, improve if one considers the compound effect of a number of RAAS polymorphisms, where each contributes a modest amount to the eventual hypertrophic phenotype.

However, the compound effect of these RAAS variants on hypertrophy might not necessarily be additive in nature. Previous studies have identified significant epistatic effects of RAAS variants on cardiovascular phenotypes [338-340]. As there is complex biological interplay between the multiple components of the RAAS, there is a need for a comprehensive analysis that focuses on the compound effect of multiple hypertrophy modifier loci within the RAAS to gain the most accurate understanding of its role in hypertrophy development.

Association studies could be a useful tool to identify hypertrophy modifier genes, but its boundaries should be understood and a very clear distinction should be made between association and causality when interpreting association studies [335]. While we report association between variants in *ACE2, AGTR1*, *AGTR2*, *NR3C2* and *SCNN1B* and indices of hypertrophy in the present HCM family cohort, this does not establish a biological link between the particular variants and hypertrophy development. Evidence for functionality is in fact still unclear in some cases, for example the ACE I/D polymorphism, while such information is lacking for most of the other significant RAAS variants. The possibility then exists that these significant variants are not in themselves functional, but that they are in LD with genetic variants that confer a true biological impact on the RAAS and consequently hypertrophy. In essence, genetic association pinpoints a genetic region that correlates significantly with a particular phenotype. The size of this region is dependent on the measure of LD in that particular study population. For instance, haplotype studies showed that aldosterone synthesis is affected by genotypes at *CYP11B2* as well as the neighbouring *CYP11B1* as LD exists across the entire CYP11B1/B2 locus in Caucasians [248;249].

In addition, the influence of epistasis where the effects of one locus is amplified, altered or masked by another locus [341], has not yet been considered extensively in HCM. It is conceivable that such an interaction should exist between RAAS variants due to their complex biological functions and such epistatic effects have been reported between RAAS variants in atrial fibrillation [338], coronary atherosclerosis [340], hypertension [342] and coronary artery disease [339].

Comprehensive studies are therefore needed to pinpoint a subset of RAAS variants that confer a measurable biological effect on hypertrophy in HCM. The use of haplotypes offers an advantage over single SNP association approaches by providing additional power for mapping disease modifier genes while factoring in the interdependency among genetic markers studies as it considers the compound effect of a number of loci [343;344].

In summary, our results show a number of RAAS variants that each exert a modest effect on HCM LVH phenotypes, including the first significant association between variants in *NR3C2* as well as *SCNN1B* and hypertrophy traits in HCM. This suggests that the eventual phenotype of HCM might be influenced by the cumulative result of a number of RAAS variants of modest effect. Future studies should take the plausible biological impact of these genes on hypertrophy into account, as a clear need exists to expand RAAS modifier studies to recently identified genes, such as the PRR as well as the MR and downstream RAAS effectors, namely the ENaCs and Na^{+}/K^{+}-ATPases. Our study then informs on the design of future HCM hypertrophy modifier studies, as these results should be replicated in larger homogenous cohorts in which the primary HCM-causal mutation is known.

5. Discussion on RAAS Variants in Hypertrophy

Previous studies have reported modest effect sizes for RAAS variants on hypertrophy [30;32;173;245], while others reported that RAAS polymorphisms collectively influence the penetrance and extent of hypertrophy in HCM [31;33;345]. This suggests that the hypertrophic phenotype of HCM is modulated by the compound effect of a number of hypertrophic RAAS modifier loci, where each polymorphism makes a modest contribution to the eventual phenotype. However, several gaps exist in our knowledge of the involvement of the RAAS in HCM hypertrophy. For now, HCM modifier studies appear to have converged on a very limited list of "pro-LVH" polymorphisms; however renin and renin-associated genes, as well as downstream RAAS effectors such as the Na^{+}/K^{+}-ATPase and ENaCs, have plausible hypertrophic effects, but their contribution to modifying the hypertrophic phenotype in HCM has received little attention. Moreover, there exists a very real possibility that genetic variation in these genes might not contribute in an equal or even additive manner to hypertrophy in HCM; to complicate matters further, the functionality of most of these polymorphisms remains unclear.

Not only do a potentially large number of susceptibility alleles contribute to hypertrophy, but environmental factors also impact on hypertrophy development. Previous studies have reported context-dependent associations between RAAS variants and hypertrophy traits, where such associations were dependent on, among others, ethnicity [167;194], salt intake [92], blood pressure [93] and the primary HCM causal mutation [33;170]. Future studies therefore should address not only the full complexity of the RAAS, but should also use adequate adjustment for known hypertrophy covariates.

In summary, it is now clear that there exists an important cross-talk between Ang II/AT_1R and aldosterone/MR, which results in activation of signalling pathways involved in cell growth, contraction, and collagen deposition [346]. These processes are of particular interest in the heart where this interdependency significantly modulates hypertrophy and adverse cardiac remodelling. Considering that a number of RAAS variants contribute significantly to LVH indices, albeit each with modest effect sizes, and considering the growing evidence for epistasis among these variants, it becomes imperative to rethink the way we analyze the involvement of the RAAS on cardiac structure. Indeed, the contribution of all of the components of the RAAS, which often signal in opposite directions, rather than only selected components, should be considered if we want to understand the role of this complex system in cardiac remodelling, as otherwise there remains a risk of overstating, or indeed understating, the effect of this pathway on hypertrophy development.

References

[1] Lorell BH, Carabello BA. Left ventricular hypertrophy: pathogenesis, detection, and prognosis. *Circulation* 2000 Jul 25;102(4):470-9.

[2] Frey N, Olson EN. Cardiac hypertrophy: the good, the bad, and the ugly. *Annu. Rev. Physiol.* 2003;65:45-79.

[3] Mathew J, Sleight P, Lonn E, Johnstone D, Pogue J, Yi Q, et al. Reduction of cardiovascular risk by regression of electrocardiographic markers of left ventricular hypertrophy by the angiotensin-converting enzyme inhibitor ramipril. *Circulation* 2001 Oct 2;104(14):1615-21.

[4] Devereux RB, Roman MJ. Inter-relationships between hypertension, left ventricular hypertrophy and coronary heart disease. *J. Hypertens Suppl.* 1993 Jun;11(4):S3-S9.

[5] Verdecchia P, Porcellati C, Reboldi G, Gattobigio R, Borgioni C, Pearson TA, et al. Left ventricular hypertrophy as an independent predictor of acute cerebrovascular events in essential hypertension. *Circulation* 2001 Oct 23;104(17):2039-44.

[6] McLenachan JM, Henderson E, Morris KI, Dargie HJ. Ventricular arrhythmias in patients with hypertensive left ventricular hypertrophy. *N. Engl. J. Med.* 1987 Sep 24;317(13):787-92.

[7] Haider AW, Larson MG, Benjamin EJ, Levy D. Increased left ventricular mass and hypertrophy are associated with increased risk for sudden death. *J. Am. Coll Cardiol.* 1998 Nov;32(5):1454-9.

[8] Sharp A, Mayet J. Regression of left ventricular hypertrophy: hoping for a longer life. *J. Renin. Angiotensin Aldosterone Syst.* 2002 Sep;3(3):141-4.

[9] Muiesan ML, Salvetti M, Rizzoni D, Castellano M, Donato F, Agabiti-Rosei E. Association of change in left ventricular mass with prognosis during long-term antihypertensive treatment. *J. Hypertens* 1995 Oct;13(10):1091-5.

[10] Verdecchia P, Schillaci G, Borgioni C, Ciucci A, Gattobigio R, Zampi I, et al. Prognostic significance of serial changes in left ventricular mass in essential hypertension. *Circulation* 1998 Jan 6;97(1):48-54.

[11] Levy D, Labib SB, Anderson KM, Christiansen JC, Kannel WB, Castelli WP. Determinants of sensitivity and specificity of electrocardiographic criteria for left ventricular hypertrophy. *Circulation* 1990 Mar;81(3):815-20.

[12] Dahlof B, Devereux RB, Kjeldsen SE, Julius S, Beevers G, de Faire U., et al. Cardiovascular morbidity and mortality in the Losartan Intervention For Endpoint reduction in hypertension study (LIFE): a randomised trial against atenolol. *Lancet* 2002 Mar 23;359(9311):995-1003.

[13] Devereux RB, Wachtell K, Gerdts E, Boman K, Nieminen MS, Papademetriou V, et al. Prognostic significance of left ventricular mass change during treatment of hypertension. *JAMA* 2004 Nov 17;292(19):2350-6.

[14] Koren MJ, Devereux RB, Casale PN, Savage DD, Laragh JH. Relation of left ventricular mass and geometry to morbidity and mortality in uncomplicated essential hypertension. *Ann. Intern. Med.* 1991 Mar 1;114(5):345-52.

[15] Schunkert H, Brockel U, Hengstenberg C, Luchner A, Muscholl MW, Kurzidim K, et al. Familial predisposition of left ventricular hypertrophy. *J. Am. Coll Cardiol.* 1999 May;33(6):1685-91.

[16] Barry SP, Davidson SM, Townsend PA. Molecular regulation of cardiac hypertrophy. *Int. J. Biochem. Cell Biol.* 2008;40(10):2023-39.

[17] Lijnen P, Petrov V. Renin-angiotensin system, hypertrophy and gene expression in cardiac myocytes. *J. Mol. Cell Cardiol.* 1999 May;31(5):949-70.

[18] Kim S, Iwao H. Molecular and cellular mechanisms of angiotensin II-mediated cardiovascular and renal diseases. *Pharmacol. Rev.* 2000 Mar;52(1):11-34.

[19] Yamazaki T, Komuro I, Yazaki Y. Role of the renin-angiotensin system in cardiac hypertrophy. *Am. J. Cardiol.* 1999 Jun 17;83(12A):53H-7H.

[20] Baker KM, Aceto JF. Angiotensin II stimulation of protein synthesis and cell growth in chick heart cells. *Am. J. Physiol.* 1990 Aug;259(2 Pt 2):H610-H618.

[21] Sadoshima J, Izumo S. Molecular characterization of angiotensin II--induced hypertrophy of cardiac myocytes and hyperplasia of cardiac fibroblasts. Critical role of the AT1 receptor subtype. *Circ. Res.* 1993 Sep;73(3):413-23.

[22] Ritchie RH, Schiebinger RJ, LaPointe MC, Marsh JD. Angiotensin II-induced hypertrophy of adult rat cardiomyocytes is blocked by nitric oxide. *Am. J. Physiol.* 1998 Oct;275(4 Pt 2):H1370-H1374.

[23] Schunkert H, Sadoshima J, Cornelius T, Kagaya Y, Weinberg EO, Izumo S, et al. Angiotensin II-induced growth responses in isolated adult rat hearts. Evidence for load-independent induction of cardiac protein synthesis by angiotensin II. *Circ. Res.* 1995 Mar;76(3):489-97.

[24] Wada H, Zile MR, Ivester CT, Cooper G, McDermott PJ. Comparative effects of contraction and angiotensin II on growth of adult feline cardiocytes in primary culture. *Am. J. Physiol.* 1996 Jul;271(1 Pt 2):H29-H37.

[25] Schluter KD, Wenzel S. Angiotensin II: a hormone involved in and contributing to pro-hypertrophic cardiac networks and target of anti-hypertrophic cross-talks. *Pharmacol. Ther.* 2008 Sep;119(3):311-25.

[26] Schunkert H, Dzau VJ, Tang SS, Hirsch AT, Apstein CS, Lorell BH. Increased rat cardiac angiotensin converting enzyme activity and mRNA expression in pressure overload left ventricular hypertrophy. Effects on coronary resistance, contractility, and relaxation. *J. Clin. Invest.* 1990 Dec;86(6):1913-20.

[27] Dostal DE, Baker KM. Angiotensin II stimulation of left ventricular hypertrophy in adult rat heart. Mediation by the AT1 receptor. *Am. J. Hypertens* 1992 May;5(5 Pt 1):276-80.

[28] Luft FC, Mervaala E, Muller DN, Gross V, Schmidt F, Park JK, et al. Hypertension-induced end-organ damage : A new transgenic approach to an old problem. *Hypertension* 1999 Jan;33(1 Pt 2):212-8.

[29] Mervaala E, Muller DN, Schmidt F, Park JK, Gross V, Bader M, et al. Blood pressure-independent effects in rats with human renin and angiotensinogen genes. *Hypertension* 2000 Feb;35(2):587-94.

[30] Carstens N, van der Merwe L, Revera M, Heradien M, Goosen A, Brink PA, et al. Genetic variation in angiotensin II type 2 receptor gene influences extent of left ventricular hypertrophy in hypertrophic cardiomyopathy independent of blood pressure. *J. Renin. Angiotensin Aldosterone Syst.* 2010 Dec 16.

[31] Ortlepp JR, Vosberg HP, Reith S, Ohme F, Mahon NG, Schroder D, et al. Genetic polymorphisms in the renin-angiotensin-aldosterone system associated with expression of left ventricular hypertrophy in hypertrophic cardiomyopathy: a study of five polymorphic genes in a family with a disease causing mutation in the myosin binding protein C gene. *Heart* 2002 Mar;87(3):270-5.

[32] Van der Merwe L, Cloete R, Revera M, Heradien M, Goosen A, Corfield VA, et al. Genetic variation in angiotensin-converting enzyme 2 gene is associated with extent of

left ventricular hypertrophy in hypertrophic cardiomyopathy. *Hum. Genet.* 2008 Aug;124(1):57-61.

[33] Perkins MJ, Van Driest SL, Ellsworth EG, Will ML, Gersh BJ, Ommen SR, et al. Gene-specific modifying effects of pro-LVH polymorphisms involving the renin-angiotensin-aldosterone system among 389 unrelated patients with hypertrophic cardiomyopathy. *Eur. Heart J.* 2005 Nov;26(22):2457-62.

[34] Watkins H, Seidman JG, Seidman CE. Familial hypertrophic cardiomyopathy: a genetic model of cardiac hypertrophy. *Hum. Mol. Genet.* 1995;4 Spec No:1721-7.

[35] Marian AJ. Modifier genes for hypertrophic cardiomyopathy. *Curr. Opin. Cardiol.* 2002 May;17(3):242-52.

[36] Seidman JG, Seidman C. The genetic basis for cardiomyopathy: from mutation identification to mechanistic paradigms. *Cell* 2001 Feb 23;104(4):557-67.

[37] Wigle ED, Rakowski H, Kimball BP, Williams WG. Hypertrophic cardiomyopathy. Clinical spectrum and treatment. *Circulation* 1995 Oct 1;92(7):1680-92.

[38] Maron BJ, Gardin JM, Flack JM, Gidding SS, Kurosaki TT, Bild DE. Prevalence of hypertrophic cardiomyopathy in a general population of young adults. Echocardiographic analysis of 4111 subjects in the CARDIA Study. Coronary Artery Risk Development in (Young) Adults. *Circulation* 1995 Aug 15;92(4):785-9.

[39] Niimura H, Patton KK, McKenna WJ, Soults J, Maron BJ, Seidman JG, et al. Sarcomere protein gene mutations in hypertrophic cardiomyopathy of the elderly. *Circulation* 2002 Jan 29;105(4):446-51.

[40] Maron BJ, McKenna WJ, Danielson GK, Kappenberger LJ, Kuhn HJ, Seidman CE, et al. American College of Cardiology/European Society of Cardiology clinical expert consensus document on hypertrophic cardiomyopathy. A report of the American College of Cardiology Foundation Task Force on Clinical Expert Consensus Documents and the European Society of Cardiology Committee for Practice Guidelines. *J. Am. Coll Cardiol.* 2003 Nov 5;42(9):1687-713.

[41] Tsoutsman T, Lam L, Semsarian C. Genes, calcium and modifying factors in hypertrophic cardiomyopathy. *Clin. Exp. Pharmacol. Physiol.* 2006 Jan;33(1-2):139-45.

[42] Klues HG, Schiffers A, Maron BJ. Phenotypic spectrum and patterns of left ventricular hypertrophy in hypertrophic cardiomyopathy: morphologic observations and significance as assessed by two-dimensional echocardiography in 600 patients. *J. Am. Coll Cardiol.* 1995 Dec;26(7):1699-708.

[43] Thierfelder L, Watkins H, MacRae C, Lamas R, McKenna W, Vosberg HP, et al. Alpha-tropomyosin and cardiac troponin T mutations cause familial hypertrophic cardiomyopathy: a disease of the sarcomere. *Cell* 1994 Jun 3;77(5):701-12.

[44] Seidman CE, Seidman JG. Identifying sarcomere gene mutations in hypertrophic cardiomyopathy: a personal history. *Circ. Res.* 2011 Mar 18;108(6):743-50.

[45] Ho CY. Genetics and clinical destiny: improving care in hypertrophic cardiomyopathy. *Circulation* 2010 Dec 7;122(23):2430-40.

[46] Spirito P, Bellone P, Harris KM, Bernabo P, Bruzzi P, Maron BJ. Magnitude of left ventricular hypertrophy and risk of sudden death in hypertrophic cardiomyopathy. *N. Engl. J. Med.* 2000 Jun 15;342(24):1778-85.

[47] Spirito P, Maron BJ. Relation between extent of left ventricular hypertrophy and occurrence of sudden cardiac death in hypertrophic cardiomyopathy. *J. Am. Coll Cardiol.* 1990 Jun;15(7):1521-6.

[48] Charron P, Dubourg O, Desnos M, Isnard R, Hagege A, Bonne G, et al. Genotype-phenotype correlations in familial hypertrophic cardiomyopathy. A comparison between mutations in the cardiac protein-C and the beta-myosin heavy chain genes. *Eur. Heart J.* 1998 Jan;19(1):139-45.

[49] Erdmann J, Raible J, Maki-Abadi J, Hummel M, Hammann J, Wollnik B, et al. Spectrum of clinical phenotypes and gene variants in cardiac myosin-binding protein C mutation carriers with hypertrophic cardiomyopathy. *J. Am. Coll Cardiol.* 2001 Aug;38(2):322-30.

[50] Lekanne Deprez RH, Muurling-Vlietman JJ, Hruda J, Baars MJ, Wijnaendts LC, Stolte-Dijkstra I, et al. Two cases of severe neonatal hypertrophic cardiomyopathy caused by compound heterozygous mutations in the MYBPC3 gene. *J. Med. Genet.* 2006 Oct;43(10):829-32.

[51] Mohiddin SA, Begley DA, McLam E, Cardoso JP, Winkler JB, Sellers JR, et al. Utility of genetic screening in hypertrophic cardiomyopathy: prevalence and significance of novel and double (homozygous and heterozygous) beta-myosin mutations. *Genet. Test* 2003;7(1):21-7.

[52] Keller DI, Schwitter J, Valsangiacomo ER, Landolt P, Attenhofer Jost CH. Hypertrophic cardiomyopathy due to beta-myosin heavy chain mutation with extreme phenotypic variability within a family. *Int. J. Cardiol.* 2009 May 29;134(3):e87-e93.

[53] Epstein ND, Cohn GM, Cyran F, Fananapazir L. Differences in clinical expression of hypertrophic cardiomyopathy associated with two distinct mutations in the beta-myosin heavy chain gene. A 908Leu----Val mutation and a 403Arg----Gln mutation. *Circulation* 1992 Aug;86(2):345-52.

[54] Fananapazir L, Epstein ND. Genotype-phenotype correlations in hypertrophic cardiomyopathy. Insights provided by comparisons of kindreds with distinct and identical beta-myosin heavy chain gene mutations. *Circulation* 1994 Jan;89(1):22-32.

[55] Posen BM, Moolman JC, Corfield VA, Brink PA. Clinical and prognostic evaluation of familial hypertrophic cardiomyopathy in two South African families with different cardiac beta myosin heavy chain gene mutations. *Br. Heart J.* 1995 Jul;74(1):40-6.

[56] Marian AJ, Mares A, Jr., Kelly DP, Yu QT, Abchee AB, Hill R, et al. Sudden cardiac death in hypertrophic cardiomyopathy. Variability in phenotypic expression of beta-myosin heavy chain mutations. *Eur. Heart J.* 1995 Mar;16(3):368-76.

[57] Marian AJ. On genetic and phenotypic variability of hypertrophic cardiomyopathy: nature versus nurture. *J. Am. Coll Cardiol.* 2001 Aug;38(2):331-4.

[58] Solomon SD, Wolff S, Watkins H, Ridker PM, Come P, McKenna WJ, et al. Left ventricular hypertrophy and morphology in familial hypertrophic cardiomyopathy associated with mutations of the beta-myosin heavy chain gene. *J. Am. Coll Cardiol.* 1993 Aug;22(2):498-505.

[59] Geisterfer-Lowrance AA, Christe M, Conner DA, Ingwall JS, Schoen FJ, Seidman CE, et al. A mouse model of familial hypertrophic cardiomyopathy. *Science* 1996 May 3;272(5262):731-4.

[60] Semsarian C, Healey MJ, Fatkin D, Giewat M, Duffy C, Seidman CE, et al. A polymorphic modifier gene alters the hypertrophic response in a murine model of familial hypertrophic cardiomyopathy. *J. Mol. Cell Cardiol.* 2001 Nov;33(11):2055-60.

[61] Moolman-Smook JC, De Lange WJ, Bruwer EC, Brink PA, Corfield VA. The origins of hypertrophic cardiomyopathy-causing mutations in two South African

subpopulations: a unique profile of both independent and founder events. *Am. J. Hum. Genet.* 1999 Nov;65(5):1308-20.

[62] Griendling KK, Murphy TJ, Alexander RW. Molecular biology of the renin-angiotensin system. *Circulation* 1993 Jun;87(6):1816-28.

[63] Paul M, Poyan Mehr A., Kreutz R. Physiology of local renin-angiotensin systems. *Physiol. Rev.* 2006 Jul;86(3):747-803.

[64] De Gasparo M, Catt KJ, Inagami T, Wright JW, Unger T. International union of pharmacology. XXIII. The angiotensin II receptors. *Pharmacol. Rev.* 2000 Sep;52(3):415-72.

[65] Chai W, Danser AH. Why are mineralocorticoid receptor antagonists cardioprotective? *Naunyn Schmiedebergs Arch. Pharmacol.* 2006 Dec;374(3):153-62.

[66] Lemarie CA, Paradis P, Schiffrin EL. New insights on signaling cascades induced by cross-talk between angiotensin II and aldosterone. *J. Mol. Med.* 2008 Jun;86(6):673-8.

[67] Tannin GM, Agarwal AK, Monder C, New MI, White PC. The human gene for 11 beta-hydroxysteroid dehydrogenase. Structure, tissue distribution, and chromosomal localization. *J. Biol. Chem.* 1991 Sep 5;266(25):16653-8.

[68] Eaton DC, Malik B, Saxena NC, Al-Khalili OK, Yue G. Mechanisms of aldosterone's action on epithelial Na + transport. *J. Membr. Biol.* 2001 Dec 1;184(3):313-9.

[69] Kamynina E, Staub O. Concerted action of ENaC, Nedd4-2, and Sgk1 in transepithelial Na(+) transport. *Am. J. Physiol. Renal Physiol* 2002 Sep;283(3):F377-F387.

[70] Rossier BC, Pradervand S, Schild L, Hummler E. Epithelial sodium channel and the control of sodium balance: interaction between genetic and environmental factors. *Annu. Rev. Physiol.* 2002;64:877-97.

[71] Stockand JD. New ideas about aldosterone signaling in epithelia. *Am. J. Physiol. Renal Physiol* 2002 Apr;282(4):F559-F576.

[72] Bader M, Ganten D. Update on tissue renin-angiotensin systems. *J. Mol. Med.* 2008 Jun;86(6):615-21.

[73] Solomon SD, Appelbaum E, Manning WJ, Verma A, Berglund T, Lukashevich V, et al. Effect of the direct Renin inhibitor aliskiren, the Angiotensin receptor blocker losartan, or both on left ventricular mass in patients with hypertension and left ventricular hypertrophy. *Circulation* 2009 Feb 3;119(4):530-7.

[74] Sever PS, Gradman AH, Azizi M. Managing cardiovascular and renal risk: the potential of direct renin inhibition. *J. Renin. Angiotensin Aldosterone Syst.* 2009 Jun;10(2):65-76.

[75] Watt GC, Harrap SB, Foy CJ, Holton DW, Edwards HV, Davidson HR, et al. Abnormalities of glucocorticoid metabolism and the renin-angiotensin system: a four-corners approach to the identification of genetic determinants of blood pressure. *J. Hypertens* 1992 May;10(5):473-82.

[76] Kim HS, Krege JH, Kluckman KD, Hagaman JR, Hodgin JB, Best CF, et al. Genetic control of blood pressure and the angiotensinogen locus. *Proc. Natl. Acad. Sci. USA* 1995 Mar 28;92(7):2735-9.

[77] Kimura S, Mullins JJ, Bunnemann B, Metzger R, Hilgenfeldt U, Zimmermann F, et al. High blood pressure in transgenic mice carrying the rat angiotensinogen gene. *EMBO J.* 1992 Mar;11(3):821-7.

[78] Tanimoto K, Sugiyama F, Goto Y, Ishida J, Takimoto E, Yagami K, et al. Angiotensinogen-deficient mice with hypotension. *J. Biol. Chem.* 1994 Dec 16;269(50):31334-7.

[79] Xu P, Wang Y, Sterner-Kock A, Bader M, Schultheiss HP, Walther T. Excessive hypertension and end-organ damage in a transgenic mouse line carrying the rat angiotensinogen gene. *J. Cardiovasc. Pharmacol.* 2009 Jan;53(1):38-43.

[80] Brand-Herrmann SM, Kopke K, Reichenberger F, Schmidt-Petersen K, Reineke T, Paul M, et al. Angiotensinogen promoter haplotypes are associated with blood pressure in untreated hypertensives. *J. Hypertens* 2004 Jul;22(7):1289-97.

[81] Jain S, Li Y, Patil S, Kumar A. A single-nucleotide polymorphism in human angiotensinogen gene is associated with essential hypertension and affects glucocorticoid induced promoter activity. *J. Mol. Med.* 2005 Feb;83(2):121-31.

[82] Jeunemaitre X, Gimenez-Roqueplo AP, Celerier J, Corvol P. Angiotensinogen variants and human hypertension. *Curr. Hypertens Rep.* 1999 Feb;1(1):31-41.

[83] Kumar A, Li Y, Patil S, Jain S. A haplotype of the angiotensinogen gene is associated with hypertension in african americans. *Clin. Exp. Pharmacol. Physiol.* 2005 May;32(5-6):495-502.

[84] Dickson ME, Sigmund CD. Genetic basis of hypertension: revisiting angiotensinogen. *Hypertension* 2006 Jul;48(1):14-20.

[85] Kurland L, Melhus H, Karlsson J, Kahan T, Malmqvist K, Ohman P, et al. Polymorphisms in the angiotensinogen and angiotensin II type 1 receptor gene are related to change in left ventricular mass during antihypertensive treatment: results from the Swedish Irbesartan Left Ventricular Hypertrophy Investigation versus Atenolol (SILVHIA) trial. *J. Hypertens* 2002 Apr;20(4):657-63.

[86] Iwai N, Shimoike H, Ohmichi N, Kinoshita M. Angiotensinogen gene and blood pressure in the Japanese population. *Hypertension* 1995 Apr;25(4 Pt 2):688-93.

[87] Jeng JR. Left ventricular mass, carotid wall thickness, and angiotensinogen gene polymorphism in patients with hypertension. *Am. J. Hypertens* 1999 May;12(5):443-50.

[88] Karjalainen J, Kujala UM, Stolt A, Mantysaari M, Viitasalo M, Kainulainen K, et al. Angiotensinogen gene M235T polymorphism predicts left ventricular hypertrophy in endurance athletes. *J. Am. Coll Cardiol.* 1999 Aug;34(2):494-9.

[89] Kauma H, Ikaheimo M, Savolainen MJ, Kiema TR, Rantala AO, Lilja M, et al. Variants of renin-angiotensin system genes and echocardiographic left ventricular mass. *Eur. Heart J.* 1998 Jul;19(7):1109-17.

[90] Staessen JA, Ginocchio G, Wang JG, Saavedra AP, Soubrier F, Vlietinck R, et al. Genetic variability in the renin-angiotensin system: prevalence of alleles and genotypes. *J. Cardiovasc. Risk* 1997 Oct;4(5-6):401-22.

[91] Staessen JA, Kuznetsova T, Wang JG, Emelianov D, Vlietinck R, Fagard R. M235T angiotensinogen gene polymorphism and cardiovascular renal risk. *J. Hypertens* 1999 Jan;17(1):9-17.

[92] Kuznetsova T, Staessen JA, Reineke T, Olszanecka A, Ryabikov A, Tikhonoff V, et al. Context-dependency of the relation between left ventricular mass and AGT gene variants. *J. Hum. Hypertens* 2005 Feb;19(2):155-63.

[93] Tang W, Devereux RB, Rao DC, Oberman A, Hopkins PN, Kitzman DW, et al. Associations between angiotensinogen gene variants and left ventricular mass and function in the HyperGEN study. *Am. Heart J.* 2002 May;143(5):854-60.

[94] Bader M. Role of the local renin-angiotensin system in cardiac damage: a minireview focussing on transgenic animal models. *J. Mol. Cell Cardiol.* 2002 Nov;34(11):1455-62.

[95] Mazzolai L, Nussberger J, Aubert JF, Brunner DB, Gabbiani G, Brunner HR, et al. Blood pressure-independent cardiac hypertrophy induced by locally activated renin-angiotensin system. *Hypertension* 1998 Jun;31(6):1324-30.

[96] Reudelhuber TL, Bernstein KE, Delafontaine P. Is angiotensin II a direct mediator of left ventricular hypertrophy? Time for another look. *Hypertension* 2007 Jun;49(6):1196-201.

[97] Kang N, Walther T, Tian XL, Bohlender J, Fukamizu A, Ganten D, et al. Reduced hypertension-induced end-organ damage in mice lacking cardiac and renal angiotensinogen synthesis. *J. Mol. Med.* 2002 Jun;80(6):359-66.

[98] Cai SY, Shi YP, Yu F, Xu G. [Association of angiotensinogen gene M235T variant with hypertrophic cardiomyopathy]. *Zhonghua Yi Xue Yi Chuan Xue Za Zhi* 2004 Jun;21(3):280-2.

[99] Ishanov A, Okamoto H, Yoneya K, Watanabe M, Nakagawa I, Machida M, et al. Angiotensinogen gene polymorphism in Japanese patients with hypertrophic cardiomyopathy. *Am. Heart J.* 1997 Feb;133(2):184-9.

[100] Kawaguchi H. Angiotensin-converting enzyme and angiotensinogen gene polymorphism in hypertrophic cardiomyopathy. *Exp. Clin. Cardiol.* 2003;8(3):155-9.

[101] Manohar Rao PP, Munshi A, Mullapudi R, Kumar PS, Sharath A, Krishna GA, et al. The M235T polymorphism of the angiotensinogen gene in South Indian patients of hypertrophic cardiomyopathy. *J. Renin. Angiotensin Aldosterone Syst.* 2010 Dec 16.

[102] Lopez-Haldon J, Garcia-Lozano JR, Martinez MA, Nunez-Roldan A, Burgos Cornejo J. [The effect of polymorphisms of the angiotensin-converting enzyme and angiotensinogen genes on the phenotypic expression of Spanish patients with hypertrophic cardiomyopathy]. *Med. Clin.* (Barc) 1999 Jul 10;113(5):161-3.

[103] Yamada Y, Ichihara S, Fujimura T, Yokota M. Lack of association of polymorphisms of the angiotensin converting enzyme and angiotensinogen genes with nonfamilial hypertrophic or dilated cardiomyopathy. *Am. J. Hypertens* 1997 Aug;10(8):921-8.

[104] Coto E, Palacin M, Martin M, Castro MG, Reguero JR, Garcia C, et al. Functional polymorphisms in genes of the Angiotensin and Serotonin systems and risk of hypertrophic cardiomyopathy: AT1R as a potential modifier. *J. Transl. Med.* 2010;8:64.

[105] Brugada R, Kelsey W, Lechin M, Zhao G, Yu QT, Zoghbi W, et al. Role of candidate modifier genes on the phenotypic expression of hypertrophy in patients with hypertrophic cardiomyopathy. *J. Investig. Med.* 1997 Dec;45(9):542-51.

[106] Sethi AA, Nordestgaard BG, Tybjaerg-Hansen A. Angiotensinogen gene polymorphism, plasma angiotensinogen, and risk of hypertension and ischemic heart disease: a meta-analysis. *Arterioscler. Thromb. Vasc. Biol.* 2003 Jul 1;23(7):1269-75.

[107] Inoue I, Nakajima T, Williams CS, Quackenbush J, Puryear R, Powers M, et al. A nucleotide substitution in the promoter of human angiotensinogen is associated with essential hypertension and affects basal transcription in vitro. *J. Clin. Invest.* 1997 Apr 1;99(7):1786-97.

[108] Danser JAH, Schunkert H. Renin-angiotensin system gene polymorphisms: potential mechanisms for their association with cardiovascular diseases. *Eur. J. Pharmacol.* 2000 Dec 27;410(2-3):303-16.

[109] Cvetkovic B, Keen HL, Zhang X, Davis D, Yang B, Sigmund CD. Physiological significance of two common haplotypes of human angiotensinogen using gene targeting in the mouse. *Physiol Genomics* 2002 Dec 3;11(3):253-62.

[110] Jain S, Tillinger A, Mopidevi B, Pandey VG, Chauhan CK, Fiering SN, et al. Transgenic mice with -6A haplotype of the human angiotensinogen gene have increased blood pressure compared with -6G haplotype. *J. Biol. Chem.* 2010 Dec 24;285(52):41172-86.

[111] Grobe JL, Dickson ME, Park S, Davis DR, Born EJ, Sigmund CD. Cardiovascular consequences of genetic variation at -6/235 in human angiotensinogen using "humanized" gene-targeted mice. *Hypertension* 2010 Nov;56(5):981-7.

[112] Verdecchia P, Angeli F, Mazzotta G, Gentile G, Reboldi G. The renin angiotensin system in the development of cardiovascular disease: role of aliskiren in risk reduction. *Vasc. Health Risk Manag.* 2008;4(5):971-81.

[113] Balakumar P, Jagadeesh G. Cardiovascular and renal pathologic implications of prorenin, renin, and the (pro)renin receptor: promising young players from the old renin-angiotensin-aldosterone system. *J. Cardiovasc. Pharmacol.* 2010 Nov;56(5):570-9.

[114] Pilz B, Shagdarsuren E, Wellner M, Fiebeler A, Dechend R, Gratze P, et al. Aliskiren, a human renin inhibitor, ameliorates cardiac and renal damage in double-transgenic rats. *Hypertension* 2005 Sep;46(3):569-76.

[115] van Esch JH, Moltzer E, van VR, Garrelds IM, Leijten F, Bouhuizen AM, et al. Beneficial cardiac effects of the renin inhibitor aliskiren in spontaneously hypertensive rats. *J. Hypertens* 2010 Oct;28(10):2145-55.

[116] Westermann D, Riad A, Lettau O, Roks A, Savvatis K, Becher PM, et al. Renin inhibition improves cardiac function and remodeling after myocardial infarction independent of blood pressure. *Hypertension* 2008 Dec;52(6):1068-75.

[117] Saris JJ, Derkx FH, Lamers JM, Saxena PR, Schalekamp MA, Danser AH. Cardiomyocytes bind and activate native human prorenin : role of soluble mannose 6-phosphate receptors. *Hypertension* 2001 Feb;37(2 Part 2):710-5.

[118] Nguyen G, Muller DN. The biology of the (pro)renin receptor. *J. Am. Soc. Nephrol.* 2010 Jan;21(1):18-23.

[119] de Lannoy LM, Danser AH, van Kats JP, Schoemaker RG, Saxena PR, Schalekamp MA. Renin-angiotensin system components in the interstitial fluid of the isolated perfused rat heart. Local production of angiotensin I. *Hypertension* 1997 Jun;29(6):1240-51.

[120] Danser JAH, Saris JJ. Prorenin uptake in the heart: a prerequisite for local angiotensin generation? *J. Mol. Cell Cardiol.* 2002 Nov;34(11):1463-72.

[121] Catanzaro DF. Physiological relevance of renin/prorenin binding and uptake. *Hypertens Res.* 2005 Feb;28(2):97-105.

[122] Nguyen G, Burckle CA, Sraer JD. Renin/prorenin-receptor biochemistry and functional significance. *Curr. Hypertens Rep.* 2004 Apr;6(2):129-32.

[123] Nguyen G, Delarue F, Burckle C, Bouzhir L, Giller T, Sraer JD. Pivotal role of the renin/prorenin receptor in angiotensin II production and cellular responses to renin. *J. Clin. Invest.* 2002 Jun;109(11):1417-27.

[124] Nguyen G, Danser AH. Prorenin and (pro)renin receptor: a review of available data from in vitro studies and experimental models in rodents. *Exp. Physiol.* 2008 May;93(5):557-63.

[125] Reudelhuber TL, Ramla D, Chiu L, Mercure C, Seidah NG. Proteolytic processing of human prorenin in renal and non-renal tissues. *Kidney Int.* 1994 Dec;46(6):1522-4.

[126] Danser AH, Derkx FH, Schalekamp MA, Hense HW, Riegger GA, Schunkert H. Determinants of interindividual variation of renin and prorenin concentrations: evidence for a sexual dimorphism of (pro)renin levels in humans. *J. Hypertens* 1998 Jun;16(6):853-62.

[127] Susic D, Zhou X, Frohlich ED, Lippton H, Knight M. Cardiovascular effects of prorenin blockade in genetically spontaneously hypertensive rats on normal and high-salt diet. *Am. J. Physiol. Heart Circ. Physiol.* 2008 Sep;295(3):H1117-H1121.

[128] Veniant M, Menard J, Bruneval P, Morley S, Gonzales MF, Mullins J. Vascular damage without hypertension in transgenic rats expressing prorenin exclusively in the liver. *J. Clin. Invest.* 1996 Nov 1;98(9):1966-70.

[129] Nguyen G, Burckle C, Sraer JD. The renin receptor: the facts, the promise and the hope. *Curr. Opin Nephrol. Hypertens* 2003 Jan;12(1):51-5.

[130] Oliver JA. Receptor-mediated actions of renin and prorenin. *Kidney Int.* 2006 Jan;69(1):13-5.

[131] Saris JJ, 't Hoen PA, Garrelds IM, Dekkers DH, den Dunnen JT, Lamers JM, et al. Prorenin induces intracellular signaling in cardiomyocytes independently of angiotensin II. *Hypertension* 2006 Oct;48(4):564-71.

[132] Cousin C, Bracquart D, Contrepas A, Nguyen G. Potential role of the (pro)renin receptor in cardiovascular and kidney diseases. *J. Nephrol.* 2010 Sep;23(5):508-13.

[133] Huang Y, Wongamorntham S, Kasting J, McQuillan D, Owens RT, Yu L, et al. Renin increases mesangial cell transforming growth factor-beta1 and matrix proteins through receptor-mediated, angiotensin II-independent mechanisms. *Kidney Int.* 2006 Jan;69(1):105-13.

[134] Huang Y, Noble NA, Zhang J, Xu C, Border WA. Renin-stimulated TGF-beta1 expression is regulated by a mitogen-activated protein kinase in mesangial cells. *Kidney Int.* 2007 Jul;72(1):45-52.

[135] Ichihara A, Kaneshiro Y, Takemitsu T, Sakoda M, Suzuki F, Nakagawa T, et al. Nonproteolytic activation of prorenin contributes to development of cardiac fibrosis in genetic hypertension. *Hypertension* 2006 May;47(5):894-900.

[136] Methot D, Silversides DW, Reudelhuber TL. In vivo enzymatic assay reveals catalytic activity of the human renin precursor in tissues. *Circ. Res.* 1999 May 14;84(9):1067-72.

[137] Nguyen G, Delarue F, Berrou J, Rondeau E, Sraer JD. Specific receptor binding of renin on human mesangial cells in culture increases plasminogen activator inhibitor-1 antigen. *Kidney Int.* 1996 Dec;50(6):1897-903.

[138] Prescott G, Silversides DW, Reudelhuber TL. Tissue activity of circulating prorenin. *Am. J. Hypertens* 2002 Mar;15(3):280-5.

[139] Paulis L, Unger T. Novel therapeutic targets for hypertension. *Nat. Rev. Cardiol.* 2010 Aug;7(8):431-41.

[140] Ichihara A, Sakoda M, Kurauchi-Mito A, Narita T, Kinouchi K, Murohashi-Bokuda K, et al. Possible roles of human (pro)renin receptor suggested by recent clinical and experimental findings. *Hypertens Res.* 2010 Mar;33(3):177-80.

[141] Cruciat CM, Ohkawara B, Acebron SP, Karaulanov E, Reinhard C, Ingelfinger D, et al. Requirement of prorenin receptor and vacuolar H+-ATPase-mediated acidification for Wnt signaling. *Science* 2010 Jan 22;327(5964):459-63.

[142] Balakumar P, Jagadeesh G. Multifarious molecular signaling cascades of cardiac hypertrophy: can the muddy waters be cleared? *Pharmacol. Res.* 2010 Nov;62(5):365-83.

[143] Connelly KA, Advani A, Kim S, Advani SL, Zhang M, White KE, et al. The cardiac (pro)renin receptor is primarily expressed in myocyte transverse tubules and is increased in experimental diabetic cardiomyopathy. *J. Hypertens* 2011 Jun;29(6):1175-84.

[144] Finckenberg P, Mervaala E. Novel regulators and drug targets of cardiac hypertrophy. *J. Hypertens* 2010 Sep;28 Suppl 1:S33-S38.

[145] Reudelhuber TL. Prorenin, Renin, and their receptor: moving targets. *Hypertension* 2010 May;55(5):1071-4.

[146] Van den Eijnden MM, Saris JJ, de Bruin RJ, de Wit E., Sluiter W, Reudelhuber TL, et al. Prorenin accumulation and activation in human endothelial cells: importance of mannose 6-phosphate receptors. *Arterioscler. Thromb. Vasc. Biol.* 2001 Jun;21(6):911-6.

[147] Van Kesteren CA, Danser AH, Derkx FH, Dekkers DH, Lamers JM, Saxena PR, et al. Mannose 6-phosphate receptor-mediated internalization and activation of prorenin by cardiac cells. *Hypertension* 1997 Dec;30(6):1389-96.

[148] Saris JJ, Derkx FH, de Bruin RJ, Dekkers DH, Lamers JM, Saxena PR, et al. High-affinity prorenin binding to cardiac man-6-P/IGF-II receptors precedes proteolytic activation to renin. *Am. J. Physiol. Heart Circ. Physiol.* 2001 Apr;280(4):H1706-H1715.

[149] Saris JJ, van den Eijnden MM, Lamers JM, Saxena PR, Schalekamp MA, Danser AH. Prorenin-induced myocyte proliferation: no role for intracellular angiotensin II. *Hypertension* 2002 Feb;39(2 Pt 2):573-7.

[150] Takahashi S, Ohsawa T, Miura R, Miyake Y. Purification of high molecular weight (HMW) renin from porcine kidney and direct evidence that the HMW renin is a complex of renin with renin binding protein (RnBP). *J. Biochem.* 1983 Jan;93(1):265-74.

[151] Takahashi S, Inoue H, Fukui K, Miyake Y. Structure and function of renin binding protein. *Kidney Int.* 1994 Dec;46(6):1525-7.

[152] Takahashi S, Takahashi K, Kaneko T, Ogasawara H, Shindo S, Kobayashi M. Human renin-binding protein is the enzyme N-acetyl-D-glucosamine 2-epimerase. *J. Biochem.* 1999 Feb;125(2):348-53.

[153] Schmitz C, Gotthardt M, Hinderlich S, Leheste JR, Gross V, Vorum H, et al. Normal blood pressure and plasma renin activity in mice lacking the renin-binding protein, a cellular renin inhibitor. *J. Biol. Chem.* 2000 May 19;275(20):15357-62.

[154] Bohlmeyer T, Ferdensi A, Bristow MR, Takahashi S, Zisman LS. Selective activation of N-acyl-D-glucosamine 2-epimerase expression in failing human heart ventricular myocytes. *J. Card Fail* 2003 Feb;9(1):59-68.

[155] Knoll A, Schunkert H, Reichwald K, Danser AH, Bauer D, Platzer M, et al. Human renin binding protein: complete genomic sequence and association of an intronic T/C polymorphism with the prorenin level in males. *Hum. Mol. Genet.* 1997 Sep;6(9):1527-34.

[156] Gu D, Kelly TN, Hixson JE, Chen J, Liu D, Chen JC, et al. Genetic variants in the renin-angiotensin-aldosterone system and salt sensitivity of blood pressure. *J. Hypertens* 2010 Jun;28(6):1210-20.

[157] Ahmad U, Saleheen D, Bokhari A, Frossard PM. Strong association of a renin intronic dimorphism with essential hypertension. *Hypertens Res.* 2005 Apr;28(4):339-44.

[158] Fleming I. Signaling by the angiotensin-converting enzyme. *Circ. Res.* 2006 Apr 14;98(7):887-96.

[159] Schunkert H, Hense HW, Muscholl M, Luchner A, Kurzinger S, Danser AH, et al. Associations between circulating components of the renin-angiotensin-aldosterone system and left ventricular mass. *Heart* 1997 Jan;77(1):24-31.

[160] Kyriakidis M, Triposkiadis F, Dernellis J, Androulakis AE, Mellas P, Kelepeshis GA, et al. Effects of cardiac versus circulatory angiotensin-converting enzyme inhibition on left ventricular diastolic function and coronary blood flow in hypertrophic obstructive cardiomyopathy. *Circulation* 1998 Apr 14;97(14):1342-7.

[161] Dahlof B, Pennert K, Hansson L. Reversal of left ventricular hypertrophy in hypertensive patients. A metaanalysis of 109 treatment studies. *Am. J. Hypertens* 1992 Feb;5(2):95-110.

[162] Klingbeil AU, Schneider M, Martus P, Messerli FH, Schmieder RE. A meta-analysis of the effects of treatment on left ventricular mass in essential hypertension. *Am. J. Med.* 2003 Jul;115(1):41-6.

[163] Schmieder RE, Martus P, Klingbeil A. Reversal of left ventricular hypertrophy in essential hypertension. A meta-analysis of randomized double-blind studies. *JAMA* 1996 May 15;275(19):1507-13.

[164] Rigat B, Hubert C, henc-Gelas F, Cambien F, Corvol P, Soubrier F. An insertion/deletion polymorphism in the angiotensin I-converting enzyme gene accounting for half the variance of serum enzyme levels. *J. Clin. Invest.* 1990 Oct;86(4):1343-6.

[165] Tiret L, Rigat B, Visvikis S, Breda C, Corvol P, Cambien F, et al. Evidence, from combined segregation and linkage analysis, that a variant of the angiotensin I-converting enzyme (ACE) gene controls plasma ACE levels. *Am. J. Hum. Genet.* 1992 Jul;51(1):197-205.

[166] Staessen JA, Wang JG, Ginocchio G, Petrov V, Saavedra AP, Soubrier F, et al. The deletion/insertion polymorphism of the angiotensin converting enzyme gene and cardiovascular-renal risk. *J. Hypertens* 1997 Dec;15(12 Pt 2):1579-92.

[167] Jin Y, Kuznetsova T, Thijs L, Richart T, Stolarz-Skrzypek K, Liu Y, et al. Association of echocardiographic left ventricular structure with the ACE D/I polymorphism: A meta-analysis. *J. Renin. Angiotensin Aldosterone Syst.* 2011 Jan 27.

[168] Lindpaintner K, Lee M, Larson MG, Rao VS, Pfeffer MA, Ordovas JM, et al. Absence of association or genetic linkage between the angiotensin-converting-enzyme gene and left ventricular mass. *N. Engl. J. Med.* 1996 Apr 18;334(16):1023-8.

[169] Marian AJ, Yu QT, Workman R, Greve G, Roberts R. Angiotensin-converting enzyme polymorphism in hypertrophic cardiomyopathy and sudden cardiac death. *Lancet* 1993 Oct 30;342(8879):1085-6.

[170] Tesson F, Dufour C, Moolman JC, Carrier L, al-Mahdawi S, Chojnowska L, et al. The influence of the angiotensin I converting enzyme genotype in familial hypertrophic

cardiomyopathy varies with the disease gene mutation. *J. Mol. Cell Cardiol.* 1997 Feb;29(2):831-8.

[171] Rai TS, Dhandapany PS, Ahluwalia TS, Bhardwaj M, Bahl A, Talwar KK, et al. ACE I/D polymorphism in Indian patients with hypertrophic cardiomyopathy and dilated cardiomyopathy. *Mol. Cell Biochem.* 2008 Apr;311(1-2):67-72.

[172] Doolan G, Nguyen L, Chung J, Ingles J, Semsarian C. Progression of left ventricular hypertrophy and the angiotensin-converting enzyme gene polymorphism in hypertrophic cardiomyopathy. *Int. J. Cardiol.* 2004 Aug;96(2):157-63.

[173] Lechin M, Quinones MA, Omran A, Hill R, Yu QT, Rakowski H, et al. Angiotensin-I converting enzyme genotypes and left ventricular hypertrophy in patients with hypertrophic cardiomyopathy. *Circulation* 1995 Oct 1;92(7):1808-12.

[174] Pfeufer A, Osterziel KJ, Urata H, Borck G, Schuster H, Wienker T, et al. Angiotensin-converting enzyme and heart chymase gene polymorphisms in hypertrophic cardiomyopathy. *Am. J. Cardiol.* 1996 Aug 1;78(3):362-4.

[175] Yoneya K, Okamoto H, Machida M, Onozuka H, Noguchi M, Mikami T, et al. Angiotensin-converting enzyme gene polymorphism in Japanese patients with hypertrophic cardiomyopathy. *Am. Heart J.* 1995 Nov;130(5):1089-93.

[176] Buck PC, Fernandes F, Arteaga E, Matsumoto AY, Araujo AQ, Oliveira EM, et al. Association of angiotensin-converting enzyme activity and polymorphism with echocardiographic measures in familial and nonfamilial hypertrophic cardiomyopathy. *Braz. J. Med. Biol. Res.* 2009 Aug;42(8):717-21.

[177] Osterop AP, Kofflard MJ, Sandkuijl LA, Ten Cate FJ, Krams R, Schalekamp MA, et al. AT1 receptor A/C1166 polymorphism contributes to cardiac hypertrophy in subjects with hypertrophic cardiomyopathy. *Hypertension* 1998 Nov;32(5):825-30.

[178] Funada A, Konno T, Fujino N, Muramoto A, Hayashi K, Tsubokawa T, et al. Impact of renin-angiotensin system polymorphisms on development of systolic dysfunction in hypertrophic cardiomyopathy. Evidence from a study of genotyped patients. *Circ. J.* 2010 Nov 25;74(12):2674-80.

[179] Kaya CT, Gurlek A, Altin T, Kilickap M, Karabulut HG, Turhan S, et al. The relationship between angiotensin converting enzyme gene I/D polymorphism and QT dispersion in patients with hypertrophic cardiomyopathy. *J. Renin. Angiotensin Aldosterone Syst.* 2010 Sep;11(3):192-7.

[180] Sayed-Tabatabaei FA, Oostra BA, Isaacs A, van Duijn CM, Witteman JC. ACE polymorphisms. *Circ. Res.* 2006 May 12;98(9):1123-33.

[181] Cox R, Bouzekri N, Martin S, Southam L, Hugill A, Golamaully M, et al. Angiotensin-1-converting enzyme (ACE) plasma concentration is influenced by multiple ACE-linked quantitative trait nucleotides. *Hum. Mol. Genet.* 2002 Nov 1;11(23):2969-77.

[182] Keavney B, McKenzie CA, Connell JM, Julier C, Ratcliffe PJ, Sobel E, et al. Measured haplotype analysis of the angiotensin-I converting enzyme gene. *Hum. Mol. Genet.* 1998 Oct;7(11):1745-51.

[183] Zhu X, McKenzie CA, Forrester T, Nickerson DA, Broeckel U, Schunkert H, et al. Localization of a small genomic region associated with elevated ACE. *Am. J. Hum. Genet.* 2000 Nov;67(5):1144-53.

[184] Kammerer CM, Gouin N, Samollow PB, VandeBerg JF, Hixson JE, Cole SA, et al. Two quantitative trait loci affect ACE activities in Mexican-Americans. *Hypertension* 2004 Feb;43(2):466-70.

[185] McKenzie CA, Sinsheimer JS, Adeyemo AA, Cox RD, Southam L, Hugill A, et al. SNP haplotypes in the angiotensin I-converting enzyme (ACE) gene: analysis of Nigerian family data using gamete competition models. *Ann. Hum. Genet.* 2005 Mar;69(Pt 2):227-32.

[186] Villard E, Tiret L, Visvikis S, Rakotovao R, Cambien F, Soubrier F. Identification of new polymorphisms of the angiotensin I-converting enzyme (ACE) gene, and study of their relationship to plasma ACE levels by two-QTL segregation-linkage analysis. *Am. J. Hum. Genet.* 1996 Jun;58(6):1268-78.

[187] Crackower MA, Sarao R, Oudit GY, Yagil C, Kozieradzki I, Scanga SE, et al. Angiotensin-converting enzyme 2 is an essential regulator of heart function. *Nature* 2002 Jun 20;417(6891):822-8.

[188] Oudit GY, Kassiri Z, Patel MP, Chappell M, Butany J, Backx PH, et al. Angiotensin II-mediated oxidative stress and inflammation mediate the age-dependent cardiomyopathy in ACE2 null mice. *Cardiovasc. Res.* 2007 Jul 1;75(1):29-39.

[189] Zhong J, Basu R, Guo D, Chow FL, Byrns S, Schuster M, et al. Angiotensin-converting enzyme 2 suppresses pathological hypertrophy, myocardial fibrosis, and cardiac dysfunction. *Circulation* 2010 Aug 17;122(7):717-28, 18.

[190] Huentelman MJ, Grobe JL, Vazquez J, Stewart JM, Mecca AP, Katovich MJ, et al. Protection from angiotensin II-induced cardiac hypertrophy and fibrosis by systemic lentiviral delivery of ACE2 in rats. *Exp. Physiol.* 2005 Sep;90(5):783-90.

[191] Tikellis C, Bernardi S, Burns WC. Angiotensin-converting enzyme 2 is a key modulator of the renin-angiotensin system in cardiovascular and renal disease. *Curr. Opin. Nephrol. Hypertens* 2011 Jan;20(1):62-8.

[192] Trask AJ, Averill DB, Ganten D, Chappell MC, Ferrario CM. Primary role of angiotensin-converting enzyme-2 in cardiac production of angiotensin-(1-7) in transgenic Ren-2 hypertensive rats. *Am. J. Physiol. Heart Circ. Physiol* 2007 Jun;292(6):H3019-H3024.

[193] Lieb W, Graf J, Gotz A, Konig IR, Mayer B, Fischer M, et al. Association of angiotensin-converting enzyme 2 (ACE2) gene polymorphisms with parameters of left ventricular hypertrophy in men. Results of the MONICA Augsburg echocardiographic substudy. *J. Mol. Med.* 2006 Jan;84(1):88-96.

[194] Wang SX, Fu CY, Zou YB, Wang H, Shi Y, Xu XQ, et al. Polymorphisms of angiotensin-converting enzyme 2 gene associated with magnitude of left ventricular hypertrophy in male patients with hypertrophic cardiomyopathy. *Chin. Med. J.* (Engl) 2008 Jan 5;121(1):27-31.

[195] Urata H, Boehm KD, Philip A, Kinoshita A, Gabrovsek J, Bumpus FM, et al. Cellular localization and regional distribution of an angiotensin II-forming chymase in the heart. *J. Clin. Invest.* 1993 Apr;91(4):1269-81.

[196] Guo C, Ju H, Leung D, Massaeli H, Shi M, Rabinovitch M. A novel vascular smooth muscle chymase is upregulated in hypertensive rats. *J. Clin. Invest.* 2001 Mar;107(6):703-15.

[197] Koga T, Urata H, Inoue Y, Hoshino T, Okamoto T, Matsunaga A, et al. Human chymase expression in a mice induces mild hypertension with left ventricular hypertrophy. *Hypertens Res.* 2003 Sep;26(9):759-68.

[198] Shiota N, Fukamizu A, Okunishi H, Takai S, Murakami K, Miyazaki M. Cloning of the gene and cDNA for hamster chymase 2, and expression of chymase 1, chymase 2 and

angiotensin-converting enzyme in the terminal stage of cardiomyopathic hearts. *Biochem. J.* 1998 Jul 15;333 (Pt 2):417-24.

[199] Shiota N, Fukamizu A, Takai S, Okunishi H, Murakami K, Miyazaki M. Activation of angiotensin II-forming chymase in the cardiomyopathic hamster heart. *J. Hypertens* 1997 Apr;15(4):431-40.

[200] Hoshino F, Urata H, Inoue Y, Saito Y, Yahiro E, Ideishi M, et al. Chymase inhibitor improves survival in hamsters with myocardial infarction. *J. Cardiovasc. Pharmacol.* 2003 Jan;41 Suppl 1:S11-S18.

[201] He H, Li LM, Cao WH, Sun NL, Liu MZ, Hu YH. A study of the relationships between angiotensin- converting enzyme gene, chymase gene polymorphisms, pharmacological treatment with ACE inhibitor and regression of left ventricular hypertrophy in essential hypertension patients treated with benazepril. *Ann. Hum. Biol.* 2005 Jan;32(1):30-43.

[202] Gumprecht J, Zychma M, Grzeszczak W, LAcka B, Burak W, Mosur M, et al. Angiotensin I-converting enzyme and chymase gene polymorphisms - relationship to left ventricular mass in type 2 diabetes patients. *Med Sci Monit* 2002 Aug;8(8):CR603-CR606.

[203] Pfeufer A, Busjahn A, Vergopoulos A, Knoblauch H, Urata H, Osterziel KJ, et al. Chymase gene locus is not associated with myocardial infarction and is not linked to heart size or blood pressure. *Am. J. Cardiol.* 1998 Oct 15;82(8):979-81.

[204] Booz GW. Cardiac angiotensin AT2 receptor: what exactly does it do? *Hypertension* 2004 Jun;43(6):1162-3.

[205] Hoffmann S, Krause T, van Geel PP, Willenbrock R, Pagel I, Pinto YM, et al. Overexpression of the human angiotensin II type 1 receptor in the rat heart augments load induced cardiac hypertrophy. *J. Mol. Med.* 2001 Oct;79(10):601-8.

[206] Hein L, Stevens ME, Barsh GS, Pratt RE, Kobilka BK, Dzau VJ. Overexpression of angiotensin AT1 receptor transgene in the mouse myocardium produces a lethal phenotype associated with myocyte hyperplasia and heart block. *Proc. Natl. Acad. Sci. USA* 1997 Jun 10;94(12):6391-6.

[207] Ainscough JF, Drinkhill MJ, Sedo A, Turner NA, Brooke DA, Balmforth AJ, et al. Angiotensin II type-1 receptor activation in the adult heart causes blood pressure-independent hypertrophy and cardiac dysfunction. *Cardiovasc. Res.* 2009 Feb 15;81(3):592-600.

[208] Dahlof B, Devereux RB, Kjeldsen SE, Julius S, Beevers G, de Faire U., et al. Cardiovascular morbidity and mortality in the Losartan Intervention For Endpoint reduction in hypertension study (LIFE): a randomised trial against atenolol. *Lancet* 2002 Mar 23;359(9311):995-1003.

[209] Okin PM, Devereux RB, Jern S, Kjeldsen SE, Julius S, Nieminen MS, et al. Regression of electrocardiographic left ventricular hypertrophy by losartan versus atenolol: The Losartan Intervention for Endpoint reduction in Hypertension (LIFE) Study. *Circulation* 2003 Aug 12;108(6):684-90.

[210] Force T, Bonow RO, Houser SR, Solaro RJ, Hershberger RE, Adhikari B, et al. Research priorities in hypertrophic cardiomyopathy: report of a Working Group of the National Heart, Lung, and Blood Institute. *Circulation* 2010 Sep 14;122(11):1130-3.

[211] Araujo AQ, Arteaga E, Ianni BM, Buck PC, Rabello R, Mady C. Effect of Losartan on left ventricular diastolic function in patients with nonobstructive hypertrophic cardiomyopathy. *Am. J. Cardiol.* 2005 Dec 1;96(11):1563-7.

[212] Kawano H, Toda G, Nakamizo R, Koide Y, Seto S, Yano K. Valsartan decreases type I collagen synthesis in patients with hypertrophic cardiomyopathy. *Circ. J.* 2005 Oct;69(10):1244-8.

[213] Penicka M, Gregor P, Kerekes R, Marek D, Curila K, Krupicka J. The effects of candesartan on left ventricular hypertrophy and function in nonobstructive hypertrophic cardiomyopathy: a pilot, randomized study. *J Mol Diagn* 2009 Jan;11(1):35-41.

[214] Yamazaki T, Suzuki J, Shimamoto R, Tsuji T, Ohmoto-Sekine Y, Ohtomo K, et al. A new therapeutic strategy for hypertrophic nonobstructive cardiomyopathy in humans. A randomized and prospective study with an Angiotensin II receptor blocker. *Int. Heart J.* 2007 Nov;48(6):715-24.

[215] Castellano M, Muiesan ML, Beschi M, Rizzoni D, Cinelli A, Salvetti M, et al. Angiotensin II type 1 receptor A/C1166 polymorphism. Relationships with blood pressure and cardiovascular structure. *Hypertension* 1996 Dec;28(6):1076-80.

[216] Hamon M, Amant C, Bauters C, Richard F, Helbecque N, McFadden E, et al. Association of angiotensin converting enzyme and angiotensin II type 1 receptor genotypes with left ventricular function and mass in patients with angiographically normal coronary arteries. *Heart* 1997 Jun;77(6):502-5.

[217] Wang X, Zhu H, Dong Y, Treiber FA, Snieder H. Effects of angiotensinogen and angiotensin II type I receptor genes on blood pressure and left ventricular mass trajectories in multiethnic youth. *Twin Res. Hum. Genet.* 2006 Jun;9(3):393-402.

[218] Ishanov A, Okamoto H, Watanabe M, Yoneya K, Nakagawa I, Kumamoto H, et al. Angiotensin II type 1 receptor gene polymorphisms in patients with cardiac hypertrophy. *Jpn Heart J.* 1998 Jan;39(1):87-96.

[219] Sethupathy P, Borel C, Gagnebin M, Grant GR, Deutsch S, Elton TS, et al. Human microRNA-155 on chromosome 21 differentially interacts with its polymorphic target in the AGTR1 3' untranslated region: a mechanism for functional single-nucleotide polymorphisms related to phenotypes. *Am. J. Hum. Genet.* 2007 Aug;81(2):405-13.

[220] Nio Y, Matsubara H, Murasawa S, Kanasaki M, Inada M. Regulation of gene transcription of angiotensin II receptor subtypes in myocardial infarction. *J. Clin. Invest.* 1995 Jan;95(1):46-54.

[221] Ohkubo N, Matsubara H, Nozawa Y, Mori Y, Murasawa S, Kijima K, et al. Angiotensin type 2 receptors are reexpressed by cardiac fibroblasts from failing myopathic hamster hearts and inhibit cell growth and fibrillar collagen metabolism. *Circulation* 1997 Dec 2;96(11):3954-62.

[222] Van Kesteren CA, van Heugten HA, Lamers JM, Saxena PR, Schalekamp MA, Danser AH. Angiotensin II-mediated growth and antigrowth effects in cultured neonatal rat cardiac myocytes and fibroblasts. *J. Mol. Cell Cardiol.* 1997 Aug;29(8):2147-57.

[223] Booz GW, Baker KM. Role of type 1 and type 2 angiotensin receptors in angiotensin II-induced cardiomyocyte hypertrophy. *Hypertension* 1996 Oct;28(4):635-40.

[224] Mukawa H, Toki Y, Miyazaki Y, Matsui H, Okumura K, Ito T. Angiotensin II type 2 receptor blockade partially negates antihypertrophic effects of type 1 receptor blockade on pressure-overload rat cardiac hypertrophy. *Hypertens Res.* 2003 Jan;26(1):89-95.

[225] Bartunek J, Weinberg EO, Tajima M, Rohrbach S, Lorell BH. Angiotensin II type 2 receptor blockade amplifies the early signals of cardiac growth response to angiotensin II in hypertrophied hearts. *Circulation* 1999 Jan 5;99(1):22-5.

[226] Zhang M, Ma H, Wang BS, Zhao YZ. Angiotensin II type 2 receptor gene polymorphisms and cardioprotective role in essential hypertension. *Heart Vessels* 2006 Mar;21(2):95-101.

[227] Alfakih K, Maqbool A, Sivananthan M, Walters K, Bainbridge G, Ridgway J, et al. Left ventricle mass index and the common, functional, X-linked angiotensin II type-2 receptor gene polymorphism (-1332 G/A) in patients with systemic hypertension. *Hypertension* 2004 Jun;43(6):1189-94.

[228] Erdmann J, Guse M, Kallisch H, Fleck E, Regitz-Zagrosek V. Novel intronic polymorphism (+1675G/A) in the human angiotensin II subtype 2 receptor gene. *Hum. Mutat.* 2000 May;15(5):487.

[229] Warnecke C, Mugrauer P, Surder D, Erdmann J, Schubert C, Regitz-Zagrosek V. Intronic ANG II type 2 receptor gene polymorphism 1675 G/A modulates receptor protein expression but not mRNA splicing. Am. J. Physiol. *Regul Integr Comp Physiol* 2005 Dec;289(6):R1729-R1735.

[230] Nishimura H, Yerkes E, Hohenfellner K, Miyazaki Y, Ma J, Hunley TE, et al. Role of the angiotensin type 2 receptor gene in congenital anomalies of the kidney and urinary tract, CAKUT, of mice and men. *Mol. Cell* 1999 Jan;3(1):1-10.

[231] Schmieder RE, Erdmann J, Delles C, Jacobi J, Fleck E, Hilgers K, et al. Effect of the angiotensin II type 2-receptor gene (+1675 G/A) on left ventricular structure in humans. *J. Am. Coll Cardiol.* 2001 Jan;37(1):175-82.

[232] Herrmann SM, Nicaud V, Schmidt-Petersen K, Pfeifer J, Erdmann J, McDonagh T, et al. Angiotensin II type 2 receptor gene polymorphism and cardiovascular phenotypes: the GLAECO and GLAOLD studies. *Eur. J. Heart Fail* 2002 Dec;4(6):707-12.

[233] Myerson SG, Montgomery HE, World MJ, Pennell DJ. Left ventricular mass: reliability of M-mode and 2-dimensional echocardiographic formulas. *Hypertension* 2002 Nov;40(5):673-8.

[234] Deinum J, van Gool JM, Kofflard MJ, ten Cate FJ, Danser AH. Angiotensin II type 2 receptors and cardiac hypertrophy in women with hypertrophic cardiomyopathy. *Hypertension* 2001 Dec 1;38(6):1278-81.

[235] Barbato JC, Rashid S, Mulrow PJ, Shapiro JI, Franco-Saenz R. Mechanisms for aldosterone and spironolactone-induced positive inotropic actions in the rat heart. *Hypertension* 2004 Nov;44(5):751-7.

[236] Okoshi MP, Yan X, Okoshi K, Nakayama M, Schuldt AJ, O'Connell TD, et al. Aldosterone directly stimulates cardiac myocyte hypertrophy. *J. Card Fail* 2004 Dec;10(6):511-8.

[237] Sato A, Funder JW. High glucose stimulates aldosterone-induced hypertrophy via type I mineralocorticoid receptors in neonatal rat cardiomyocytes. *Endocrinology* 1996 Oct;137(10):4145-53.

[238] Tsybouleva N, Zhang L, Chen S, Patel R, Lutucuta S, Nemoto S, et al. Aldosterone, through novel signaling proteins, is a fundamental molecular bridge between the genetic defect and the cardiac phenotype of hypertrophic cardiomyopathy. *Circulation* 2004 Mar 16;109(10):1284-91.

[239] Pojoga L, Gautier S, Blanc H, Guyene TT, Poirier O, Cambien F, et al. Genetic determination of plasma aldosterone levels in essential hypertension. *Am. J. Hypertens* 1998 Jul;11(7):856-60.

[240] Kupari M, Hautanen A, Lankinen L, Koskinen P, Virolainen J, Nikkila H, et al. Associations between human aldosterone synthase (CYP11B2) gene polymorphisms and left ventricular size, mass, and function. *Circulation* 1998 Feb 17;97(6):569-75.

[241] White PC, Hautanen A, Kupari M. Aldosterone synthase (CYP11B2) polymorphisms and cardiovascular function. *J. Steroid Biochem. Mol. Biol.* 1999 Apr;69(1-6):409-12.

[242] Bassett MH, Zhang Y, Clyne C, White PC, Rainey WE. Differential regulation of aldosterone synthase and 11beta-hydroxylase transcription by steroidogenic factor-1. *J. Mol. Endocrinol.* 2002 Apr;28(2):125-35.

[243] Schunkert H, Hengstenberg C, Holmer SR, Broeckel U, Luchner A, Muscholl MW, et al. Lack of association between a polymorphism of the aldosterone synthase gene and left ventricular structure. *Circulation* 1999 May 4;99(17):2255-60.

[244] Sookoian S, Gianotti TF, Pirola CJ. Role of the C-344T aldosterone synthase gene variant in left ventricular mass and left ventricular structure-related phenotypes. *Heart* 2008 Jul;94(7):903-10.

[245] Mayosi BM, Keavney B, Watkins H, Farrall M. Measured haplotype analysis of the aldosterone synthase gene and heart size. *Eur. J. Hum. Genet.* 2003 May;11(5):395-401.

[246] Ganapathipillai S, Laval G, Hoffmann IS, Castejon AM, Nicod J, Dick B, et al. CYP11B2-CYP11B1 haplotypes associated with decreased 11 beta-hydroxylase activity. *J. Clin. Endocrinol. Metab.* 2005 Feb;90(2):1220-5.

[247] Keavney B, Mayosi B, Gaukrodger N, Imrie H, Baker M, Fraser R, et al. Genetic variation at the locus encompassing 11-beta hydroxylase and aldosterone synthase accounts for heritability in cortisol precursor (11-deoxycortisol) urinary metabolite excretion. *J. Clin. Endocrinol. Metab.* 2005 Feb;90(2):1072-7.

[248] Imrie H, Freel M, Mayosi BM, Davies E, Fraser R, Ingram M, et al. Association between aldosterone production and variation in the 11beta-hydroxylase (CYP11B1) gene. *J. Clin. Endocrinol. Metab.* 2006 Dec;91(12):5051-6.

[249] varez-Madrazo S, Padmanabhan S, Mayosi BM, Watkins H, Avery P, Wallace AM, et al. Familial and phenotypic associations of the aldosterone Renin ratio. *J. Clin. Endocrinol. Metab.* 2009 Nov;94(11):4324-33.

[250] Patel R, Lim DS, Reddy D, Nagueh SF, Lutucuta S, Sole MJ, et al. Variants of trophic factors and expression of cardiac hypertrophy in patients with hypertrophic cardiomyopathy. *J. Mol. Cell Cardiol.* 2000 Dec;32(12):2369-77.

[251] Chai W, Hoedemaekers Y, van Schaik RH, van Fessem M., Garrelds IM, Saris JJ, et al. Cardiac aldosterone in subjects with hypertrophic cardiomyopathy. *J. Renin. Angiotensin Aldosterone Syst.* 2006 Dec;7(4):225-30.

[252] Lombes M, Alfaidy N, Eugene E, Lessana A, Farman N, Bonvalet JP. Prerequisite for cardiac aldosterone action. Mineralocorticoid receptor and 11 beta-hydroxysteroid dehydrogenase in the human heart. *Circulation* 1995 Jul 15;92(2):175-82.

[253] Edelheit O, Hanukoglu I, Gizewska M, Kandemir N, Tenenbaum-Rakover Y, Yurdakok M, et al. Novel mutations in epithelial sodium channel (ENaC) subunit genes and phenotypic expression of multisystem pseudohypoaldosteronism. *Clin. Endocrinol. (Oxf)* 2005 May;62(5):547-53.

[254] Geller DS, Rodriguez-Soriano J, Vallo BA, Schifter S, Bayer M, Chang SS, et al. Mutations in the mineralocorticoid receptor gene cause autosomal dominant pseudohypoaldosteronism type I. *Nat. Genet.* 1998 Jul;19(3):279-81.

[255] Le Menuet D, Viengchareun S, Muffat-Joly M, Zennaro MC, Lombes M. Expression and function of the human mineralocorticoid receptor: lessons from transgenic mouse models. *Mol. Cell Endocrinol.* 2004 Mar 31;217(1-2):127-36.
[256] Yoshida Y, Morimoto T, Takaya T, Kawamura T, Sunagawa Y, Wada H, et al. Aldosterone signaling associates with p300/GATA4 transcriptional pathway during the hypertrophic response of cardiomyocytes. *Circ. J.* 2010 Jan;74(1):156-62.
[257] Nagata K, Obata K, Xu J, Ichihara S, Noda A, Kimata H, et al. Mineralocorticoid receptor antagonism attenuates cardiac hypertrophy and failure in low-aldosterone hypertensive rats. *Hypertension* 2006 Apr;47(4):656-64.
[258] Michea L, Villagran A, Urzua A, Kuntsmann S, Venegas P, Carrasco L, et al. Mineralocorticoid receptor antagonism attenuates cardiac hypertrophy and prevents oxidative stress in uremic rats. *Hypertension* 2008 Aug;52(2):295-300.
[259] Fraccarollo D, Berger S, Galuppo P, Kneitz S, Hein L, Schutz G, et al. Deletion of cardiomyocyte mineralocorticoid receptor ameliorates adverse remodeling after myocardial infarction. *Circulation* 2011 Feb 1;123(4):400-8.
[260] Lother A, Berger S, Gilsbach R, Rosner S, Ecke A, Barreto F, et al. Ablation of mineralocorticoid receptors in myocytes but not in fibroblasts preserves cardiac function. *Hypertension* 2011 Apr;57(4):746-54.
[261] Ouvrard-Pascaud A, Sainte-Marie Y, Benitah JP, Perrier R, Soukaseum C, Nguyen Dinh CA, et al. Conditional mineralocorticoid receptor expression in the heart leads to life-threatening arrhythmias. *Circulation* 2005 Jun 14;111(23):3025-33.
[262] Taillefer M, Di Fruscia R. Benazepril and subclinical feline hypertrophic cardiomyopathy: a prospective, blinded, controlled study. *Can. Vet. J.* 2006 May;47(5):437-45.
[263] Di Zhang A, Nguyen Dinh CA, Soukaseum C, Escoubet B, Cherfa A, Messaoudi S, et al. Cross-talk between mineralocorticoid and angiotensin II signaling for cardiac remodeling. *Hypertension* 2008 Dec;52(6):1060-7.
[264] Stas S, Whaley-Connell A, Habibi J, Appesh L, Hayden MR, Karuparthi PR, et al. Mineralocorticoid receptor blockade attenuates chronic overexpression of the renin-angiotensin-aldosterone system stimulation of reduced nicotinamide adenine dinucleotide phosphate oxidase and cardiac remodeling. *Endocrinology* 2007 Aug;148(8):3773-80.
[265] Pitt B, Zannad F, Remme WJ, Cody R, Castaigne A, Perez A, et al. The effect of spironolactone on morbidity and mortality in patients with severe heart failure. Randomized Aldactone Evaluation Study Investigators. *N. Engl. J. Med.* 1999 Sep 2;341(10):709-17.
[266] Pitt B, Remme W, Zannad F, Neaton J, Martinez F, Roniker B, et al. Eplerenone, a selective aldosterone blocker, in patients with left ventricular dysfunction after myocardial infarction. *N. Engl. J. Med.* 2003 Apr 3;348(14):1309-21.
[267] Marian AJ. Experimental therapies in hypertrophic cardiomyopathy. *J. Cardiovasc. Transl. Res.* 2009 Dec;2(4):483-92.
[268] Geller DS, Farhi A, Pinkerton N, Fradley M, Moritz M, Spitzer A, et al. Activating mineralocorticoid receptor mutation in hypertension exacerbated by pregnancy. *Science* 2000 Jul 7;289(5476):119-23.

[269] Martinez F, Mansego ML, Escudero JC, Redon J, Chaves FJ. Association of a mineralocorticoid receptor gene polymorphism with hypertension in a Spanish population. *Am. J. Hypertens* 2009 Jun;22(6):649-55.

[270] Van Leeuwen N, Caprio M, Blaya C, Fumeron F, Sartorato P, Ronconi V, et al. The functional c.-2G>C variant of the mineralocorticoid receptor modulates blood pressure, renin, and aldosterone levels. *Hypertension* 2010 Nov;56(5):995-1002.

[271] Farman N, Bocchi B. Mineralocorticoid selectivity: molecular and cellular aspects. *Kidney Int.* 2000 Apr;57(4):1364-9.

[272] Dave-Sharma S, Wilson RC, Harbison MD, Newfield R, Azar MR, Krozowski ZS, et al. Examination of genotype and phenotype relationships in 14 patients with apparent mineralocorticoid excess. *J. Clin. Endocrinol. Metab.* 1998 Jul;83(7):2244-54.

[273] Qin W, Rudolph AE, Bond BR, Rocha R, Blomme EA, Goellner JJ, et al. Transgenic model of aldosterone-driven cardiac hypertrophy and heart failure. *Circ. Res.* 2003 Jul 11;93(1):69-76.

[274] Takeda M, Tatsumi T, Matsunaga S, Hayashi H, Kimata M, Honsho S, et al. Spironolactone modulates expressions of cardiac mineralocorticoid receptor and 11beta-hydroxysteroid dehydrogenase 2 and prevents ventricular remodeling in post-infarct rat hearts. *Hypertens Res.* 2007 May;30(5):427-37.

[275] Bailey MA, Craigie E, Livingstone DE, Kotelevtsev YV, Al-Dujaili EA, Kenyon CJ, et al. Hsd11b2 haploinsufficiency in mice causes salt sensitivity of blood pressure. *Hypertension* 2011 Mar;57(3):515-20.

[276] Ferrari P. The role of 11beta-hydroxysteroid dehydrogenase type 2 in human hypertension. *Biochim. Biophys. Acta* 2010 Dec;1802(12):1178-87.

[277] Glorioso N, Filigheddu F, Parpaglia PP, Soro A, Troffa C, Argiolas G, et al. 11beta-Hydroxysteroid dehydrogenase type 2 activity is associated with left ventricular mass in essential hypertension. *Eur. Heart J.* 2005 Mar;26(5):498-504.

[278] Gu JW, Anand V, Shek EW, Moore MC, Brady AL, Kelly WC, et al. Sodium induces hypertrophy of cultured myocardial myoblasts and vascular smooth muscle cells. *Hypertension* 1998 May;31(5):1083-7.

[279] Verdonck F, Volders PG, Vos MA, Sipido KR. Intracellular Na+ and altered Na+ transport mechanisms in cardiac hypertrophy and failure. *J. Mol. Cell Cardiol.* 2003 Jan;35(1):5-25.

[280] Kaplan JH. Biochemistry of Na,K-ATPase. *Annu. Rev. Biochem.* 2002;71:511-35.

[281] Shull GE, Schwartz A, Lingrel JB. Amino-acid sequence of the catalytic subunit of the (Na+ + K+)ATPase deduced from a complementary DNA. *Nature* 1985 Aug 22;316(6030):691-5.

[282] Rajasekaran SA, Barwe SP, Rajasekaran AK. Multiple functions of Na,K-ATPase in epithelial cells. *Semin Nephrol* 2005 Sep;25(5):328-34.

[283] Blanco G, Mercer RW. Isozymes of the Na-K-ATPase: heterogeneity in structure, diversity in function. *Am. J. Physiol.* 1998 Nov;275(5 Pt 2):F633-F650.

[284] Malik N, Canfield V, Sanchez-Watts G, Watts AG, Scherer S, Beatty BG, et al. Structural organization and chromosomal localization of the human Na,K-ATPase beta 3 subunit gene and pseudogene. *Mamm. Genome* 1998 Feb;9(2):136-43.

[285] Schwinger RH, Wang J, Frank K, Muller-Ehmsen J, Brixius K, McDonough AA, et al. Reduced sodium pump alpha1, alpha3, and beta1-isoform protein levels and Na+,K+-

ATPase activity but unchanged Na+-Ca2+ exchanger protein levels in human heart failure. *Circulation* 1999 Apr 27;99(16):2105-12.

[286] Wang J, Schwinger RH, Frank K, Muller-Ehmsen J, Martin-Vasallo P, Pressley TA, et al. Regional expression of sodium pump subunits isoforms and Na+-Ca++ exchanger in the human heart. *J. Clin. Invest.* 1996 Oct 1;98(7):1650-8.

[287] Baek M, Weiss M. Down-regulation of Na+ pump alpha 2 isoform in isoprenaline-induced cardiac hypertrophy in rat: evidence for increased receptor binding affinity but reduced inotropic potency of digoxin. *J. Pharmacol. Exp. Ther.* 2005 May;313(2):731-9.

[288] Xie Z, Kometiani P, Liu J, Li J, Shapiro JI, Askari A. Intracellular reactive oxygen species mediate the linkage of Na+/K+-ATPase to hypertrophy and its marker genes in cardiac myocytes. *J. Biol. Chem.* 1999 Jul 2;274(27):19323-8.

[289] Yamamoto T, Shirayama T, Takahashi T, Matsubara H. Altered expression of Na+ transporters at the mRNA level in rat normal and hypertrophic myocardium. *Heart Vessels* 2009 Jan;24(1):54-62.

[290] Zwadlo C, Borlak J. Disease-associated changes in the expression of ion channels, ion receptors, ion exchangers and Ca(2+)-handling proteins in heart hypertrophy. *Toxicol. Appl. Pharmacol.* 2005 Sep 15;207(3):244-56.

[291] Allen PD, Schmidt TA, Marsh JD, Kjeldsen K. Na,K-ATPase expression in normal and failing human left ventricle. *Basic. Res. Cardiol.* 1992;87 Suppl 1:87-94.

[292] Shamraj OI, Grupp IL, Grupp G, Melvin D, Gradoux N, Kremers W, et al. Characterisation of Na/K-ATPase, its isoforms, and the inotropic response to ouabain in isolated failing human hearts. *Cardiovasc. Res.* 1993 Dec;27(12):2229-37.

[293] Muller-Ehmsen J, Wang J, Schwinger RH, McDonough AA. Region specific regulation of sodium pump isoform and Na,Ca-exchanger expression in the failing human heart--right atrium vs left ventricle. *Cell Mol. Biol.* (Noisy -le-grand) 2001 Mar;47(2):373-81.

[294] Akera T, Ng YC. Digitalis sensitivity of Na+,K(+)-ATPase, myocytes and the heart. *Life Sci.* 1991;48(2):97-106.

[295] Huang L, Li H, Xie Z. Ouabain-induced hypertrophy in cultured cardiac myocytes is accompanied by changes in expression of several late response genes. *J. Mol. Cell Cardiol.* 1997 Feb;29(2):429-37.

[296] Fedorova OV, Talan MI, Agalakova NI, Lakatta EG, Bagrov AY. Coordinated shifts in Na/K-ATPase isoforms and their endogenous ligands during cardiac hypertrophy and failure in NaCl-sensitive hypertension. *J. Hypertens* 2004 Feb;22(2):389-97.

[297] Kometiani P, Li J, Gnudi L, Kahn BB, Askari A, Xie Z. Multiple signal transduction pathways link Na+/K+-ATPase to growth-related genes in cardiac myocytes. The roles of Ras and mitogen-activated protein kinases. *J. Biol. Chem.* 1998 Jun 12;273(24):15249-56.

[298] James PF, Grupp IL, Grupp G, Woo AL, Askew GR, Croyle ML, et al. Identification of a specific role for the Na,K-ATPase alpha 2 isoform as a regulator of calcium in the heart. *Mol. Cell* 1999 May;3(5):555-63.

[299] Magyar JP, Bartsch U, Wang ZQ, Howells N, Aguzzi A, Wagner EF, et al. Degeneration of neural cells in the central nervous system of mice deficient in the gene for the adhesion molecule on Glia, the beta 2 subunit of murine Na,K-ATPase. *J. Cell Biol.* 1994 Nov;127(3):835-45.

[300] Barwe SP, Jordan MC, Skay A, Inge L, Rajasekaran SA, Wolle D, et al. Dysfunction of ouabain-induced cardiac contractility in mice with heart-specific ablation of Na,K-ATPase beta1-subunit. *J. Mol. Cell Cardiol.* 2009 Oct;47(4):552-60.

[301] Glorioso N, Herrera VL, Bagamasbad P, Filigheddu F, Troffa C, Argiolas G, et al. Association of ATP1A1 and dear single-nucleotide polymorphism haplotypes with essential hypertension: sex-specific and haplotype-specific effects. *Circ. Res.* 2007 May 25;100(10):1522-9.

[302] Rice T, Rankinen T, Province MA, Chagnon YC, Perusse L, Borecki IB, et al. Genome-wide linkage analysis of systolic and diastolic blood pressure: the Quebec Family Study. *Circulation* 2000 Oct 17;102(16):1956-63.

[303] Chang YP, Liu X, Kim JD, Ikeda MA, Layton MR, Weder AB, et al. Multiple genes for essential-hypertension susceptibility on chromosome 1q. *Am. J. Hum. Genet.* 2007 Feb;80(2):253-64.

[304] Xiao B, Zhang Y, Niu W, Gao P, Zhu D. Association of ATP1B1 single-nucleotide polymorphisms with blood pressure and hypertension in a Chinese population. *Clin. Chim. Acta* 2009 Sep;407(1-2):47-50.

[305] Pfeufer A, Sanna S, Arking DE, Muller M, Gateva V, Fuchsberger C, et al. Common variants at ten loci modulate the QT interval duration in the QTSCD Study. *Nat. Genet.* 2009 Apr;41(4):407-14.

[306] Canessa CM, Schild L, Buell G, Thorens B, Gautschi I, Horisberger JD, et al. Amiloride-sensitive epithelial Na+ channel is made of three homologous subunits. *Nature* 1994 Feb 3;367(6462):463-7.

[307] Hansson JH, Schild L, Lu Y, Wilson TA, Gautschi I, Shimkets R, et al. A de novo missense mutation of the beta subunit of the epithelial sodium channel causes hypertension and Liddle syndrome, identifying a proline-rich segment critical for regulation of channel activity. *Proc. Natl. Acad. Sci. USA* 1995 Dec 5;92(25):11495-9.

[308] Jeunemaitre X, Bassilana F, Persu A, Dumont C, Champigny G, Lazdunski M, et al. Genotype-phenotype analysis of a newly discovered family with Liddle's syndrome. *J. Hypertens* 1997 Oct;15(10):1091-100.

[309] Rossi E, Farnetti E, Nicoli D, Sazzini M, Perazzoli F, Regolisti G, et al. A Clinical Phenotype Mimicking Essential Hypertension in a Newly Discovered Family With Liddle's Syndrome. *Am. J. Hypertens* 2011 Apr 28.

[310] Shi PP, Cao XR, Sweezer EM, Kinney TS, Williams NR, Husted RF, et al. Salt-sensitive hypertension and cardiac hypertrophy in mice deficient in the ubiquitin ligase Nedd4-2. *Am. J. Physiol. Renal Physiol* 2008 Aug;295(2):F462-F470.

[311] Spence JD. Physiologic tailoring of treatment in resistant hypertension. *Curr. Cardiol. Rev.* 2010 May;6(2):119-23.

[312] Su YR, Menon AG. Epithelial sodium channels and hypertension. *Drug Metab. Dispos.* 2001 Apr;29(4 Pt 2):553-6.

[313] Ji Y, Huang Y, Han Y, Xu Y, Ferro A. Cardiac effects of amiloride and of enalapril in the spontaneously hypertensive rat. *J. Hypertens* 2003 Aug;21(8):1583-9.

[314] Mirkovic S, Seymour AM, Fenning A, Strachan A, Margolin SB, Taylor SM, et al. Attenuation of cardiac fibrosis by pirfenidone and amiloride in DOCA-salt hypertensive rats. *Br. J. Pharmacol.* 2002 Feb;135(4):961-8.

[315] Teiwes J, Toto RD. Epithelial sodium channel inhibition in cardiovascular disease. A potential role for amiloride. *Am. J. Hypertens* 2007 Jan;20(1):109-17.

[316] Wang Q, Hummler E, Maillard M, Nussberger J, Rossier BC, Brunner HR, et al. Compensatory up-regulation of angiotensin II subtype 1 receptors in alpha ENaC knockout heterozygous mice. *Kidney Int.* 2001 Jun;59(6):2216-21.

[317] Beutler KT, Masilamani S, Turban S, Nielsen J, Brooks HL, Ageloff S, et al. Long-term regulation of ENaC expression in kidney by angiotensin II. *Hypertension* 2003 May;41(5):1143-50.

[318] Moolman-Smook JC, De Lange WJ, Bruwer EC, Brink PA, Corfield VA. The origins of hypertrophic cardiomyopathy-causing mutations in two South African subpopulations: a unique profile of both independent and founder events. *Am. J. Hum. Genet.* 1999 Nov;65(5):1308-20.

[319] Schiller NB, Shah PM, Crawford M, DeMaria A, Devereux R, Feigenbaum H, et al. Recommendations for quantitation of the left ventricle by two-dimensional echocardiography. American Society of Echocardiography Committee on Standards, Subcommittee on Quantitation of Two-Dimensional Echocardiograms. *J. Am. Soc. Echocardiogr.* 1989 Sep;2(5):358-67.

[320] Revera M, van der Merwe L., Heradien M, Goosen A, Corfield VA, Brink PA, et al. Troponin T and beta-myosin mutations have distinct cardiac functional effects in hypertrophic cardiomyopathy patients without hypertrophy. *Cardiovasc. Res.* 2008 Mar 1;77(4):687-94.

[321] Wigginton JE, Abecasis GR. PEDSTATS: descriptive statistics, graphics and quality assessment for gene mapping data. *Bioinformatics* 2005 Aug 15;21(16):3445-7.

[322] Abecasis GR, Cardon LR, Cookson WO. A general test of association for quantitative traits in nuclear families. *Am. J. Hum. Genet.* 2000 Jan;66(1):279-92.

[323] Pilia G, Chen WM, Scuteri A, Orru M, Albai G, Dei M, et al. Heritability of cardiovascular and personality traits in 6,148 sardinians. *Plos Genetics* 2006 Aug;2(8):1207-23.

[324] Mayosi BM, Keavney B, Kardos A, Davies CH, Ratcliffe PJ, Farrall M, et al. Electrocardiographic measures of left ventricular hypertrophy show greater heritability than echocardiographic left ventricular mass. *Eur. Heart J.* 2002 Dec;23(24):1963-71.

[325] Swan L, Birnie DH, Padmanabhan S, Inglis G, Connell JM, Hillis WS. The genetic determination of left ventricular mass in healthy adults. *Eur. Heart J.* 2003 Mar;24(6):577-82.

[326] Bella JN, MacCluer JW, Roman MJ, Almasy L, North KE, Best LG, et al. Heritability of left ventricular dimensions and mass in American Indians: The Strong Heart Study. *J. Hypertens* 2004 Feb;22(2):281-6.

[327] de Simone G, Tang W, Devereux RB, Hunt SC, Kitzman DW, Rao DC, et al. Assessment of the interaction of heritability of volume load and left ventricular mass: the HyperGEN offspring study. *J. Hypertens* 2007 Jul;25(7):1397-402.

[328] Juo SH, Di Tullio MR, Lin HF, Rundek T, Boden-Albala B, Homma S, et al. Heritability of left ventricular mass and other morphologic variables in Caribbean Hispanic subjects: the Northern Manhattan Family Study. *J. Am. Coll Cardiol.* 2005 Aug 16;46(4):735-7.

[329] Kotchen TA, Kotchen JM, Grim CE, George V, Kaldunski ML, Cowley AW, et al. Genetic determinants of hypertension: identification of candidate phenotypes. *Hypertension* 2000 Jul;36(1):7-13.

[330] Post WS, Larson MG, Myers RH, Galderisi M, Levy D. Heritability of left ventricular mass: the Framingham Heart Study. *Hypertension* 1997 Nov;30(5):1025-8.

[331] Busjahn CA, Schulz-Menger J, bdel-Aty H, Rudolph A, Jordan J, Luft FC, et al. Heritability of left ventricular and papillary muscle heart size: a twin study with cardiac magnetic resonance imaging. *Eur. Heart J.* 2009 Jul;30(13):1643-7.

[332] Hirschhorn JN, Lohmueller K, Byrne E, Hirschhorn K. A comprehensive review of genetic association studies. *Genet. Med.* 2002 Mar;4(2):45-61.

[333] Gordon D, Finch SJ. Factors affecting statistical power in the detection of genetic association. *J. Clin. Invest.* 2005 Jun;115(6):1408-18.

[334] Colhoun HM, McKeigue PM, Davey SG. Problems of reporting genetic associations with complex outcomes. *Lancet* 2003 Mar 8;361(9360):865-72.

[335] Donahue MP, Allen AS. Genetic association studies in cardiology. Am Heart J 2005 Jun;149(6):964-70.

[336] Perneger TV. What's wrong with Bonferroni adjustments. *BMJ* 1998 Apr 18;316(7139):1236-8.

[337] Campbell H, Rudan I. Interpretation of genetic association studies in complex disease. *Pharmacogenomics J.* 2002;2(6):349-60.

[338] Tsai CT, Lai LP, Lin JL, Chiang FT, Hwang JJ, Ritchie MD, et al. Renin-angiotensin system gene polymorphisms and atrial fibrillation. *Circulation* 2004 Apr 6;109(13):1640-6.

[339] Tsai CT, Hwang JJ, Ritchie MD, Moore JH, Chiang FT, Lai LP, et al. Renin-angiotensin system gene polymorphisms and coronary artery disease in a large angiographic cohort: detection of high order gene-gene interaction. *Atherosclerosis* 2007 Nov;195(1):172-80.

[340] Ye S, Dhillon S, Seear R, Dunleavey L, Day LB, Bannister W, et al. Epistatic interaction between variations in the angiotensin I converting enzyme and angiotensin II type 1 receptor genes in relation to extent of coronary atherosclerosis. *Heart* 2003 Oct;89(10):1195-9.

[341] Cordell HJ. Epistasis: what it means, what it doesn't mean, and statistical methods to detect it in humans. *Hum. Mol. Genet.* 2002 Oct 1;11(20):2463-8.

[342] Williams SM, Ritchie MD, Phillips JA, III, Dawson E, Prince M, Dzhura E, et al. Multilocus analysis of hypertension: a hierarchical approach. *Hum. Hered.* 2004;57(1):28-38.

[343] Clark AG. The role of haplotypes in candidate gene studies. *Genet Epidemiol.* 2004 Dec;27(4):321-33.

[344] Liu N, Zhang K, Zhao H. Haplotype-association analysis. *Adv. Genet.* 2008;60:335-405.

[345] Kaufman BD, Auerbach S, Reddy S, Manlhiot C, Deng L, Prakash A, et al. RAAS gene polymorphisms influence progression of pediatric hypertrophic cardiomyopathy. *Hum. Genet.* 2007 Dec;122(5):515-23.

[346] Montezano AC, Touyz RM. Networking between systemic angiotensin II and cardiac mineralocorticoid receptors. *Hypertension* 2008 Dec;52(6):1016-8.

In: Angiotensin: New Research
Editors: S. Harada, I. Moi, pp. 59-91
ISBN: 978-1-62100-773-9

Chapter 2

CARDIAC RENIN ANGIOTENSIN SYSTEM AND EXERCISE TRAINING

V.G. Barauna, T. Fernandes and E.M. Oliveira
University of Sao Paulo, Brazil.

INTRODUCTION

Cardiac hypertrophy is a central feature in both pathological and physiological remodeling. In cardiovascular disease, pathological remodeling with hypertrophy or dilatation leads to heart dysfunction and failure, and is at least partly caused by altered cardiac gene expression and molecular phenotype (Beisvag et al., 2009). Although the response compensates for reduced contractility in the short term, the long term effect is progressive dysfunction. In contrast, physiological hypertrophy and remodeling induced by exercise training (also known as athletes' heart) is considered beneficial, as it supports the increased O_2 demand. Exercise induces functional and structural changes in the cardiovascular system and the type of training (endurance vs. strength training) is of special importance as shown in the meta-analysis by Pluim et al. (Pluim, Zwinderman, van der Laarse, & van der Wall, 2000), which confirmed the hypothesis of two different forms: the endurance trained and the strength trained heart. Endurance-trained hearts show an eccentric hypertrophy, whereas a concentric hypertrophy develops in strength-trained hearts (Pluim et al., 2000). Within a few weeks of training such structural changes may occur but in both cases there is no sign of loss of ventricular function as observed in decompensated cardiac hypertrophy. As a result of these structural adaptations cardiac output rises significantly when compared with that of untrained individuals. The structural cardiac remodeling induced by exercise training can be dependent of local or systemic factors (Figure 1).

The renin-angiotensin system (RAS), an important system for blood pressure and intravascular volume control, is one of the hormonal systems that play relevant role in left ventricular hypertrophy (LVH) and fibrosis. The main mechanism is the increase in blood pressure, which leads to increased left ventricular wall stress; however, aldosterone release from the adrenals and the direct action of angiotensin (Ang) II on the cardiomyocytes and fibroblasts also play a role (Kim & Iwao, 2000).

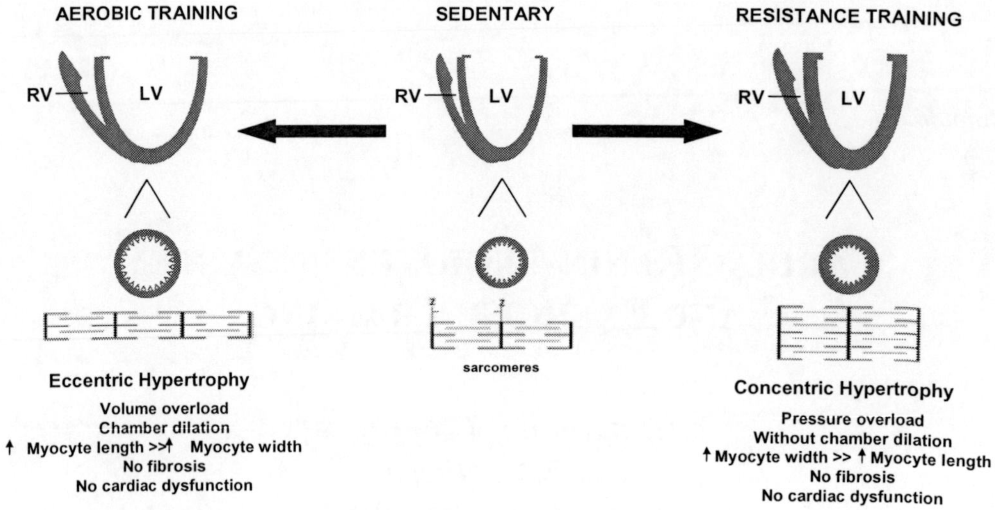

From Fernandes et al., Braz J Med Biol Res 2011 (In press).

Figure 1. Effect of exercise training on cardiac hypertrophy. Physiological hypertrophy is characterized by a uniform profile of ventricular wall and septum growth, without fibrosis and cardiac dysfunction. Aerobic exercise training, such as long-distance running or swimming, is matched with an increased volume overload accompanied by cardiac chamber dilation, referred to as eccentric hypertrophy. This phenotype is associated with the addition of sarcomeres in series to lengthen the cardiomyocyte and to increase the width of the cell in parallel. In contrast, resistance training, such as weight lifting and wrestling, results in an increased pressure overload without chamber dilation, referred to as concentric hypertrophy. This phenotype is associated with the addition of sarcomeres in parallel to an increase in the cross-sectional cardiac area. LV = left ventricle; RV = right ventricle.

The RAS has been at the centre of intensive research activities for several decades. As a result, our knowledge of cardiovascular, renal, and atherosclerotic diseases has substantially increased and our therapeutic approaches have become more efficient, taking into account the comorbidities of individual patients. Blockade of the RAS is now an evidence based strategy for the protection of cardiovascular, cerebrovascular, and renal systems (Re, 2004; Unger, 2002).

In the classic RAS paradigm, renin is released from juxtaglomerular cells of the kidney into the circulation where it converts angiotensinogen from the liver to Ang I. Ang I is subsequently hydrolyzed by angiotensin-converting enzyme (ACE) from the lung to form Ang II. While ACE has the potential to hydrolyze many proteins or even to transduce its own cell signaling, it is most appreciated for its enzymatic processing of Ang I to Ang II (Fleming, 2006). In addition, ACE mediates the hydrolysis of bradykinin, which is typically considered to have blood pressure–lowering effects. Bradykinin may also act as regulator of cardiac function (Sharma, 2009). Interestingly, ACE more readily hydrolyze bradykinin than it does to Ang I. Therefore, the net physiological effect of ACE is to increase the production of a vasoconstrictor hypertrophic peptide and decrease the availability of a vasodilator and anti-proliferative peptide.

There are two major subtypes of Ang II receptors, AT1 and AT2. In rodents, The AT1 receptor is further subdivided into AT1a and AT1b receptors. Most of the well-known Ang II functions in the cardiovascular system are mediated through the AT1 receptor, such as, sympathetic nervous system activation- resulting in vasoconstriction and increased rate and force of heart contraction, as well as, promoting cardiac hypertrophy and fibrosis, while AT2 receptor counteracts AT1 receptor effects (Dostal, 2000; Dostal & Baker, 1999).

Considering the rapid progress in understanding the molecular physiology of RAS and its many complexities, it should not be surprising that details would continue to emerge. Recently it was discovered that a distinct isoform of ACE is expressed in humans, and it was named ACE2 (Pagliaro & Penna, 2005).

In 2000, ACE2 was discovered and was characterized as an enzyme similar to ACE (Tipnis et al., 2000). Unlike ACE, ACE2 hydrolyzes Ang I to Ang 1-9, Ang II to Ang (1-7), and Bradykinin to [des-Arg^9] BK (an inactive metabolite). In marked contrast to ACE, ACE2 does not convert Ang I to Ang II, and its enzymatic activity is not inhibited by ACE inhibitors. Therefore, ACE2 is effectively an inhibitor of the formation of Ang II by stimulating alternative pathways for its precursor, Ang I, degradation. ACE2 has also been localized in cardiac tissue (Donoghue et al., 2000). It is well-know that the preferred pathway by ACE2 with 500-fold greater efficiency is Ang II to generate Ang (1-7), responsible by cardioprotective role, such as anti-proliferative, vasodilator and anti-fibrosis effects (Crackower et al., 2002; Ferrario, 2010). Mas is the functional receptor for Ang (1-7) and provides molecular basis for these physiological actions (Sharma, 2009). In fact, Santos et al. (R. A. Santos et al., 2006; R. A. Santos et al., 2003) found that hearts from Mas-deficient mice exhibited a marked change in extracellular matrix protein expression to a profibrotic profile, accompanied by an important cardiac dysfunction.

Since many studies have already demonstrated that hemodynamic overload (pressure or volume) activates the RAS in the heart in pathological states (Dahlof, Herlitz, Aurell, & Hansson, 1992; Julius, 2007) and that exercise training is a well-recognized stressor to the cardiovascular system (Taylor; Wang, Wisloff, & Kemi, 2010), here we review the literature over the last 5 years with reference to animals models that have focused on the role of the RAS in cardiovascular adaptations induced by a physiological hemodynamic overload.

Cardiac RAS and Aerobic Training: Role in Hypertrophy and Physical Performance

Exercise is known to be a potent cardiac hypertrophic stimulus, but the magnitude and pattern of left ventricular hypertrophy is dependent on the nature, duration, and intensity of exercise (Dorn, 2007; Pluim et al., 2000; Wang et al., 2010). Aerobically trained athletes show increased left ventricular mass and chamber size which is defined as eccentric cardiac hypertrophy. The increased cross-sectional area contributes to increased ventricular stroke volume and cardiac output. This physiological adaptation helps the myocardium to support the increased demands of exercise while maintaining or enhancing normal function and is not related to collagen accumulation in the extracellular matrix (Dorn, 2007; Pluim et al., 2000; Wang et al., 2010).

A large number of researches have been focused on the molecular mechanisms responsible for transducing hemodynamic load into cardiac growth induced by aerobic exercise training (Dorn, 2007). Several studies have indicated that the cardiac RAS is activated by hemodynamic overload and that the AT1 receptor might play a crucial role in the development of cardiac hypertrophy induced by load (Dorn, 2007; Paul, Poyan Mehr, & Kreutz, 2006).

In the heart, Ang II has been shown to play a role in the development of cardiac fibrosis via induction of fibroblast proliferation and collagen deposition (Dorn, 2007; Paul et al., 2006; Sadoshima & Izumo, 1993; Sadoshima, Xu, Slayter, & Izumo, 1993). In addition, Ang II, as a growth factor, may contribute to the development of both smooth muscle and cardiac cell hypertrophies (Dorn, 2007; Paul et al., 2006; Sadoshima & Izumo, 1993; Sadoshima et al., 1993). In fact, studies showed that the mechanical stretch *in vitro* may causes acute release of Ang II from cardiomyocytes (Sadoshima et al., 1993). In addition, it also showed that Ang II acts as an initial mediator of stretch-induced hypertrophic response. The prevention of stretch-induced hypertrophy response by AT1 receptor blockade suggests that Ang II plays a critical role in cardiac growth (Dostal, 2000; Paul et al., 2006) .The role and mechanisms of Ang II via the AT1 receptor in cardiac hypertrophy have been associated with increased expression of many immediate-early genes (c-fos, c-jun, junB, Egr-1 and c-myc) and fetal marker genes of cardiac hypertrophy (ANF, skeletal α-actin, β-MHC) conferring a pathological phenotype (Sadoshima et al., 1993).

It is well-known that cardiomyocyte contractility depends on the expression of α and β-MHC, since MHC is the major contractile protein of the heart and is crucial to the efficiency of cardiac performance. The α/β-MHC ratio varies in response to physiological and pathological signaling. Studies have shown a shift from α- toward β-MHC composition of the adult heart under pathological conditions accompanied by higher expression of fetal gene reprogramming (ANF and skeletal α-actin), which correlates with impaired cardiac performance (Izumo, Nadal-Ginard, & Mahdavi, 1988). In contrast, physiological cardiac hypertrophy induced by aerobic training results in an increased biosynthesis of contractile components and in higher expression of α-MHC isoform and lower of β-MHC. Such changes are not concomitant with expression of fetal reprogramming genes. The α-MHC has been associated with increased myosin ATPase activity and enhancement of contractility, thus this data corroborates the improvement of ventricular function observed with aerobic training (Rafalski, Abdourahman, & Edwards, 2007; Soci et al., 2011).

In spite of many studies having attempted to clarify the issue, it is still unclear whether activation of the cardiac RAS in response to hemodynamic overload predominantly occurs in cardiomyocytes, fibroblasts or both. Studies with transgenic mice have provided the tools for exploring many biological questions. With the use of transgenic animal models for RAS components it has been shown that accentuated formation of local Ang II in the heart was not responsible for the development of the hypertrophy (van Kats, Methot, Paradis, Silversides, & Reudelhuber, 2001), suggesting that the cardiac Ang II levels are implicated in the induction of fibrosis, but not for left ventricle hypertrophy (Reudelhuber, Bernstein, & Delafontaine, 2007; van Kats et al., 2001). In addition, transgenic mice harboring one, two, three or four ACE gene copies showed that the magnitude of physiological cardiac hypertrophy induced by swimming training was not associated with different ACE levels (Evangelista & Krieger, 2006).

On the other hand, several studies have implied that animal models overexpressing the AT1 receptor demonstrated the induction of cardiac hypertrophy (Zhai et al., 2005). Zou et al. (Zou et al., 2004) showed in vitro and in vivo that the AT1 receptor is a mechanical sensor and that it converts mechanical stress into a biochemical signal inducing left ventricle hypertrophy without the involvement of Ang II.

Nevertheless, the role of RAS in non-pressure overload hypertrophy models, such as aerobic exercise training, has not been extensively investigated. The first study demonstrating the cardiac hypertrophic response of the adult rat heart to chronic exercise conditioning in the presence and absence of an AT1 receptor antagonist showed that AT1 receptor blockade did not prevent physiological cardiac hypertrophy induced by a chronic swimming training program (Geenen, Malhotra, & Buttrick, 1996). However, the authors treated the animals with an AT1 receptor inhibitor only twice a week, probably not enough to induce cardiac hypertrophy blockade. Another potential weakness in this study is that exercise-associated adaptations that reflect integrative cardiovascular physiology, such as an increase in peak oxygen consumption and a decrease in resting heart rate, or those that may occur in skeletal muscle, such as increases in muscle succinate dehydrogenase and citrate synthase activities, were not determined which allows doubtful interpretation of the efficiency of the exercise training protocol.

In contrast, Oliveira et al. (Oliveira, Sasaki, Cerencio, Barauna, & Krieger, 2009) showed that the treatment with an AT1 receptor blocker (Losartan) prevented left ventricle hypertrophy induced by two different aerobic training protocols (first protocol: swimming training consisted of 60 min duration, 5 days a week, for 10 weeks; second protocol: the same as first protocol until 8th week, in the 9th week rats trained 2x/day and in the 10th week 3x/day). The aim of increasing training frequency (second protocol) was to induce robust cardiac hypertrophy. In fact, the left ventricle hypertrophy observed by the authors was 13% and 27% for the first and the second swimming training protocol, respectively. Interestingly, cardiac hypertrophy was not decreased when the systemic RAS was inhibited by chronic salt treatment, which suggests that the left ventricle hypertrophy induced by swimming training depends on the local RAS activity instead of the systemic RAS (Oliveira et al., 2009). This was the first report of a detailed study conducted to investigate the participation of local versus systemic RAS in cardiac hypertrophy induced by aerobic exercise training, since all the markers of aerobic exercise training were confirmed in these protocols (Figure 2).

In the last decade, researches have pointed out a cardioprotective role played by the novel branch of the RAS. The recently discovered member of the RAS, ACE2, is an essential regulator of heart function (Crackower et al., 2002) and has been used as a negative indicator of cardiovascular disease due its pivotal role in Ang (1-7) formation, which it has several biological effects that are appositive to those elicited by Ang II (20, 82).

The first study to find the role of cardiac Ang (1-7) in normotensive (Wistar) and hypertensive (SHR) rats submitted to aerobic training showed increased left ventricular Ang (1-7) levels in swimming-trained SHR, but not in trained Wistar rats. In parallel, it was observed that exercise increased both Mas mRNA and protein levels in the heart was observed, suggesting that an overall activation of the Ang (1-7) – Mas axis may be involved in the beneficial effects of physical training in hearts. The authors suggested that the cardiac Ang (1-7) - Mas axis is particularly activated by exercise in pathological conditions such as hypertension. The reason for the absence of changes in left ventricular Ang (1-7) levels in normotensive rats remains to be clarified and may be related to the intensity and/or duration of the exercise. They indicated that the training protocol should be repeated using other normotensive strains, including Wistar–Kyoto rats, to establish whether the responses observed in the study are restricted to SHR or not (Filho et al., 2008). In addition, the mechanisms underlying the left ventricular Ang (1-7) levels, such as ACE2 levels and the cardiac ACE-Ang II-AT1 receptor axis induced by swimming training were not investigated in this study.

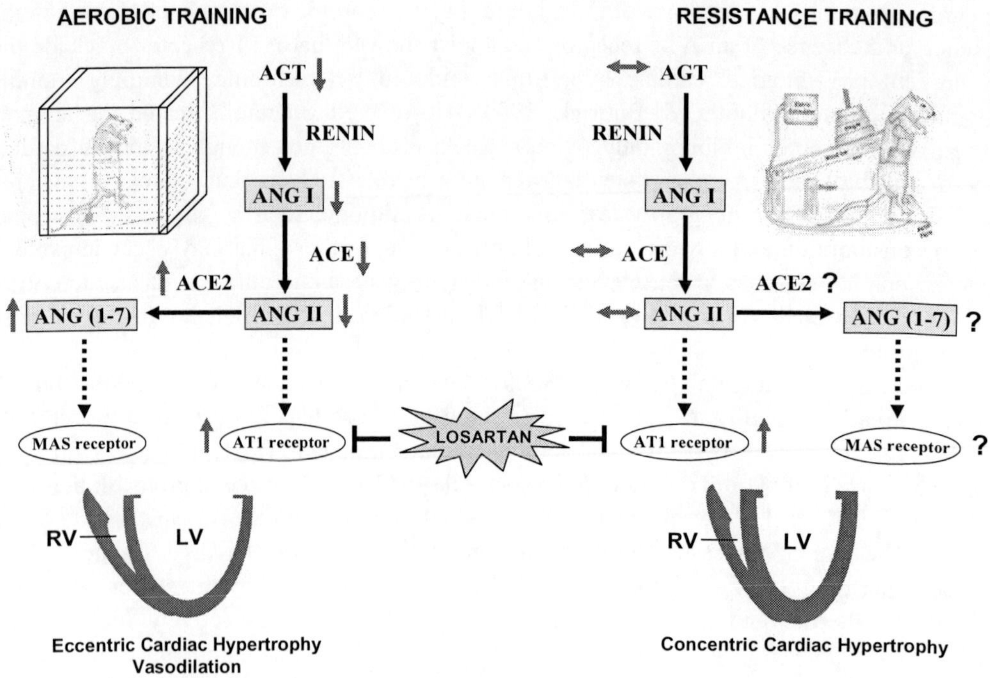

From Fernandes et al., Braz J Med Biol Res 2011 (In press).

Figure 2. Schematic presentation of the effects of exercise training on the cardiac renin-angiotensin system (RAS). Aerobic and resistance training induced eccentric and concentric cardiac hypertrophy, respectively, via the angiotensin II type 1 (AT1) receptor, and both types of physiological cardiac hypertrophy were prevented by AT1 receptor blockade (Losartan). We suggest that aerobic training shifts the generation of angiotensin peptides away from angiotensin II (Ang II) and towards Ang-(1-7), implicated in vasodilation and anti-fibrosis. In contrast, resistance training did not modify these cardiac RAS components. Arrows indicate points of up-regulation, down-regulation or maintenance of RAS components induced by exercise training. ACE = angiotensin-converting enzyme; ACE2 = angiotensin-converting enzyme 2; Ang-(1-7) = angiotensin-(1-7); AGT = angiotensinogen; RV = right ventricle; LV = left ventricle.

In a recent study, Fernandes et al. (T. Fernandes et al., 2011) showed that cardiac angiotensinogen expression, Ang I levels, ACE activity and protein expression, as well as Ang II levels were lower in swimming-trained Wistar rats, however, cardiac AT1 receptor levels increased after training. In addition, ACE2 and Ang (1-7) levels were also increased in the hearts of swimming-trained rats. Therefore, the authors suggested that the non classic cardiac RAS (ACE2 - Ang (1-7) axis) counteracts the classic cardiac RAS. The counterbalancing effect increases vasodilatation and cardiac hypertrophy in response to the demands of aerobic capacity for greater transport of blood and oxygen supply to the exercising cardiac muscle. Recently, Soci et al. (Soci et al., 2011) showed that the LVH is a strong and independent predictor of peak oxygen uptake or maximal work capacity, since the authors revealed there is a close positive correlation ($r=0.68$; $P<0.05$) between LVH and oxygen uptake. In addition, the authors, as expected, showed that swimming training increased exercise tolerance and muscle oxidative enzyme activity and this increase was proportional to the volume of training, modulated by a greater number of exercise sessions. These finding suggest that the physiological cardiac hypertrophy phenotype depends of increased aerobic performance.

Interestingly, Fernandes et al. (T. Fernandes et al., 2011) showed new mechanisms through microRNAs (miRNAs) regulation by which aerobic training can act on the cardiac RAS. MiRNAs are endogenous small, and noncoding RNAs, targeted to specific genes and function as negative regulators of gene expression by inhibiting translation or promoting degradation of target mRNAs. Recent studies have shown the roles played by miRNAs in different forms of cardiovascular disease (Small & Olson, 2011; van Rooij & Olson, 2007). MiRNAs- 29, 1, 133a and 133b has been shown to play significant roles in cardiac remodeling, hypertrophy and function. Caré et al. (Care et al., 2007) showed that both miRNA-1 and miRNA-133 were downregulated in three models of cardiac hypertrophy, such as, transverse aortic constriction, Akt transgenic mice and high intensity interval training. In agreement, Soci et al. (Soci et al., 2011) demonstrated that aerobic training caused a reduction of expression pattern to miRNAs- 1, 133a and 133b in the heart, indicating that these miRNAs are valid for both physiological and pathological cardiac hypertrophy. On the other hand, increased of cardiac miRNA-29 levels mediated a decrease of cardiac collagen expression involved in the improvement of ventricular compliance induced by aerobic training.

Regarding miRNAs and cardiac RAS, Fernandes et al. (36) showed that exercise training alters specific miRNAs that regulate cardiac RAS genes and tip the balance of classic RAS genes in favor of the novel RAS genes to contribute to physiological cardiac hypertrophy. The results showed that exercise increased miRNA-27a and 27b levels, responsible for decreased ACE protein expression in the heart, in comparison with the control group. In parallel, the authors also observed decreased microRNA-143 targeting ACE2 while there was increased ACE2 protein expression in the heart compared with the control group (T. Fernandes et al., 2011). Thus, the results suggest that a decrease in miRNA-143 could upregulate cardioprotective genes (ACE2), and an increase of miRNA-27 expression inhibits damage genes (such ACE gene) in the heart induced by aerobic training corroborating with physiological cardiac hypertrophy and higher physical performance.

Cardiac RAS and Resistance Training: Role in Hypertrophy and Cell Signaling

Resistance or Strength training (RT) refers to training programs that involve weight, static and/or isometric exercises designed specifically to increase muscular strength, power and/or endurance (Howley, 2001). It is one of the most widely practiced forms of physical activity used to enhance athletic performance, augment musculo-skeletal health and alter body aesthetics. Chronic exposure to this type of activity produces marked increases in muscular strength, which are attributed to a range of neurological and morphological adaptations (Folland & Williams, 2007).

We could find only 2 papers published using animal models in the last 5 years that systematically studied the role of the RAS on the cardiovascular adaptation induced by this exercise type.

Resistance Training is another way of inducing physiological cardiac hypertrophy (Baggish et al., 2008; Barbier, Ville, Kervio, Walther, & Carre, 2006). However, differently from the aerobic training such as swimming or running, RT is a known hypertrophic stimulus for cardiac enlargement due to pressure overload imposed on the heart during training when blood pressure may reach peaks of 480/350 mmHg (Lentini, McKelvie, McCartney, Tomlinson, & MacDougall, 1993; MacDougall, Tuxen, Sale, Moroz, & Sutton, 1985). The studies on the effects of RT at molecular level are not as deeply explored as aerobic training are because the lack of animal model available.

There are some models described in the literature, but none of them have focused on the cardiovascular system adaptations. (Klitgaard, 1988; Krisan et al., 2004; Notomi, Lee et al., 2000; Notomi, Okazaki et al., 2000; Tamaki et al., 1997; Wong & Booth, 1988; Yaspelkis, Singh, Trevino, Krisan, & Collins, 2002). The great majority of the studies focused on skeletal muscle adaptations such as the cellular and molecular mechanisms of skeletal muscle hypertrophy (Lowe & Alway, 2002). One of the major advantages of using animal models is the ability to precisely control environmental and food intake conditions for all animals. Furthermore, the animals can be killed and tissue samples harvested and used for physiological, histological, biochemical and molecular analyses.

In 2005 and 2007, Barauna et al. (Barauna et al., 2005; Barauna, Rosa, Irigoyen, & de Oliveira, 2007), using a well-documented squat-training apparatus for rats first described the cardiovascular adaptations in an animal model of RT. Among the results observed this exercise training model induced concentric cardiac hypertrophy without ventricular dysfunction or left ventricular cavity reduction. Also, using the same animal model, de Pinter et al. (de Cassia Cypriano Ervati Pinter, Padilha, de Oliveira, Vassallo, & de Fucio Lizardo, 2008) found that RT induced improvement in contractility of cardiac muscle and of cardiac myosin ATPase activity.

Later, in 2008, Barauna et al. (Barauna, Magalhaes, Krieger, & Oliveira, 2008) used the same apparatus model to study the role of the RAS in exercise training-induced cardiac hypertrophy. In this study the authors first showed that RT does not activate the systemic or any local RAS. However, RT training increased the expression of cardiac AT1a receptor which suggested that, although the enzymatic components were not altered, cardiac hypertrophy could nevertheless be induced by RAS.

Increase in AT1 expression in overloaded cardiomyocytes was first described in 1995 by Zhang et al. (X. Zhang et al., 1995), however the study by Barauna et al. (2008) was the first to show this upregulation *in vivo* in response to a exercise-induced cardiac hypertrophy.

Based on experimental data that the receptor could also be activated by mechanical stimuli, such as stretching of cardiomyocytes independent of the ligand Ang II (Zou et al., 2004), animals were trained concomitantly with ARB, Losartan, treatment. AT1 receptor blockade prevented the RT-induced cardiac hypertrophy, demonstrating the essential role of this receptor in the adaptation of the heart. Moreover, to show that the cardiac hypertrophy was independent of the systemic RAS, another group of animals were treated with 1% salt-overload, a well known maneuver to inhibit renin enzyme activity (Oliveira & Krieger, 2005;

Oliveira et al., 2009). The treatment did not alter the cardiac hypertrophy induced by the RT, confirming the role of local cardiac AT1 receptor instead of systemic and circulating components of the RAS.

In summary, this study showed that AT1 receptor stimulation is necessary for the development of cardiac hypertrophy in response to RT even in the absence of increased Ang II levels (Figure 2).

Among the signaling events mediating an adaptive hypertrophic mechanism, of emerging importance is the pathway that causes activation of the PI3K (phosphatidylinositol 3-kinase)/Akt cascade (Matsui, Nagoshi, & Rosenzweig, 2003). This pathway is regulated through several classes of transmembrane receptors, including receptor protein tyrosine kinases, such as the IGF-I receptor, and G protein-coupled receptors, such as α- and β-adrenergic receptors (Cantley, 2002). It has been demonstrated that the overexpression of constitutively active PI3K or Akt in the hearts of transgenic mice induces an increase in cardiomyocyte size and concentric hypertrophy in the absence of fibrosis, with preserved systolic function (Matsui et al., 2002). In particular, Akt promotes cell survival by inhibiting apoptosis at multiple points through transcription-independent and -dependent mechanisms. According to this 'adaptive' role of the PI3K pathway in hypertrophic growth, McMullen et al. (McMullen et al., 2003) recently discovered the role of p110a isoform of PI3K in the transduction of a biochemical pathway in 'physiological' exercise-induced hypertrophy by using transgenic mice expressing a dominant negative PI3K(p110a) (McMullen et al., 2003). These mice developed hypertrophy as a consequence of pressure overload but not in exercise training, suggesting the specific role of this molecule in the 'physiological' hypertrophy. This is very interesting because, as mentioned above, all authors agree on the compensatory role of cardiac hypertrophy in athletes, which allows their hearts to develop enhanced force.

To demonstrate the role of the AT1 receptor activation by RT in this intracellular signaling pathway by RT, the same research group studied the activation of signaling cascades after an acute bout of RT (Melo et al., 2010). The authors focused on the activation state of myocardial Akt-mTOR signaling and downstream substrates as it has been proposed that this is the divergent pathway between pathological and physiological cardiac hypertrophies (Kemi et al., 2008). After 5' and 30' of one set of squat exercise an increase of 60% and 62% in the p-AKT^{473} was observed, but increase of 74% in p-mTOR was only observed in the latter time point group. Both activations were blocked in Losartan-treated animals, confirming that the cardiac AT1 receptor is activated by a single RT session.

Altogether, these two studies clearly demonstrated the role of the RAS in the RT-induced cardiac hypertrophy. This is a very interestingly observation since it is attributed to the same hormonal system involved in the pathological and physiological cardiac hypertrophy but through different cardiac structural and functional changes.

Deleterious Effects of Anabolic Steroids on Cardiac RAS: Role of Exercise Training

Anabolic steroids (AS) are synthetic derivatives of testosterone initially used for therapeutic ends. However, in view of their effect on increasing protein synthesis, improving energy reserves and reducing the recovery time after exercise training, AS have been used by athletes to improve their physical performance (Medei et al., 2010; Urhausen, Albers, & Kindermann, 2004), currently appearing as the most used ergogenic substance in doping situations (Krieg, Scharhag, Albers, Kindermann, & Urhausen, 2007; Medei et al., 2010; Urhausen et al., 2004). The most commonly AS used is Nandrolone Decanoate, which has higher anabolic effects and less androgenic activity than testosterone (Krieg et al., 2007; Medei et al., 2010; Urhausen et al., 2004).

On the other hand, several researches have questioned the anabolic effects of testosterone, since its derivatives do not increase muscle size or strength in normal men and have discounted positive results as unduly influenced by the positive expectations of athletes. These conflicting data may be related to the difficulty of finding athletes who admit the exact pattern of AS administration. Moreover, not only the type and regimen of AS administration, but the additional influence of dietary intake and patterns and/or training intensity may have different effects on individual subjects (Krieg et al., 2007; Medei et al., 2010; Nascimento & Medei, 2011; Urhausen et al., 2004). Since it is difficult to dissociate the metabolic supplements or the abusive use of drugs in athletes, experimental models can be used, and one of the major advantages is the capability of precisely control environmental and food intake conditions for all animals.

Although the increase in muscle mass and power induced by AS is still questionable, it has been well established that AS abuse is associated with detrimental side-effects (do Carmo et al.; Krieg et al., 2007; Medei et al., 2010; Nascimento & Medei, 2011; Nottin, Nguyen, Terbah, & Obert, 2006; Rocha et al., 2007; Urhausen et al., 2004). Studies have shown that AS induce adverse effects on the cardiovascular system, including electrical and structural changes in the myocardium, and cardiac hypertrophy associated with impaired ventricular compliance and increased susceptibility to ischemic injuries. All of these factors contribute to an increased risk of ventricular arrhythmias and sudden cardiac death (do Carmo et al.; Krieg et al., 2007; Medei et al., 2010; Nascimento & Medei, 2011; Nottin et al., 2006; Rocha et al., 2007; Urhausen et al., 2004). Interestingly, exercise training associated with AS causes loss of the beneficial effects on cardiac function induced by exercise characterized by maladaptive remodeling and deterioration in cardiac performance (do Carmo et al.; Nottin et al., 2006; Rocha et al., 2007).

Previous findings indicate that the combination of exercise training and AS, causes disproportional extracellular collagen accumulation and interstitial fibrosis accompanied by diastolic dysfunction, suggesting pathological cardiac hypertrophy (do Carmo et al.; Rocha et al., 2007). In fact, signals of diastolic dysfunction by echocardiography such as decreased peak velocity during early diastolic filling have been observed in weight lifters who used AS when compared to non-users (Nascimento & Medei, 2011; Pearson, Schiff, Mrosek, Labovitz, & Williams, 1986). Recently, Alves et al. (Alves et al., 2010) showed that AS increases muscle sympathetic nerve activity and reduces muscle blood flow in young individuals, suggesting that AS increases the susceptibility for cardiovascular disease in humans. In addition, several years after chronic misuse of AS, power athletes showed both impaired systolic and diastolic myocardial function, strongly associated with mean dosage and duration of AS use (D'Andrea et al., 2007). On the other hand, reports have shown no differences in left ventricular morphofunction between AS users and non-users (Parssinen, Kujala, Vartiainen, Sarna, & Seppala, 2000).

The diastolic dysfunction has been strongly associated with increased interstitial collagen. Fibrillar collagens, types I and III, are the major structural proteins of the myocardial collagen matrix (Krieg et al., 2007) and are responsible for distributing the forces working on the heart, exerting an important influence on ventricular compliance (Soci et al., 2011). Rocha et al. (Rocha et al., 2007) showed that exposure to supraphysiological AS doses may lead to tissue necrosis and diastolic dysfunction, resulting in structural changes similar to those observed in the early stages of heart failure. These data led to the suggestion that the diastolic dysfunction observed in exercise training associated with AS is correlated with a higher amount of collagen, as determined by the hydroxyproline method and histological quantification of collagen volumetric fraction (Figure 3). The authors also observed that the AS group had an increase in cardiac collagen type I and type III gene expression compared with the trained group (Rocha et al., 2007). Thus, the left ventricular dysfunction observed is related to the structural remodeling of the myocardium, and particularly to the development of myocardial fibrosis. It is important to mention that other myocardial structural alterations, such as destroyed mitochondria, aberrant myofibrils, and necrotic cells in the myocardium may also account for the dysfunction (Melchert, Herron, & Welder, 1992).

The mechanisms by which AS can act on the cardiovascular system are diverse and can vary from mechanical stimuli to circulating humoral factors released by the heart and peripheral organs, however the molecular mechanisms are still poorly understood (Riezzo et al., 2011). Rocha et al.(Rocha et al., 2007) suggested, for the first time, that the change from physiological to pathological cardiac hypertrophy in rats treated with AS associated with physical training is directly correlated to the higher activation of cardiac RAS. In fact, it is well known that the RAS is of primary regulatory importance for cardiac extracellular matrix remodeling, since higher cardiac Ang II levels contribute to hyperplasia of cardiac fibroblasts and to development of cardiac fibrosis (Brilla, 2000). Studies performed in animal models have suggested that blockade of AT1 receptor with specific AT1 receptor antagonist, Losartan, was effective in reducing cardiac remodeling, and this was associated with the reduction in interstitial fibrosis (Brilla, 2000; do Carmo et al.; Kawano et al., 2005; Rocha et al., 2007) (Figure 4).

An important result observed by the authors was the higher local ACE activity found in the hearts from the AS and exercise training + AS groups compared with control and trained groups and the close, positive correlation between left ventricle-ACE activity and collagen type III (r^2=0.88; $P< 0.05$). Moreover, the AT1a receptor gene expression was increased by 60% in the hearts from the AS and exercise training + AS groups compared with control group, and the Ang II level was increased in the hearts from the AS (60%) and exercise training + AS (40%) compared with control group. This is an evidence of the local RAS participation in the development of cardiac remodeling in this model. These findings were reinforced by the fact that AT1-receptor antagonist prevented these effects induce by AS(Rocha et al., 2007).

Considering that ACE also inactivates bradykinin, the higher AS-induced ACE activity increased the degradation of bradykinin, which can reduce nitric oxide production, independent of Ang II action, impairing the vasodilatation induced by exercise training (Rocha et al., 2007). Recently, it was demonstrated that exercise training induces enhancement of nitric oxide production; however, AS treatment blocked this effect promoted by exercise training, probably because this treatment damages endothelial function in trained animals (Cunha, Moura, Bernardes, Tanno, & Marcondes, 2005).

On the other hand, the effect of blockade of AT1 receptor on cardiac fibrosis can be related to the reduction in aldosterone (Kawano et al., 2005), since Ang II, by means of AT1 receptor, is one of main factors responsible for the regulation of aldosterone secretion, which plays important role in collagen synthesis (do Carmo et al.; Kawano et al., 2005).

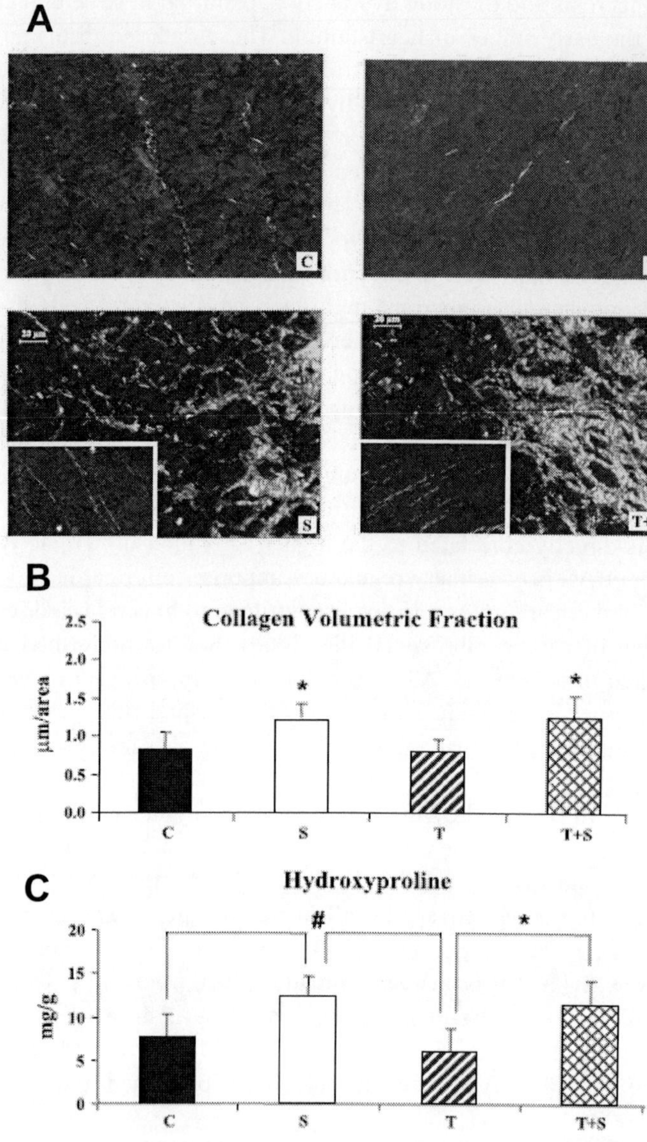

From Rocha et al. Am J Physiol Heart Circ Physiol 293: H3575-3583, 2007.

Figure 3. Effects of anabolic steroids (S), swimming training (T), and swimming training associated with anabolic steroids (T+S) compared with control (C) on collagen fibers in the myocardium. A: representative histological sections of the myocardium under polarized light. Representative section of collagen fibers in the LV of C and T groups (top) and S and T+S groups (bottom insets) are shown. Bottom: regions with patched cardiac (reparative fibrosis) in the LV of the S and T+S groups. **B:** quantitative analysis of collagen fibers in myocardium. * Significant difference vs. C and T groups, $P < 0.05$. **C:** hydroxyproline concentration in the LV of C, S, T, and T+S groups. Significant difference vs. $^{\#}$C and T groups, and * T group: $P < 0.05$.

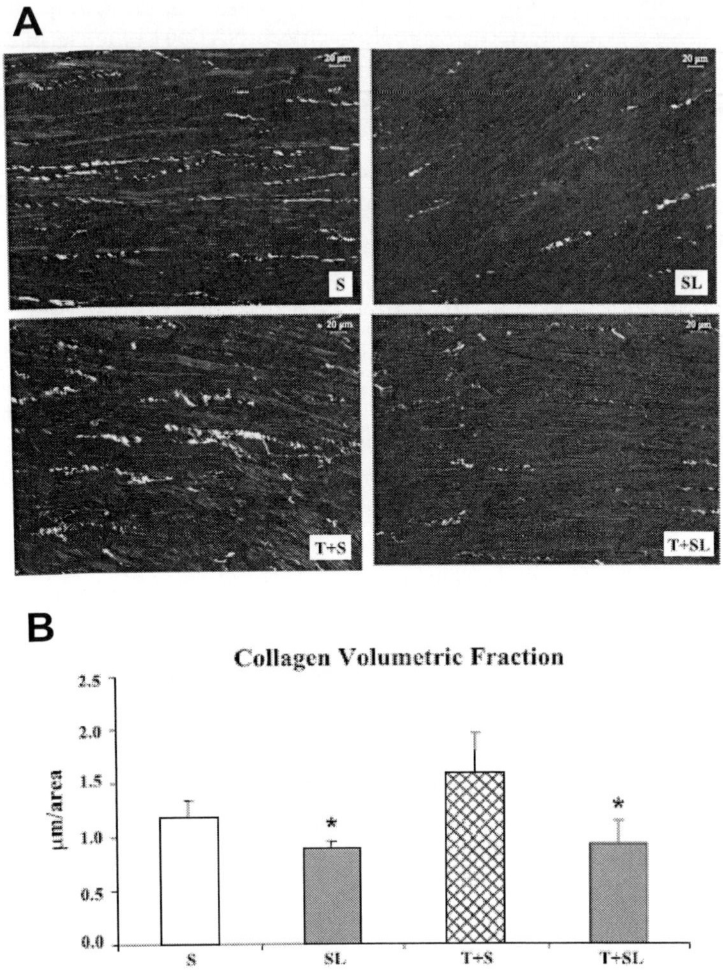

From Rocha et al. Am J Physiol Heart Circ Physiol 293: H3575-3583, 2007.

Figure 4. Effects of Losartan treatment on collagen fibers in the myocardium induced by chronic anabolic steroid use. A: representative histological sections of the myocardium under polarized light. Representative section of collagen fibers in the LV of anabolic steroids (S) and S treated with Losartan [angiotensin type 1 (AT1)-receptor blocker; 20 $mgkg^{-1}$ day^{-1} as drinking water] (SL) groups (top panels), and swimming training associated with anabolic steroid (T+S) and T+S treated with Losartan (T+SL) groups (bottom panels) are shown. **B:** quantitative analysis of collagen fibers in myocardium of S, SL, T+S, and T+SL groups. Results are presented as means SD. *Significant difference vs. S and T+S groups, $P < 0.05$.

In addition to its synthesis in the adrenal glands, aldosterone has also been shown to be synthesized in the heart, the aldosterone synthase gene (CYP11B2) being the key enzyme in this process. Aldosterone acts by binding to the mineralocorticoid receptors inducing inflammatory responses, collagen synthesis and cardiac remodeling (do Carmo et al.; Qin et al., 2003).

Aldosterone can exert its action in non-genomic ways, in which interaction with the mineralocorticoid receptor induces phosphorylation of signaling molecules such as PKC, c-

Src and MAP kinase which directly contributes to cardiac remodeling and inflammatory processes. By these ways, aldosterone can also activate NADPH oxidase in different tissues, including the heart, inducing an increase in oxidative stress and fibrosis (Johar, Cave, Narayanapanicker, Grieve, & Shah, 2006; Riezzo et al., 2011). In addition, studies have demonstrated that chronic treatment with AS causes an impairment of exercise induction of antioxidant enzyme activities, leading to reduced cardioprotection upon ischemic events, since the activities of superoxide dismutase, glutathione peroxidase and glutathione reductase were significantly higher in trained animals compared with control, AS and exercise training + AS groups (Chaves et al., 2006).

In accordance, do Carmo et al. (do Carmo et al., 2011) investigated the hypothesis that cardiac aldosterone could also be associated with deleterious effects induced by treatment with AS and its association to exercise training. Interestingly, expression of mineralocorticoid receptors was not modified by AS treatment; however CYP11B2 levels were increased by AS treatment, indicating that the use of AS may lead to an increase in cardiac aldosterone synthesis. In addition, a positive correlation has been shown between the expression of CYP11B2 and the expression of collagen type III in animals treated with AS, confirming that increased expression of the CYP11B2 gene is also related to increase in cardiac collagen synthesis induced by Nandrolone Decanoate.

In addition, higher expression of inflammatory factors, such as transforming growth factor beta (TGFβ) and osteopontin was detected, and positive correlation with increased CYP11B2 expression observed with AS treatment, demonstrating that higher cardiac aldosterone levels in cardiac collagen induced by AS could be related to high TGFβ and osteopontin expression (do Carmo et al., 2011).

Aldosterone actions on myocardial fibrosis and cardiac remodeling mediated by osteopontin have also been shown in studies with Ang II and aldosterone blockers that were effective inhibiting osteopontin expression in the myocardium infarcted area, reducing collagen and preventing the cardiac remodeling (Y. L. Zhang, Zhou, Lei, Yuan, & Wang, 2008). TGFβ has also been shown to be released by aldosterone, leading to an increase in the expression of growth factors and connective tissue (Satoh et al., 2002).

Interestingly, do Carmo et al. (do Carmo et al., 2011) showed that Spironolactone treatment, an aldosterone inhibitor, were also effective in preventing collagen expression. Spironolactone prevented increase in collagen volumetric fraction and in cardiac collagen type I and type III gene expression in the AS and exercise training + AS groups compared with their respective controls, confirming the involvement of mineracorticoid receptors and aldosterone in the increased cardiac collagen induced by AS.

Losartan and Spironolactone treatment prevented increase in left ventricle-ACE activity, CYP11B2 cardiac expression and inflammatory factors TGFβ and osteopontin in the AS and exercise training + AS groups. Thus, the lower expression of these genes observed with these therapies can also be responsible for the lower degree of cardiac fibrosis found, confirming the participation of Ang II and aldosterone participation in cardiac fibroses induced by the AS treatment (do Carmo et al., 2011). In fact, a mechanism of cross-talk between the mineralocorticoid and the AT1 receptors have been proposed in which, when Ang II and aldosterone act simultaneously on their respective receptors, there were different effects from those observed when only one of them is acting. It was demonstrated that in order to be activated, signaling pathways such as ERK1/2, JNK and NF-kB need aldosterone and AT1 receptor, suggesting that the effects of aldosterone on cardiac fibroses depend in part on activation of AT1 receptor mediated pathway. In parallel, it has been shown that Ang II induced ventricular damage is mediated by a mechanism dependent on signaling via mineracorticoid receptor-aldosterone (Lemarie, Paradis, & Schiffrin, 2008).

Taken together, these results showed that the Ang II and aldosterone can synergistically promote deleterious cardiac effects via the interaction of the AT1 and mineralocorticoid receptors by use of AS and its association with swimming training.

Exercise Training as Cardiovascular Therapy: Role of RAS Inhibition

Cardiovascular diseases such as heart failure, coronary artery disease, cerebrovascular disease and others continue to be one of the leading causes of morbidity and mortality (Pipilis et al., 2007; Stefanadis, 2008). They account for over 17 million deaths worldwide each year, representing nearly one-third of the total annual deaths (WHO, 2009). Although genetic factors and age are important in determining cardiovascular risk, other factors, including hypertension, hypercholesterolemia, insulin resistance, diabetes, and lifestyle factors such as smoking, diet and physical activity level are also major risk factors associated with the disease.

The RAS plays a key role in the regulation of cardiovascular function, with Ang II being involved in hemodynamic and non-hemodynamic mechanisms in the pathophysiology of cardiovascular disease. A number of studies have demonstrated that pharmacological modulation of the RAS, either with ACE inhibitor or an Ang II receptor blocker (ARB), provides cardiovascular protection decreasing cardiovascular morbidity and mortality in high risk patients. ACE inhibitors and ARBs are the preferred drugs of choice in the management of many cardiovascular diseases since it was first described and even nowadays, researchers are still looking for ways to improve this therapy especially testing the effects of combined RAS blockade with ACE inhibitors and ARBs and developing new blockers for the system such as the renin inhibitors.

It is well established that physical activity reduces the risk of cardiovascular disease. Data collected over the past 40 years have shown that exercise training is safe, and can induce many health-related adaptations both in humans and rodents (Franco, Cooper, Bilal, & Fuster, 2011). The effectiveness of cardiac rehabilitation programs has been well documented by some research groups (Nelson et al., 2007; Rodriguez, Di Marco, & Langley, 2009) and the most recent position statement on exercise prescription was published last year by the American College of Sports Medicine (ACSM, 2010).

Since both the inhibition of the RAS and practice of exercise training have effects on cardiovascular prevention or therapy, in this section, we have sought to review whether the effects of the exercise training are related to inhibition of the RAS.

Heart Failure

Heart failure (HF) in a progressive disorder characterized by reduced cardiac output associated with neurohumoral changes, including activation of the RAS and the sympathetic nervous system (Barki-Harrington, Luttrell, & Rockman, 2003; Brum, Rolim, Bacurau, & Medeiros, 2006). It is well known also, that increased sympathetic activity also leads to activation of the RAS (Dostal & Baker, 1999; Sauzeau et al., 2006). Prolonged RAS and sympathetic nervous system hyperactivation in HF exerts a direct deleterious effect on the heart independently of their hemodynamic actions (Grassi et al., 1997; Mann, Florek, & Reiter, 1992). Neurohumoral imbalance leads to altered cardiac function and hypertrophy, which culminates in cardiac remodeling and development of HF.

Therapeutic strategies that modulate neurohormonal activation in HF are valuable and its benefits need to be better understood. Using genetically modified mice lacking both α2A/α2C adrenergic receptors (ARKO), Ferreira et al. (Ferreira et al., 2008) demonstrated that chronic sympathetic hyperactivity is associated with local RAS activation and that the deleterious cardiac effects can be counteracted by ARB treatment underscoring the role of local RAS activation in this process.

Aerobic exercise training reduces sympathetic nerve activity in both experimental and human HF (Medeiros et al., 2008; Roveda et al., 2003) and is recognized as an important and safe strategy for prevention and treatment of HF, since it improves patient outcome and quality of life (Jonsdottir, Andersen, Sigurosson, & Sigurosson, 2006; Medeiros et al., 2008; Roveda et al., 2003; Wisloff et al., 2007). To test the role of exercise training on the RAS during heart failure progression, Pereira et al. (Pereira et al., 2009) also used the α2A/α2C ARKO mouse model at 3 to 5 months of age, prior to the development of heart failure in a attempt to delay the onset of cardiac dysfunction.

After 8 weeks of exercise training on a treadmill running at 60% of maximal speed, molecular and structural cardiovascular benefits were observed. Wild-type mice improved their exercise capacity and systolic function, while the α2A/α2C ARKO mice overcame exercise intolerance and the decreased fractional shortening observed in the sedentary group, and reached the same levels as those of the wild-type group. As regards RAS modulation, exercise training in α2A/α2C ARKO mice reduced cardiac Ang II expression and cardiac ACE activity to age-matched wild-type animals, and increased cardiac ACE2 expression. These responses were observed only in the exercise-trained α2A/α2C ARKO mice but not in WT, which suggest that training effects are restricted to RAS components with altered baseline levels or activity in mice.

Due to the positive feedback between the RAS and the SNS in producing Ang II (Leenen, White, & Yuan, 2001; Nagano et al., 1992), and the reduced plasma noradrenaline in α2A/α2C ARKO trained mice (Medeiros et al., 2008), the reduction in sympathetic hyperactivity may, at least in part, contribute to decreased cardiac Ang II levels. Furthermore, as cardiac ACE is decreased while ACE2 is elevated in exercise-trained α2A/α2C ARKO mice, one could speculate that there would be an increase in cardiac Ang (1-7) formation in exercise-trained α2A/α2C ARKO mice, which would be beneficial since it attenuates the development of HF (Grobe et al., 2007; Mendes, Ferreira, Pinheiro, & Santos, 2005). Notwithstanding all these molecular modulations, exercise training had little impact on ventricular remodeling, while an impressive effect was previously observed in the same mouse lineage treated with Losartan (Ferreira et al., 2008).

In 2010, Kar et al. (Kar, Gao, & Zucker, 2011), found similar results using a rabbit model of HF (chronic ventricular pacing model) but in the brain components of the RAS. The same group previously showed that the brain RAS is hyperactive in HF and contributes to an increase in SNA and vasoconstriction, which exacerbates HF (Gao et al., 2004; McKinley et al., 2003; Zucker, 2002). The purpose of the study was to investigate the balance between ACE and ACE2 during heart failure progression and the effects of exercise training on a treadmill. First, the authors show that ACE is upregulated in the brain of rabbits with HF while ACE2 is downregulated. However, similar to the results of Pereira et al. (Pereira et al., 2009) in cardiac tissue, exercise-trained rabbits had the expression of ACE and ACE2 normalized to their age-matched sedentary animals, but exercise training did not significantly change the brain RAS components of the sham animals. Once again, these data suggest that exercise training may activate the Ang (1-7) axis while it inhibits the Ang II axis only when there is a change in the normal condition of the system, such as in the HF.

In 2008, Mousa et al. (Mousa, Liu, Cornish, & Zucker, 2008) showed that exercise training decreases plasma Ang II and central AT1 receptor expression to control levels in the same rabbit model of HF used by Kar et al. (Kar et al., 2011). In another group of animals, elevated plasma Ang II levels were maintained through minipumps and the beneficial effects of exercise training such as lowered sympathetic nerve activity and normalized baroreflex control were no longer observed, consistent with the idea of the importance of RAS modulation by exercise training in pathological states.

In addition to decrease Ang II and increase Ang (1-7) formation, lower ACE activity also modulates the Kallikrein-kinin system (KSS) by decreasing bradykinin degradation. The cardiac KSS exerts anti-proliferative effects on cardiomyocytes and preserves the metabolic state of the heart, while a dysfunctional KKS is associated with dilated cardiomyopathy and heart failure. The involvement of KSS in cardiac adaptations induced by exercise training are not completely established although a decreased in B2 receptor gene expression in humans was related with exaggerated left ventricular hypertrophy in response to exercise training (Brull et al., 2001; Zuraw, 2001).

The role of KSS in exercise-induced cardiac hypertrophy was studied in B2 KO mice submitted to swimming training (Batista et al., 2008). B2 receptor deficiency by itself induces cardiac hypertrophy and HF, and exercise training increased pathological cardiac hypertrophy in B2 KO mice. Although no functional analyses were performed, increased interstitial fibrosis was observed, which is a marked sign of pathological hypertrophy. These data again confirm that exercise training has its beneficial effects on cardiac diseases by inhibition of the RAS (decreased Ang II and increased bradykinin formation) and consequently activating the KSS, because B2 KO mice loose the therapeutic effects of exercise training.

On the basis of the present data, it may also be possible to design an exercise regimen to normalize ACE and ACE2 levels in HF without pharmacological interventions.

Myocardial Infarction

After Myocardial Infarction (MI), the injured heart undergoes compensatory remodeling to repair depressed cardiac function. Circulating RAS is activated to maintain blood volume, blood pressure and organ perfusion but it is also involved in the post-MI remodeling of the heart (Pearson et al., 1986; Sun & Weber, 2003). There are clinical evidences that exercise training may improve cardiac function and remodeling after MI. However, there is no evidence of these beneficial effects of exercise training and the modulation of the RAS after MI.

Wan et al., in 2007 (Wan et al., 2007), sought to determine whether the onset of exercise training (1 week vs. 6 weeks after MI) would affect RAS, myocardial remodeling and cardiac function. Experimental MI was created in rats by left anterior descending coronary artery ligation, and the animals were trained for 8 weeks on a treadmill.

The main finding of the study was that post-MI exercise lowered circulating RAS, which was suggested by decreased plasma renin and serum ACE activities, and reduced aldosterone levels in animals that started the exercise training either 1 week or 6 weeks after MI. However, circulating Ang II levels were only normalized in the non-infarcted group in the animals that started exercise training earlier. In spite of the difference in circulating angiotensin II levels, exercise starting early or late after MI affects myocardial remodeling and function similarly.

Hypertension

Left ventricular hypertrophy (LVH) and diastolic dysfunction are the early manifestations of cardiac damage in patients with arterial hypertension characterizing hypertensive heart disease (Diamond & Phillips, 2005). It has been reported that increased BP and blood pressure variability (BPV) are both important determinants of heart damage (Parati et al., 1994; Su & Miao, 2005). The importance of the RAS for the pathogenesis of hypertension is underscored by pharmacological interventions. ACE inhibitors and ARBs have been used to attenuate or prevent the development of hypertension and its consequences on target organs (Oddie, Dilley, & Bobik, 1992; Wu & Berecek, 1993).

In 2010, Zamo et al. (Zamo et al., 2010) using the SHR model, described local and systemic RAS activation during the time course of hypertension development by comparing young and adult animals. Young animals (3 months old) still show progressive increase in blood pressure, while adult animals (5 months old) have the established hypertension. The authors showed that some components are activated in young SHR, at the onset of hypertension, and these activations, such as the serum ACE activity and the Ang II levels, are unchanged in adult rats. On the other hand plasma renin activity is increased in adult rats due to the well-described neurogenic hypertension in SHR(Irigoyen & Krieger, 1998; Krieger, 1964).

After this description, the same group investigated the effects of exercise training on the modulation of the RAS in these two time points of the hypertension development (Zamo, Barauna, Chiavegatto, Irigoyen, & Oliveira, 2011). Young and adult SHR were submitted to swimming training protocol for 8 weeks. The main finding of the study was that although swimming training had induced hemodynamic adjustments in SHR, irrespective of the animal's age, cardiac hypertrophy and RAS modulation were distinctive. Young SHR had decreased blood pressure, downregulated local RAS components and did not develop LVH; while in adult SHR, the swimming training protocol also decreased blood pressure but did not downregulate cardiac RAS and did not prevent LVH. The decrease in circulating Ang II content may help the blood pressure lowering effect due to exercise training, but cardiac remodeling was only prevented when the local RAS was also inhibited. These distinctive roles of local and RAS proposed by these results are in agreement with previous results also found in exercise-training models or pathophysiological states.

Although this review is focused on the roles of RAS in the development of cardiac hypertrophy induced by exercise training, and high blood pressure is a predictor of cardiac hypertrophy, it is also appropriate to review the exercise modulation of blood pressure. The group headed by Michelini LC, has shown the association between increased angiotensinogen and AT1 receptor expression in central areas and elevated blood pressure and the permissive role of angiotensin II to orchestrate, via AT1 receptors, detrimental cardiovascular responses during the development of hypertension (Bezerra, dos Santos, Moreira, Krieger, & Michelini, 2001; Michelini, de Oliveira, & dos Santos, 1992; Sangaleti, Crescenzi, & Michelini, 2004; C. M. Santos, Pontieri, Leomil Neto, & Michelini, 1995). It was also shown that Ang II acts centrally to depress reflex control of circulation and to increase volemia and sympathetic outflow, thus contributing increasing blood pressure (Johnston, 1990; McKinley et al., 2003).

Since exercise training has been associated with a variety of adjustments in hypertension, Felix JVC and Michelini LC, in 2007 (Felix & Michelini, 2007), sought to investigate the effects of exercise training on RAS components in central areas involved in cardiovascular control. For this purpose, SHR and Wistar rats were trained on a treadmill over 3 months. Exercise training did not change AT1a mRNA receptor expression in the nucleus tratu solitarius in hypertensive or normotensive rats but it completely normalizes the increased angiotensinogen expression within this area in the SHR group. The reduced angiotensinogen mRNA density after training was correlated with decreased arterial pressure. It should be noted that the blunting effect of training on brain RAS overactivity is specific for areas involved in cardiovascular control such as the NTS and area postrema (but not in the gracilis nucleus). One could expect that Angiotensinogen reduction might not be enough to blunt the brain RAS overactivity but angiotensiongen has already been shown to be the main limiting factor for brain angiotensin II production, central regulation of blood pressure, and for the pathogenesis of hypertension (Schinke et al., 1999).

Skeletal Muscle RAS and Exercise Training: Implications for Physical Performance

Skeletal muscle represents 40-50% of the total corporal weight and is mainly responsible for the generation of force for locomotion and breathing. Skeletal muscle is further divided into fibers of type I, IIa, IIx/d and IIb and their distribution is genetically determined and recognized by their high adaptive capacity in the face of physiological and environmental factors, with variations in type of fiber, size and metabolism. Exercise training is an important physiological stimulus capable of influencing genetic predisposition, promoting optimization of mechanisms for the metabolic pathways that will predominantly be requested. Thus, differentiated performance in a sport modality seems to be the product of a genetic predisposition associated with specific exercise training (Koulmann & Bigard, 2006; Stewart & Rittweger, 2006).

Skeletal muscle adaptation to aerobic training includes an increase in oxidative enzymes activity as well as the number and size of mitochondria, development of muscle capillary network, and transition in myosin heavy chain isoforms (MHC). Such training-induced changes contribute to improved aerobic capacity and reliance on oxidative metabolism to provide energy (Koulmann & Bigard, 2006). In contrast, resistance training has a greater effect on muscle glycolytic capacity involved in skeletal muscle hypertrophy with an increased number of sarcomeres in series (Brentano & Martins Kruel, 2011). Advanced researches in molecular biology have supported the hypothesis that genetic components may be involved in physical performance and skeletal muscle function. More recently the ACE insertion/deletion (I/D) polymorphism has become the most intensely studied gene polymorphism known to affect skeletal muscle adaptation to exercise training (Jones & Woods, 2003; Stewart & Rittweger, 2006). The absence (deletion, D allele) of a 287-bp fragment in intron 16 of the ACE gene is associated with increased ACE activity, known to influence blood pressure through both the generation of the vasoconstrictor factor Ang II deriving from Ang I, and inactivation of the vasodilatator bradykinin. Conversely, the presence (insertion, I allele) of this fragment is associated with lower ACE activity in serum (Jones & Woods, 2003; Stewart & Rittweger, 2006).

Moreover, local RAS exist in many tissues including skeletal muscle, and these systems might affect muscle metabolic efficiency. Skeletal muscle RAS has recently been investigated and the occurrence of an intrinsic, physiologically active ACE has been demonstrated (Jones & Woods, 2003). The first study that identified ACE activity in the skeletal muscle showed that ACE activity does not correlated with that of serum ACE, suggesting local RAS regulation (Reneland & Lithell, 1994). In addition, skeletal muscle membrane fractions from rats, dogs, cultured myoblasts and rabbit skeletal muscle membranes display ACE activity (Ward, Russell, & Vaghy, 1995). Moreover, RAS components are present throughout the skeletal muscle microcirculation, including endothelial cells, vascular smooth muscle cells, and other vessel-associated cells (Agoudemos & Greene, 2005).

Human studies have identified an increased frequency of the I allele in elite endurance athletes, long-distance runners, rowers, and mountaineers, as well as augmented occurrence of the D allele with strength gains in power performance athletes (Hruskovicova et al., 2006; Jones & Woods, 2003; Williams et al., 2005). An excess of the I allele is associated with decreased ACE activity and prevalence of type I fibers, revealing a relationship between this type of polymorphism and performance in endurance sports (Hruskovicova et al., 2006; Jones & Woods, 2003). On the other hand, the D allele is associated with increased ACE activity and a higher proportion of type II fibers, so this type of polymorphism may be related to power performance sports (Jones & Woods, 2003; Williams et al., 2005).

Fast (type II) and slow (type I) twitch muscle fibers exhibit different characteristics with respect to functional properties due to differences in the isoforms and level of expression of most muscle proteins. The prevalence of oxidative metabolism in red muscle, in which type I fibers predominate, and the larger number of capillaries as well as higher oxygen support, are important for maintenance of the aerobic capacity of this muscle. The lower ACE levels in red muscle compared with white muscle might contribute to decreased bradykinin degradation, thereby potentiating bradykinin concentration, a potent activator of the L-arginine-Nitric Oxide (NO) pathway. This may promote vasodilation and angiogenesis. Indeed, low ACE levels have previously been shown to cause NO accumulation, thus inducing vasodilation and angiogenesis by bradykinin receptors (Dietze & Henriksen, 2008; Jones & Woods, 2003; Momken et al., 2003; Onder, Vedova, & Pahor, 2006; Zoll et al., 2006).

Fernandes et al. (T. Fernandes, Hashimoto, & Oliveira, 2010) showed that lower ACE activity and protein levels are detected in the soleus (red) muscle compared with the plantaris (white) muscle, which could attenuate Ang II production as well as reduce bradykinin degradation favoring vasodilation, formation of new vessels, and oxygen and substrate delivery. Together, these effects should enhance the aerobic capacity necessary for oxidative muscle activity.

On the other hand, studies have indicated that ACE inhibition failed to affect the endurance capacity during running exercise and/or the maximal oxidative capacity of skeletal muscles in sedentary rats (Bahi et al., 2004). In a recent study, Habouzit et al. (Habouzit et al., 2009) investigated the effects of ACE inhibition on training-related changes in the capacity of muscle mitochondria to oxidize energetic substrates via oxidative phosphorylation and on the shift toward type I fibers, since the authors hypothesized that chronic ACE inhibition combined with endurance training could improve endurance performance more than training alone and that this association could positively affect skeletal muscle metabolic efficiency. However, the authors demonstrated that the enhancement in physical performance observed in perindopril-treated (ACE inhibitor) animals cannot be explained by changes in mitochondrial respiration and/or MHC distribution within muscles involved in running exercise.

It is well known that white muscle contains a larger proportion of type II fibers and is responsible for producing greater force per unit of cross-sectional area, thereby affecting muscle strength thorough elevated ACE-Ang II levels (Jones & Woods, 2003; Williams et al., 2005). Previous data regarding the role of Ang II in skeletal muscle mass control are controversial. Ang II has been shown to promote muscle atrophy (Sanders, Russell, & Tisdale, 2005); nevertheless, others studies have reported that Ang II induces skeletal muscle hypertrophy associated with strength gain (Gordon, Davis, Carlson, & Booth, 2001; McBride, 2006). Gordon et al. (Gordon et al., 2001) showed that in surgically-induced plantaris and/or soleus muscle overload, inhibiting endogenous Ang II production by ACE inhibition markedly attenuated muscle hypertrophy which was restored by local Ang II perfusion. In agreement, another study demonstrated that Losartan treatment prevented training-induced increases in muscle wet and dry weights compared with untreated rats. Both low and high doses of Losartan also prevented an increase in muscle contractile force following training when compared with the untreated group. Thus, functional AT1 receptors are necessary for muscle hypertrophy and increased contractile force associated with training (McBride, 2006).

The RAS is well known to be implicated in the development of peripheral abnormalities. Its key effector peptide Ang II, a strong vasoconstrictor augmenting vascular tone, reduces cardiac and muscle perfusions, and modulates angiogenesis. Long-term ACE inhibition enhances blood flow to skeletal muscle during exercise, probably in relation to vascular mechanisms and improved oxygen utilization (Dietze & Henriksen, 2008; Onder et al., 2006). Accordingly, ACE inhibitor has been shown to prevent vascular alterations, protect the mitochondrial function of skeletal muscle and to restore the abnormal MHC profile in skeletal muscle in the model of myocardial infarction (Momken et al., 2003; Onder et al., 2006; Zoll et al., 2006).

On the other hand, Ang II has also been demonstrated to play a critical role in angiogenesis or growth of new capillaries in skeletal muscle. Chronic infusion of Ang II at a dose that has no effect on blood pressure has been demonstrated to cause significant capillary growth (Petersen, Munzenmaier, & Greene, 2006). Moreover, reports have shown that the RAS can also modulate the angiogenic response to electrical stimulation in the skeletal muscle of rats, and the authors proposed a pathway involving Ang II and vascular endothelial growth factor (VEGF) expression (Amaral, Linderman, Morse, & Greene, 2001; de Resende,

Amaral, Moreno, & Greene, 2008; de Resende & Greene, 2008). Although several studies have demonstrated that ACE-Ang II axis increases vessel density in the skeletal muscle of rats, its role in angiogenesis is still controversial. Knockout mice of the ACE gene increased capillary density as expressed by the number of capillaries around type IIa fibers without significant difference in the cross-sectional area or type of fiber composition (Onder et al., 2006; B. Zhang et al., 2005).

Only one study has investigated the role of the RAS on skeletal muscle angiogenic response of normotensive rats to exercise. Interestingly, Amaral et al. (Amaral et al., 2001) showed that Ang II, acting through the AT1 receptor, increased VEGF protein expression and consequently induced skeletal muscle angiogenesis by short-term exercise training (3 days of running). This hypothesis was confirmed when the VEGF protein expression and angiogenesis were completely inhibited after treatment with ACE inhibitor (Captopril) or AT1 receptor blocker (Losartan).

In agreement, Fernandes et al. (Tiago Fernandes et al., 2008) reported that 10 weeks of swimming training increased ACE, Ang II and AT1 receptor levels in the soleus muscle. These results were related to exercise training-induced angiogenesis due an increase in capillaries observed. These findings were reinforced by the fact that AT1-receptor antagonist (Losartan) prevented these effects induced by exercise training. These mechanisms that enhance perfusion reflect a vital adaptation to exercise, contributing to the improved aerobic capacity of skeletal muscle.

Thus, the local RAS (ACE-Ang II axis), and ACE genotype are all variables that may impact the skeletal muscle responses to exercise training, but the responses of most of these variables to regular exercise training and the mechanisms responsible for these have not been systematically studied. In addition, although evidences suggest a beneficial role of ACE2 in cardiovascular function, the role played by the ACE2-Ang 1-7 axis in skeletal muscle function remains unknown. Interestingly, for the first time, Fernandes et al. (T. Fernandes et al., 2010) identified this enzyme in the skeletal muscle, broadening the concept of tissue RAS. The authors demonstrated that: ACE2 is expressed in the skeletal muscle of rats and there is no difference between the soleus and the plantaris muscle related ACE2 activity and protein levels.

The significance of the present findings is that, through characterization of ACE2 in the skeletal muscle, future therapeutics strategies targeting ACE2 might be developed for the treatment of peripheral abnormalities in skeletal muscle mediated cardiovascular disease such as vasomotor tonus imbalance induced by high peripheral vasoconstriction, increased wall-to-lumen vascular ratio, and microvascular rarefaction. Moreover, the present results might have implications for sports performance.

In summary, these results bring new insight into the role of RAS in the skeletal muscle induced by exercise training. In addition, as ACE2 differs in its specificity and physiological role from ACE, the signals responsible for these chronic adaptations are not clearly understood, and may include changes in skeletal muscle RAS components prompted by exercise.

Concluding Remark

There is no doubt in the literature that exercise training induces positive cardiovascular adaptations such as left ventricular hypertrophy with improved cardiac function. However, little is known about the role of RAS in these adaptations.

In this review we have shown data from studies using animal models, which have been published on this subject over the last 5 years. In conclusion, we may summarize the findings as follows:

- Cardiac Hypertrophy induced by exercise training (either aerobic or resistance) is regulated by the local RAS. Exercise training increases cardiac AT1 receptor expression and the blockade of AT1 receptor inhibits this response, while inhibition of the plasma renin activity has no effect;
- ACE2-Ang (1-7) axis counteracts the cardiac ACE-Ang II axis induced by aerobic training controlling vascular tonus and fibrosis in the heart;
- Expression of cardiac miRNAs is modulated by exercise training and may be responsible for the regulation of some RAS components;
- Aerobic training induces skeletal muscle angiogenesis by Ang II action and the blockade of AT1 receptor prevented this response;
- Both exercise training types do not significantly modulate the circulating components of RAS in a normal condition;

Benefits of exercise training on cardiac function and blood pressure in pathological states may at least partially be mediated by the normalization of expression and activity of many RAS components in different target organs, such as the heart, brain and skeletal muscle.

Acknowledgments

The present investigation was supported by Grants from Brazil: FAPESP (#2009/18370-3 and #2010/50048-1) and MCT-CNPq (# 485720/07-8).

References

ACSM. (2010). *ACSM's Guidelines for Exercise Testing and Prescription*: Lippincott Williams & Wilkins.

Agoudemos, M. M., & Greene, A. S. (2005). Localization of the renin-angiotensin system components to the skeletal muscle microcirculation. *Microcirculation, 12*(8), 627-636.

Alves, M. J., Dos Santos, M. R., Dias, R. G., Akiho, C. A., Laterza, M. C., Rondon, M. U., et al. (2010). Abnormal neurovascular control in anabolic androgenic steroids users. *Med Sci Sports Exerc, 42*(5), 865-871.

Amaral, S. L., Linderman, J. R., Morse, M. M., & Greene, A. S. (2001). Angiogenesis induced by electrical stimulation is mediated by angiotensin II and VEGF. *Microcirculation, 8*(1), 57-67.

Baggish, A. L., Wang, F., Weiner, R. B., Elinoff, J. M., Tournoux, F., Boland, A., et al. (2008). Training-specific changes in cardiac structure and function: a prospective and longitudinal assessment of competitive athletes. *J Appl Physiol, 104*(4), 1121-1128.

Bahi, L., Koulmann, N., Sanchez, H., Momken, I., Veksler, V., Bigard, A. X., et al. (2004). Does ACE inhibition enhance endurance performance and muscle energy metabolism in rats? *J Appl Physiol, 96*(1), 59-64.

Barauna, V. G., Batista, M. L., Jr., Costa Rosa, L. F., Casarini, D. E., Krieger, J. E., & Oliveira, E. M. (2005). Cardiovascular adaptations in rats submitted to a resistance-training model. *Clin Exp Pharmacol Physiol, 32*(4), 249-254.

Barauna, V. G., Magalhaes, F. C., Krieger, J. E., & Oliveira, E. M. (2008). AT1 receptor participates in the cardiac hypertrophy induced by resistance training in rats. *Am J Physiol Regul Integr Comp Physiol, 295*(2), R381-387.

Barauna, V. G., Rosa, K. T., Irigoyen, M. C., & de Oliveira, E. M. (2007). Effects of resistance training on ventricular function and hypertrophy in a rat model. *Clin Med Res, 5*(2), 114-120.

Barbier, J., Ville, N., Kervio, G., Walther, G., & Carre, F. (2006). Sports-specific features of athlete's heart and their relation to echocardiographic parameters. *Herz, 31*(6), 531-543.

Barki-Harrington, L., Luttrell, L. M., & Rockman, H. A. (2003). Dual inhibition of beta-adrenergic and angiotensin II receptors by a single antagonist: a functional role for receptor-receptor interaction in vivo. *Circulation, 108*(13), 1611-1618.

Batista, E. C., Ramalho, J. D., Reis, F. C., Barros, C. C., Moraes, M. R., Pesquero, J. L., et al. (2008). Swimming training exacerbates pathological cardiac hypertrophy in kinin B2 receptor-deficient mice. *Int Immunopharmacol, 8*(2), 271-275.

Beisvag, V., Kemi, O. J., Arbo, I., Loennechen, J. P., Wisloff, U., Langaas, M., et al. (2009). Pathological and physiological hypertrophies are regulated by distinct gene programs. *Eur J Cardiovasc Prev Rehabil, 16*(6), 690-697.

Bezerra, S. M., dos Santos, C. M., Moreira, E. D., Krieger, E. M., & Michelini, L. C. (2001). Chronic AT(1) receptor blockade alters autonomic balance and sympathetic responses in hypertension. *Hypertension, 38*(3 Pt 2), 569-575.

Brentano, M. A., & Martins Kruel, L. F. (2011). A review on strength exercise-induced muscle damage: applications, adaptation mechanisms and limitations. *J Sports Med Phys Fitness, 51*(1), 1-10.

Brilla, C. G. (2000). Renin-angiotensin-aldosterone system and myocardial fibrosis. *Cardiovasc Res, 47*(1), 1-3.

Brull, D., Dhamrait, S., Myerson, S., Erdmann, J., Woods, D., World, M., et al. (2001). Bradykinin B2BKR receptor polymorphism and left-ventricular growth response. *Lancet, 358*(9288), 1155-1156.

Brum, P. C., Rolim, N. P., Bacurau, A. V., & Medeiros, A. (2006). Neurohumoral activation in heart failure: the role of adrenergic receptors. *An Acad Bras Cienc, 78*(3), 485-503.

Cantley, L. C. (2002). The phosphoinositide 3-kinase pathway. *Science, 296*(5573), 1655-1657.

Care, A., Catalucci, D., Felicetti, F., Bonci, D., Addario, A., Gallo, P., et al. (2007). MicroRNA-133 controls cardiac hypertrophy. *Nat Med, 13*(5), 613-618.

Chaves, E. A., Pereira-Junior, P. P., Fortunato, R. S., Masuda, M. O., de Carvalho, A. C., de Carvalho, D. P., et al. (2006). Nandrolone decanoate impairs exercise-induced cardioprotection: role of antioxidant enzymes. *J Steroid Biochem Mol Biol, 99*(4-5), 223-230.

Crackower, M. A., Sarao, R., Oudit, G. Y., Yagil, C., Kozieradzki, I., Scanga, S. E., et al. (2002). Angiotensin-converting enzyme 2 is an essential regulator of heart function. *Nature, 417*(6891), 822-828.

Cunha, T. S., Moura, M. J., Bernardes, C. F., Tanno, A. P., & Marcondes, F. K. (2005). Vascular sensitivity to phenylephrine in rats submitted to anaerobic training and nandrolone treatment. *Hypertension, 46*(4), 1010-1015.

D'Andrea, A., Caso, P., Salerno, G., Scarafile, R., De Corato, G., Mita, C., et al. (2007). Left ventricular early myocardial dysfunction after chronic misuse of anabolic androgenic steroids: a Doppler myocardial and strain imaging analysis. *Br J Sports Med, 41*(3), 149-155.

Dahlof, B., Herlitz, H., Aurell, M., & Hansson, L. (1992). Reversal of cardiovascular structural changes when treating essential hypertension. The importance of the renin-angiotensin-aldosterone system. *Am J Hypertens, 5*(12 Pt 1), 900-911.

de Cassia Cypriano Ervati Pinter, R., Padilha, A. S., de Oliveira, E. M., Vassallo, D. V., & de Fucio Lizardo, J. H. (2008). Cardiovascular adaptive responses in rats submitted to moderate resistance training. *Eur J Appl Physiol, 103*(5), 605-613.

de Resende, M. M., Amaral, S. L., Moreno, C., & Greene, A. S. (2008). Congenic strains reveal the effect of the renin gene on skeletal muscle angiogenesis induced by electrical stimulation. *Physiol Genomics, 33*(1), 33-40.

de Resende, M. M., & Greene, A. S. (2008). Effect of ANG II on endothelial cell apoptosis and survival and its impact on skeletal muscle angiogenesis after electrical stimulation. *Am J Physiol Heart Circ Physiol, 294*(6), H2814-2821.

Diamond, J. A., & Phillips, R. A. (2005). Hypertensive heart disease. *Hypertens Res, 28*(3), 191-202.

Dietze, G. J., & Henriksen, E. J. (2008). Angiotensin-converting enzyme in skeletal muscle: sentinel of blood pressure control and glucose homeostasis. *J Renin Angiotensin Aldosterone Syst, 9*(2), 75-88.

do Carmo, E. C., Fernandes, T., Koike, D., da Silva, N. D. J., Mattos, K. C., Rosa, K. T., et al. (2011). Anabolic Steroid Associated To Physical Training Induces Deleterious Cardiac Effects. *Med Sci Sports Exerc.*

Donoghue, M., Hsieh, F., Baronas, E., Godbout, K., Gosselin, M., Stagliano, N., et al. (2000). A novel angiotensin-converting enzyme-related carboxypeptidase (ACE2) converts angiotensin I to angiotensin 1-9. *Circ Res, 87*(5), E1-9.

Dorn, G. W., 2nd. (2007). The fuzzy logic of physiological cardiac hypertrophy. *Hypertension, 49*(5), 962-970.

Dostal, D. E. (2000). The cardiac renin-angiotensin system: novel signaling mechanisms related to cardiac growth and function. *Regul Pept, 91*(1-3), 1-11.

Dostal, D. E., & Baker, K. M. (1999). The cardiac renin-angiotensin system: conceptual, or a regulator of cardiac function? *Circ Res, 85*(7), 643-650.

Evangelista, F. S., & Krieger, J. E. (2006). Small gene effect and exercise training-induced cardiac hypertrophy in mice: an Ace gene dosage study. *Physiol Genomics, 27*(3), 231-236.

Felix, J. V., & Michelini, L. C. (2007). Training-induced pressure fall in spontaneously hypertensive rats is associated with reduced angiotensinogen mRNA expression within the nucleus tractus solitarii. *Hypertension, 50*(4), 780-785.

Fernandes, T., Hashimoto, N., Cachofeiro, V., Lahera, V., Krieger, J. E., & Oliveira, E. M. d. (2008). *Aerobic exercise training promotes angiogenesis by angiotensin II and ACE2-Ang (1-7) axis can activates vasodilatation pathways in the skeletal muscle.* Paper presented at the J Hypertens Suppl.

Fernandes, T., Hashimoto, N. Y., Magalhaes, F. C., Fernandes, F. B., Casarini, D. E., Carmona, A. K., et al. (2011). Aerobic Exercise Training-Induced Left Ventricular Hypertrophy Involves Regulatory MicroRNAs, Decreased Angiotensin-Converting Enzyme-Angiotensin II, and Synergistic Regulation of Angiotensin-Converting Enzyme 2-Angiotensin (1-7). *Hypertension, 58*(2), 182-189.

Fernandes, T., Hashimoto, N. Y., & Oliveira, E. M. (2010). Characterization of angiotensin-converting enzymes 1 and 2 in the soleus and plantaris muscles of rats. *Braz J Med Biol Res, 43*(9), 837-842.

Ferrario, C. M. (2010). ACE2: more of Ang-(1-7) or less Ang II? *Curr Opin Nephrol Hypertens, 20*(1), 1-6.

Ferreira, J. C., Bacurau, A. V., Evangelista, F. S., Coelho, M. A., Oliveira, E. M., Casarini, D. E., et al. (2008). The role of local and systemic renin angiotensin system activation in a genetic model of sympathetic hyperactivity-induced heart failure in mice. *Am J Physiol Regul Integr Comp Physiol, 294*(1), R26-32.

Filho, A. G., Ferreira, A. J., Santos, S. H., Neves, S. R., Silva Camargos, E. R., Becker, L. K., et al. (2008). Selective increase of angiotensin(1-7) and its receptor in hearts of spontaneously hypertensive rats subjected to physical training. *Exp Physiol, 93*(5), 589-598.

Fleming, I. (2006). Signaling by the angiotensin-converting enzyme. *Circ Res, 98*(7), 887-896.

Folland, J. P., & Williams, A. G. (2007). The adaptations to strength training : morphological and neurological contributions to increased strength. *Sports Med, 37*(2), 145-168.

Franco, M., Cooper, R. S., Bilal, U., & Fuster, V. (2011). Challenges and opportunities for cardiovascular disease prevention. *Am J Med, 124*(2), 95-102.

Gao, L., Wang, W., Li, Y. L., Schultz, H. D., Liu, D., Cornish, K. G., et al. (2004). Superoxide mediates sympathoexcitation in heart failure: roles of angiotensin II and NAD(P)H oxidase. *Circ Res, 95*(9), 937-944.

Geenen, D. L., Malhotra, A., & Buttrick, P. M. (1996). Angiotensin receptor 1 blockade does not prevent physiological cardiac hypertrophy in the adult rat. *J Appl Physiol, 81*(2), 816-821.

Gordon, S. E., Davis, B. S., Carlson, C. J., & Booth, F. W. (2001). ANG II is required for optimal overload-induced skeletal muscle hypertrophy. *Am J Physiol Endocrinol Metab, 280*(1), E150-159.

Grassi, G., Cattaneo, B. M., Seravalle, G., Lanfranchi, A., Pozzi, M., Morganti, A., et al. (1997). Effects of chronic ACE inhibition on sympathetic nerve traffic and baroreflex control of circulation in heart failure. *Circulation, 96*(4), 1173-1179.

Grobe, J. L., Mecca, A. P., Lingis, M., Shenoy, V., Bolton, T. A., Machado, J. M., et al. (2007). Prevention of angiotensin II-induced cardiac remodeling by angiotensin-(1-7). *Am J Physiol Heart Circ Physiol, 292*(2), H736-742.

Habouzit, E., Richard, H., Sanchez, H., Koulmann, N., Serrurier, B., Monnet, R., et al. (2009). Decreased muscle ACE activity enhances functional response to endurance training in rats, without change in muscle oxidative capacity or contractile phenotype. *J Appl Physiol, 107*(1), 346-353.

Howley, E. T. (2001). Type of activity: resistance, aerobic and leisure versus occupational physical activity. *Med Sci Sports Exerc, 33*(6 Suppl), S364-369; discussion S419-320.

Hruskovicova, H., Dzurenkova, D., Selingerova, M., Bohus, B., Timkanicova, B., & Kovacs, L. (2006). The angiotensin converting enzyme I/D polymorphism in long distance runners. *J Sports Med Phys Fitness, 46*(3), 509-513.

Irigoyen, M. C., & Krieger, E. M. (1998). Baroreflex control of sympathetic activity in experimental hypertension. *Braz J Med Biol Res, 31*(9), 1213-1220.

Izumo, S., Nadal-Ginard, B., & Mahdavi, V. (1988). Protooncogene induction and reprogramming of cardiac gene expression produced by pressure overload. *Proc Natl Acad Sci U S A, 85*(2), 339-343.

Johar, S., Cave, A. C., Narayanapanicker, A., Grieve, D. J., & Shah, A. M. (2006). Aldosterone mediates angiotensin II-induced interstitial cardiac fibrosis via a Nox2-containing NADPH oxidase. *FASEB J, 20*(9), 1546-1548.

Johnston, C. I. (1990). Biochemistry and pharmacology of the renin-angiotensin system. *Drugs, 39 Suppl 1*, 21-31.

Jones, A., & Woods, D. R. (2003). Skeletal muscle RAS and exercise performance. *Int J Biochem Cell Biol, 35*(6), 855-866.

Jonsdottir, S., Andersen, K. K., Sigurosson, A. F., & Sigurosson, S. B. (2006). The effect of physical training in chronic heart failure. *Eur J Heart Fail, 8*(1), 97-101.

Julius, S. (2007). Blood pressure lowering only or more? Has the jury reached its verdict? *Am J Cardiol, 100*(3A), 32J-37J.

Kar, S., Gao, L., & Zucker, I. H. (2011). Exercise training normalizes ACE and ACE2 in the brain of rabbits with pacing-induced heart failure. *J Appl Physiol, 108*(4), 923-932.

Kawano, H., Toda, G., Nakamizo, R., Koide, Y., Seto, S., & Yano, K. (2005). Valsartan decreases type I collagen synthesis in patients with hypertrophic cardiomyopathy. *Circ J, 69*(10), 1244-1248.

Kemi, O. J., Ceci, M., Wisloff, U., Grimaldi, S., Gallo, P., Smith, G. L., et al. (2008). Activation or inactivation of cardiac Akt/mTOR signaling diverges physiological from pathological hypertrophy. *J Cell Physiol, 214*(2), 316-321.

Kim, S., & Iwao, H. (2000). Molecular and cellular mechanisms of angiotensin II-mediated cardiovascular and renal diseases. *Pharmacol Rev, 52*(1), 11-34.

Klitgaard, H. (1988). A model for quantitative strength training of hindlimb muscles of the rat. *J Appl Physiol, 64*(4), 1740-1745.

Koulmann, N., & Bigard, A. X. (2006). Interaction between signalling pathways involved in skeletal muscle responses to endurance exercise. *Pflugers Arch, 452*(2), 125-139.

Krieg, A., Scharhag, J., Albers, T., Kindermann, W., & Urhausen, A. (2007). Cardiac tissue Doppler in steroid users. *Int J Sports Med, 28*(8), 638-643.

Krieger, E. M. (1964). Neurogenic Hypertension in the Rat. *Circ Res, 15*, 511-521.

Krisan, A. D., Collins, D. E., Crain, A. M., Kwong, C. C., Singh, M. K., Bernard, J. R., et al. (2004). Resistance training enhances components of the insulin signaling cascade in normal and high-fat-fed rodent skeletal muscle. *J Appl Physiol, 96*(5), 1691-1700.

Leenen, F. H., White, R., & Yuan, B. (2001). Isoproterenol-induced cardiac hypertrophy: role of circulatory versus cardiac renin-angiotensin system. *Am J Physiol Heart Circ Physiol, 281*(6), H2410-2416.

Lemarie, C. A., Paradis, P., & Schiffrin, E. L. (2008). New insights on signaling cascades induced by cross-talk between angiotensin II and aldosterone. *J Mol Med (Berl), 86*(6), 673-678.

Lentini, A. C., McKelvie, R. S., McCartney, N., Tomlinson, C. W., & MacDougall, J. D. (1993). Left ventricular response in healthy young men during heavy-intensity weight-lifting exercise. *J Appl Physiol, 75*(6), 2703-2710.

Lowe, D. A., & Alway, S. E. (2002). Animal models for inducing muscle hypertrophy: are they relevant for clinical applications in humans? *J Orthop Sports Phys Ther, 32*(2), 36-43.

MacDougall, J. D., Tuxen, D., Sale, D. G., Moroz, J. R., & Sutton, J. R. (1985). Arterial blood pressure response to heavy resistance exercise. *J Appl Physiol, 58*(3), 785-790.

Mann, D. E., Florek, R. C., & Reiter, M. J. (1992). Effect of pacing drive cycle length on induction of sustained monomorphic ventricular tachycardia. *J Electrocardiol, 25*(1), 33-38.

Matsui, T., Li, L., Wu, J. C., Cook, S. A., Nagoshi, T., Picard, M. H., et al. (2002). Phenotypic spectrum caused by transgenic overexpression of activated Akt in the heart. *J Biol Chem, 277*(25), 22896-22901.

Matsui, T., Nagoshi, T., & Rosenzweig, A. (2003). Akt and PI 3-kinase signaling in cardiomyocyte hypertrophy and survival. *Cell Cycle, 2*(3), 220-223.

McBride, T. A. (2006). AT1 receptors are necessary for eccentric training-induced hypertrophy and strength gains in rat skeletal muscle. *Exp Physiol, 91*(2), 413-421.

McKinley, M. J., Albiston, A. L., Allen, A. M., Mathai, M. L., May, C. N., McAllen, R. M., et al. (2003). The brain renin-angiotensin system: location and physiological roles. *Int J Biochem Cell Biol, 35*(6), 901-918.

McMullen, J. R., Shioi, T., Zhang, L., Tarnavski, O., Sherwood, M. C., Kang, P. M., et al. (2003). Phosphoinositide 3-kinase(p110alpha) plays a critical role for the induction of physiological, but not pathological, cardiac hypertrophy. *Proc Natl Acad Sci U S A, 100*(21), 12355-12360.

Medei, E., Marocolo, M., Rodrigues Dde, C., Arantes, P. C., Takiya, C. M., Silva, J., et al. (2010). Chronic treatment with anabolic steroids induces ventricular repolarization disturbances: cellular, ionic and molecular mechanism. *J Mol Cell Cardiol, 49*(2), 165-175.

Medeiros, A., Rolim, N. P., Oliveira, R. S., Rosa, K. T., Mattos, K. C., Casarini, D. E., et al. (2008). Exercise training delays cardiac dysfunction and prevents calcium handling abnormalities in sympathetic hyperactivity-induced heart failure mice. *J Appl Physiol, 104*(1), 103-109.

Melchert, R. B., Herron, T. J., & Welder, A. A. (1992). The effect of anabolic-androgenic steroids on primary myocardial cell cultures. *Med Sci Sports Exerc, 24*(2), 206-212.

Melo, S., Amadeu, M., Fernandes, T., Carmo, E. C., Magalhaes, F., Barreti, D., et al. (2010). *A session of strength exercise induced cardiac hypertrophy by AT1 receptor-Akt-mTOR signaling pathway.* Paper presented at the FASEB J.

Mendes, A. C., Ferreira, A. J., Pinheiro, S. V., & Santos, R. A. (2005). Chronic infusion of angiotensin-(1-7) reduces heart angiotensin II levels in rats. *Regul Pept, 125*(1-3), 29-34.

Michelini, L. C., de Oliveira, M., & dos Santos, M. (1992). Baroreceptor reflex control of heart rate during development of coarctation hypertension. *Hypertension, 19*(2 Suppl), II159-163.

Momken, I., Kahapip, J., Bahi, L., Badoual, T., Hittinger, L., Ventura-Clapier, R., et al. (2003). Does angiotensin-converting enzyme inhibition improve the energetic status of cardiac and skeletal muscles in heart failure induced by aortic stenosis in rats? *J Mol Cell Cardiol, 35*(4), 399-407.

Mousa, T. M., Liu, D., Cornish, K. G., & Zucker, I. H. (2008). Exercise training enhances baroreflex sensitivity by an angiotensin II-dependent mechanism in chronic heart failure. *J Appl Physiol, 104*(3), 616-624.

Nagano, M., Higaki, J., Nakamura, F., Higashimori, K., Nagano, N., Mikami, H., et al. (1992). Role of cardiac angiotensin II in isoproterenol-induced left ventricular hypertrophy. *Hypertension, 19*(6 Pt 2), 708-712.

Nascimento, J. H., & Medei, E. (2011). Cardiac effects of anabolic steroids: hypertrophy, ischemia and electrical remodelling as potential triggers of sudden death. *Mini Rev Med Chem, 11*(5), 425-429.

Nelson, M. E., Rejeski, W. J., Blair, S. N., Duncan, P. W., Judge, J. O., King, A. C., et al. (2007). Physical activity and public health in older adults: recommendation from the American College of Sports Medicine and the American Heart Association. *Med Sci Sports Exerc, 39*(8), 1435-1445.

Notomi, T., Lee, S. J., Okimoto, N., Okazaki, Y., Takamoto, T., Nakamura, T., et al. (2000). Effects of resistance exercise training on mass, strength, and turnover of bone in growing rats. *Eur J Appl Physiol, 82*(4), 268-274.

Notomi, T., Okazaki, Y., Okimoto, N., Saitoh, S., Nakamura, T., & Suzuki, M. (2000). A comparison of resistance and aerobic training for mass, strength and turnover of bone in growing rats. *Eur J Appl Physiol, 83*(6), 469-474.

Nottin, S., Nguyen, L. D., Terbah, M., & Obert, P. (2006). Cardiovascular effects of androgenic anabolic steroids in male bodybuilders determined by tissue Doppler imaging. *Am J Cardiol, 97*(6), 912-915.

Oddie, C. J., Dilley, R. J., & Bobik, A. (1992). Long-term angiotensin II antagonism in spontaneously hypertensive rats: effects on blood pressure and cardiovascular amplifiers. *Clin Exp Pharmacol Physiol, 19*(5), 392-395.

Oliveira, E. M., & Krieger, J. E. (2005). Chronic beta-adrenoceptor stimulation and cardiac hypertrophy with no induction of circulating renin. *Eur J Pharmacol, 520*(1-3), 135-141.

Oliveira, E. M., Sasaki, M. S., Cerencio, M., Barauna, V. G., & Krieger, J. E. (2009). Local renin-angiotensin system regulates left ventricular hypertrophy induced by swimming training independent of circulating renin: a pharmacological study. *J Renin Angiotensin Aldosterone Syst, 10*(1), 15-23.

Onder, G., Vedova, C. D., & Pahor, M. (2006). Effects of ACE inhibitors on skeletal muscle. *Curr Pharm Des, 12*(16), 2057-2064.

Pagliaro, P., & Penna, C. (2005). Rethinking the renin-angiotensin system and its role in cardiovascular regulation. *Cardiovasc Drugs Ther, 19*(1), 77-87.

Parati, G., Ravogli, A., Frattola, A., Groppelli, A., Ulian, L., Santucciu, C., et al. (1994). Blood pressure variability: clinical implications and effects of antihypertensive treatment. *J Hypertens Suppl, 12*(5), S35-40.

Parssinen, M., Kujala, U., Vartiainen, E., Sarna, S., & Seppala, T. (2000). Increased premature mortality of competitive powerlifters suspected to have used anabolic agents. *Int J Sports Med, 21*(3), 225-227.

Paul, M., Poyan Mehr, A., & Kreutz, R. (2006). Physiology of local renin-angiotensin systems. *Physiol Rev, 86*(3), 747-803.

Pearson, A. C., Schiff, M., Mrosek, D., Labovitz, A. J., & Williams, G. A. (1986). Left ventricular diastolic function in weight lifters. *Am J Cardiol, 58*(13), 1254-1259.

Pereira, M. G., Ferreira, J. C., Bueno, C. R., Jr., Mattos, K. C., Rosa, K. T., Irigoyen, M. C., et al. (2009). Exercise training reduces cardiac angiotensin II levels and prevents cardiac dysfunction in a genetic model of sympathetic hyperactivity-induced heart failure in mice. *Eur J Appl Physiol, 105*(6), 843-850.

Petersen, M. C., Munzenmaier, D. H., & Greene, A. S. (2006). Angiotensin II infusion restores stimulated angiogenesis in the skeletal muscle of rats on a high-salt diet. *Am J Physiol Heart Circ Physiol, 291*(1), H114-120.

Pipilis, A., Kaliambakos, S., Xenodochidis, C., Tsakonas, G., Sourlas, N., & Mallios, K. (2007). Overestimation and underestimation of cardiovascular risk in clinical practice: usefulness of risk estimation charts. *Hellenic J Cardiol, 48*(6), 341-345.

Pluim, B. M., Zwinderman, A. H., van der Laarse, A., & van der Wall, E. E. (2000). The athlete's heart. A meta-analysis of cardiac structure and function. *Circulation, 101*(3), 336-344.

Qin, W., Rudolph, A. E., Bond, B. R., Rocha, R., Blomme, E. A., Goellner, J. J., et al. (2003). Transgenic model of aldosterone-driven cardiac hypertrophy and heart failure. *Circ Res, 93*(1), 69-76.

Rafalski, K., Abdourahman, A., & Edwards, J. G. (2007). Early adaptations to training: upregulation of alpha-myosin heavy chain gene expression. *Med Sci Sports Exerc, 39*(1), 75-82.

Re, R. N. (2004). Mechanisms of disease: local renin-angiotensin-aldosterone systems and the pathogenesis and treatment of cardiovascular disease. *Nat Clin Pract Cardiovasc Med, 1*(1), 42-47.

Reneland, R., & Lithell, H. (1994). Angiotensin-converting enzyme in human skeletal muscle. A simple in vitro assay of activity in needle biopsy specimens. *Scand J Clin Lab Invest, 54*(2), 105-111.

Reudelhuber, T. L., Bernstein, K. E., & Delafontaine, P. (2007). Is angiotensin II a direct mediator of left ventricular hypertrophy? Time for another look. *Hypertension, 49*(6), 1196-1201.

Riezzo, I., De Carlo, D., Neri, M., Nieddu, A., Turillazzi, E., & Fineschi, V. (2011). Heart disease induced by AAS abuse, using experimental mice/rats models and the role of exercise-induced cardiotoxicity. *Mini Rev Med Chem, 11*(5), 409-424.

Rocha, F. L., Carmo, E. C., Roque, F. R., Hashimoto, N. Y., Rossoni, L. V., Frimm, C., et al. (2007). Anabolic steroids induce cardiac renin-angiotensin system and impair the beneficial effects of aerobic training in rats. *Am J Physiol Heart Circ Physiol, 293*(6), H3575-3583.

Rodriguez, N. R., Di Marco, N. M., & Langley, S. (2009). American College of Sports Medicine position stand. Nutrition and athletic performance. *Med Sci Sports Exerc, 41*(3), 709-731.

Roveda, F., Middlekauff, H. R., Rondon, M. U., Reis, S. F., Souza, M., Nastari, L., et al. (2003). The effects of exercise training on sympathetic neural activation in advanced heart failure: a randomized controlled trial. *J Am Coll Cardiol, 42*(5), 854-860.

Sadoshima, J., & Izumo, S. (1993). Molecular characterization of angiotensin II--induced hypertrophy of cardiac myocytes and hyperplasia of cardiac fibroblasts. Critical role of the AT1 receptor subtype. *Circ Res, 73*(3), 413-423.

Sadoshima, J., Xu, Y., Slayter, H. S., & Izumo, S. (1993). Autocrine release of angiotensin II mediates stretch-induced hypertrophy of cardiac myocytes in vitro. *Cell, 75*(5), 977-984.

Sanders, P. M., Russell, S. T., & Tisdale, M. J. (2005). Angiotensin II directly induces muscle protein catabolism through the ubiquitin-proteasome proteolytic pathway and may play a role in cancer cachexia. *Br J Cancer, 93*(4), 425-434.

Sangaleti, C. T., Crescenzi, A., & Michelini, L. C. (2004). Endogenous angiotensin and pressure modulate brain angiotensinogen and AT1A mRNA expression. *Hypertension, 43*(2), 317-323.

Santos, C. M., Pontieri, V., Leomil Neto, M., & Michelini, L. C. (1995). Losartan improves baroreflex control of heart rate of coarcted hypertensive rats. *Am J Physiol, 269*(3 Pt 2), H812-818.

Santos, R. A., Castro, C. H., Gava, E., Pinheiro, S. V., Almeida, A. P., Paula, R. D., et al. (2006). Impairment of in vitro and in vivo heart function in angiotensin-(1-7) receptor MAS knockout mice. *Hypertension, 47*(5), 996-1002.

Santos, R. A., Simoes e Silva, A. C., Maric, C., Silva, D. M., Machado, R. P., de Buhr, I., et al. (2003). Angiotensin-(1-7) is an endogenous ligand for the G protein-coupled receptor Mas. *Proc Natl Acad Sci U S A, 100*(14), 8258-8263.

Satoh, M., Nakamura, M., Saitoh, H., Satoh, H., Akatsu, T., Iwasaka, J., et al. (2002). Aldosterone synthase (CYP11B2) expression and myocardial fibrosis in the failing human heart. *Clin Sci (Lond), 102*(4), 381-386.

Sauzeau, V., Sevilla, M. A., Rivas-Elena, J. V., de Alava, E., Montero, M. J., Lopez-Novoa, J. M., et al. (2006). Vav3 proto-oncogene deficiency leads to sympathetic hyperactivity and cardiovascular dysfunction. *Nat Med, 12*(7), 841-845.

Schinke, M., Baltatu, O., Bohm, M., Peters, J., Rascher, W., Bricca, G., et al. (1999). Blood pressure reduction and diabetes insipidus in transgenic rats deficient in brain angiotensinogen. *Proc Natl Acad Sci U S A, 96*(7), 3975-3980.

Sharma, J. N. (2009). Hypertension and the bradykinin system. *Curr Hypertens Rep, 11*(3), 178-181.

Small, E. M., & Olson, E. N. (2011). Pervasive roles of microRNAs in cardiovascular biology. *Nature, 469*(7330), 336-342.

Soci, U. P., Fernandes, T., Hashimoto, N. Y., Mota, G. F., Amadeu, M. A., Rosa, K. T., et al. (2011). MicroRNAs 29 are involved in the improvement of ventricular compliance promoted by aerobic exercise training in rats. *Physiol Genomics, 43*(11), 665-673.

Stefanadis, C. I. (2008). The future of antihypertensive treatment: from myth to imminent reality. *Hellenic J Cardiol, 49*(5), 377-378.

Stewart, C. E., & Rittweger, J. (2006). Adaptive processes in skeletal muscle: molecular regulators and genetic influences. *J Musculoskelet Neuronal Interact, 6*(1), 73-86.

Su, D. F., & Miao, C. Y. (2005). Reduction of blood pressure variability: a new strategy for the treatment of hypertension. *Trends Pharmacol Sci, 26*(8), 388-390.

Sun, Y., & Weber, K. T. (2003). RAS and connective tissue in the heart. *Int J Biochem Cell Biol, 35*(6), 919-931.

Tamaki, T., Akatsuka, A., Tokunaga, M., Ishige, K., Uchiyama, S., & Shiraishi, T. (1997). Morphological and biochemical evidence of muscle hyperplasia following weight-lifting exercise in rats. *Am J Physiol, 273*(1 Pt 1), C246-256.

Taylor, J. (2011). Sports and cardiac function 1: exercise is a potent stressor on the heart. *Eur Heart J, 31*(1), 6-8.

Tipnis, S. R., Hooper, N. M., Hyde, R., Karran, E., Christie, G., & Turner, A. J. (2000). A human homolog of angiotensin-converting enzyme. Cloning and functional expression as a captopril-insensitive carboxypeptidase. *J Biol Chem, 275*(43), 33238-33243.

Unger, T. (2002). The role of the renin-angiotensin system in the development of cardiovascular disease. *Am J Cardiol, 89*(2A), 3A-9A; discussion 10A.

Urhausen, A., Albers, T., & Kindermann, W. (2004). Are the cardiac effects of anabolic steroid abuse in strength athletes reversible? *Heart, 90*(5), 496-501.

van Kats, J. P., Methot, D., Paradis, P., Silversides, D. W., & Reudelhuber, T. L. (2001). Use of a biological peptide pump to study chronic peptide hormone action in transgenic mice. Direct and indirect effects of angiotensin II on the heart. *J Biol Chem, 276*(47), 44012-44017.

van Rooij, E., & Olson, E. N. (2007). MicroRNAs: powerful new regulators of heart disease and provocative therapeutic targets. *J Clin Invest, 117*(9), 2369-2376.

Wan, W., Powers, A. S., Li, J., Ji, L., Erikson, J. M., & Zhang, J. Q. (2007). Effect of post-myocardial infarction exercise training on the renin-angiotensin-aldosterone system and cardiac function. *Am J Med Sci, 334*(4), 265-273.

Wang, Y., Wisloff, U., & Kemi, O. J. (2010). Animal models in the study of exercise-induced cardiac hypertrophy. *Physiol Res, 59*(5), 633-644.

Ward, P. E., Russell, J. S., & Vaghy, P. L. (1995). Angiotensin and bradykinin metabolism by peptidases identified in skeletal muscle. *Peptides, 16*(6), 1073-1078.

WHO, S. (2009). http://www.who.int/healthinfo/statistics/. from http://www.who.int/healthinfo/statistics/

Williams, A. G., Day, S. H., Folland, J. P., Gohlke, P., Dhamrait, S., & Montgomery, H. E. (2005). Circulating angiotensin converting enzyme activity is correlated with muscle strength. *Med Sci Sports Exerc, 37*(6), 944-948.

Wisloff, U., Stoylen, A., Loennechen, J. P., Bruvold, M., Rognmo, O., Haram, P. M., et al. (2007). Superior cardiovascular effect of aerobic interval training versus moderate continuous training in heart failure patients: a randomized study. *Circulation, 115*(24), 3086-3094.

Wong, T. S., & Booth, F. W. (1988). Skeletal muscle enlargement with weight-lifting exercise by rats. *J Appl Physiol, 65*(2), 950-954.

Wu, J. N., & Berecek, K. H. (1993). Prevention of genetic hypertension by early treatment of spontaneously hypertensive rats with the angiotensin converting enzyme inhibitor captopril. *Hypertension, 22*(2), 139-146.

Yaspelkis, B. B., 3rd, Singh, M. K., Trevino, B., Krisan, A. D., & Collins, D. E. (2002). Resistance training increases glucose uptake and transport in rat skeletal muscle. *Acta Physiol Scand, 175*(4), 315-323.

Zamo, F. S., Barauna, V. G., Chiavegatto, S., Irigoyen, M. C., & Oliveira, E. M. (2011). The renin-angiotensin system is modulated by swimming training depending on the age of spontaneously hypertensive rats. *Life Sci, 89*(3-4), 93-99.

Zamo, F. S., Lacchini, S., Mostarda, C., Chiavegatto, S., Silva, I. C., Oliveira, E. M., et al. (2010). Hemodynamic, morphometric and autonomic patterns in hypertensive rats - Renin-Angiotensin system modulation. *Clinics (Sao Paulo), 65*(1), 85-92.

Zhai, P., Yamamoto, M., Galeotti, J., Liu, J., Masurekar, M., Thaisz, J., et al. (2005). Cardiac-specific overexpression of AT1 receptor mutant lacking G alpha q/G alpha i coupling causes hypertrophy and bradycardia in transgenic mice. *J Clin Invest, 115*(11), 3045-3056.

Zhang, B., Shono, N., Fan, P., Ando, S., Xu, H., Jimi, S., et al. (2005). Histochemical characteristics of soleus muscle in angiotensin-converting enzyme gene knockout mice. *Hypertens Res, 28*(8), 681-688.

Zhang, X., Dostal, D. E., Reiss, K., Cheng, W., Kajstura, J., Li, P., et al. (1995). Identification and activation of autocrine renin-angiotensin system in adult ventricular myocytes. *Am J Physiol, 269*(5 Pt 2), H1791-1802.

Zhang, Y. L., Zhou, S. X., Lei, J., Yuan, G. Y., & Wang, J. F. (2008). Blockades of angiotensin and aldosterone reduce osteopontin expression and interstitial fibrosis infiltration in rats with myocardial infarction. *Chin Med J (Engl), 121*(21), 2192-2196.

Zoll, J., Monassier, L., Garnier, A., N'Guessan, B., Mettauer, B., Veksler, V., et al. (2006). ACE inhibition prevents myocardial infarction-induced skeletal muscle mitochondrial dysfunction. *J Appl Physiol, 101*(2), 385-391.

Zou, Y., Akazawa, H., Qin, Y., Sano, M., Takano, H., Minamino, T., et al. (2004). Mechanical stress activates angiotensin II type 1 receptor without the involvement of angiotensin II. *Nat Cell Biol, 6*(6), 499-506.

Zucker, I. H. (2002). Brain angiotensin II: new insights into its role in sympathetic regulation. *Circ Res, 90*(5), 503-505.

Zuraw, B. (2001). Bradykinin in protection against left-ventricular hypertrophy. *Lancet, 358*(9288), 1116-1118.

In: Angiotensin: New Research
Editors: S. Harada, I. Moi, pp. 93-111

ISBN: 978-1-62100-773-9

Chapter 3

THE ROLE OF THE COUNTER-REGULATORY RENIN ANGIOTENSIN SYSTEM IN THE HEART

Monica Flores-Muñoz and Stuart A. Nicklin*
Institute of Cardiovascular and Medical Sciences, BHF GCRC,
University of Glasgow, 126 University Place, Glasgow, UK.

ABSTRACT

The counter-regulatory renin angiotensin system (RAS) is centred around the angiotensin converting enzyme (ACE) homologue ACE2. ACE2 metabolizes angiotensin (Ang) II to Ang-(1-7), decreasing AngII and increasing Ang-(1-7) levels. ACE2 also converts AngI to Ang-(1-9), which can be further converted to Ang-(1-7) via ACE-mediated metabolism. Ang-(1-7) has been shown to counteract AngII actions mainly via stimulating the protooncogene Mas receptor. Thus the ACE2/Ang-(1-7)/Mas axis has received much recent focus as a potential therapeutic target in cardiovascular disease. In experimental models the heart has been a major focus of this research in pathophysiologies such as cardiac remodelling following experimental myocardial infarction, ischaemia reperfusion injury, cardiac hypertrophy in aortic banding and AngII infusion models and heart failure. In these settings administration of the peptide Ang-(1-7), or over-expression of ACE2 via somatic gene transfer or transgenic strategies mediates clear therapeutic benefit in reversing many of the phenotypes in these models. This experimental evidence is supported by clinical research which has shown that in patients on ACE inhibitors or angiotensin type 1 receptor antagonists ACE2 and Ang-(1-7) levels are upregulated, suggesting they may contribute to the therapeutic benefit of these drugs in patients following myocardial infarction and in heart failure. While these studies have provided clear evidence for ACE2 and Ang-(1-7) as potential therapeutic targets there still remains much to be understood about the counter-regulatory RAS in the heart. Certain studies using transgenic or somatic overexpression of ACE2 in the heart have demonstrated a severe effect on cardiac conduction and promotion of cardiac fibrosis. Furthermore, recent new discoveries in the RAS may also play a role in the counter-regulatory RAS. For example, Ang-(1-9) may inhibit ACE-mediated generation of AngII by binding the same catalytic site as AngI. Furthermore, Ang-(1-9) reduces

* Correspondence to: Stuart A Nicklin Email: stuart.nicklin@glasgow.ac.uk

cardiac hypertrophy in rat myocardial infarction and has also been demonstrated to inhibit cardiomyocyte hypertrophy directly via the angiotensin type 2 receptor. Ang-(1-9) is produced at enhanced levels in cardiac lysates from heart failure patients. The role of the AngI metabolite Ang-(1-12) in cardiac pathophysiology is still unknown, however it has been shown to be a substrate for the production of AngII and Ang-(1-7) from cardiomyocytes. In this article we will review the current status of knowledge regarding the role of the counter-regulatory RAS in the heart and focus on the future of exciting research in this field which may further our understanding of cardiovascular disease and identify new targets for the development of novel therapies.

INTRODUCTION

The concept of the counter-regulatory renin angiotensin system (RAS) stems from the identification of novel RAS peptide hormones that in general are thought to antagonize the actions of angiotensin II (AngII) in different organs. The counter-regulatory RAS was defined through the initial concept of a local RAS in specific organs and tissues which was based on two fundamental discoveries. First, expression of almost all components of the RAS in specific tissues was highlighted by the recognition that the generation of the final effector peptide AngII could be performed locally and not just via recruitment from the systemic circulation. For example, in the heart a new form of cytosolic renin and angiotensinogen have been shown to be expressed, although the levels are very low compared to those found in the kidney and liver, respectively (Paul *et al.*, 1993). Angiotensin converting enzyme (ACE) expression has also been detected in the myocardium of rats and humans (Hirsch *et al.*, 1991; Paul *et al.*, 1993; Burrell *et al.*, 2005). The presence of endogenous angiotensin I (AngI) and AngII in cardiomyocytes was demonstrated by van Kats *et al.*, who by measuring plasma and tissue levels of infused radiolabeled angiotensin peptides were able to show cardiac synthesis of both AngI and AngII (van Kats *et al.*, 1998). Both the angiotensin type 1 receptor (AT_1R) and the angiotensin type 2 receptor (AT_2R) have also been shown to be expressed in ventricular cardiomyocytes (Booz and Baker, 1996). All these findings suggested that local AngII generation and consequent AngII-mediated signalling could be initiated directly in individual tissues without the requirement for AngII generation from systemic, circulating RAS components. The second discovery was the identification of new novel components of the RAS expressed in specific tissues, predominantly the enzyme angiotensin converting enzyme 2 (ACE 2), a homologue of ACE with different substrate specificity (Donoghue *et al.*, 2000). ACE 2 metabolizes AngII to Angiotensin 1-7 [Ang-(1-7)], decreasing AngII and increasing Ang-(1-7) levels (Donoghue *et al.*, 2000). ACE 2 also converts AngI to Angiotensin 1-9 [Ang-(1-9)], which can be further converted to Ang-(1-7) via ACE-mediated metabolism (Donoghue *et al.*, 2000; Vickers *et al.*, 2002).

There are also alternative routes to form both Ang-(1-7) and Ang-(1-9), AngI can also be cleaved by cathepsin A (CpA) and carboxypeptidase A (Cx A) to form Ang-(1-9) (Kokkonen *et al.*, 1997; Jackman *et al.*, 2002; Garabelli *et al.*, 2008); or by prolyl endopeptidase (POP), neutral endopeptidase (NEP) and thimet oligopeptidase (TOP) to form Ang-(1-7) (Welches *et al.*, 1993; Keidar *et al.*, 2007). Ang-(1-7) has been shown to counteract the actions of AngII mainly via stimulating the protooncogene Mas receptor (Santos *et al.*, 2003). These findings resulted in the theory of a "local and tissue-specific" RAS. Since the recognition of this local tissue-specific RAS many studies have been described in order to elucidate the actions and mechanisms of their components and to attempt to segregate these actions from those mediated by circulating AngII produced via the classical pathway. This has led to the characterization of the physiological and pathophysiological action of the RAS in different organs. A local tissue-specific RAS centred around the ACE2/Ang-(1-7)/Mas axis has been defined in many different organs including the heart, blood vessels, kidney, adrenal gland, nervous system, reproductive system, skin, digestive system, lymphatic and adipose tissue (Figure 1). Thus the ACE 2/Ang-(1-7)/Mas axis has received much recent focus as a potential therapeutic target in cardiovascular disease.

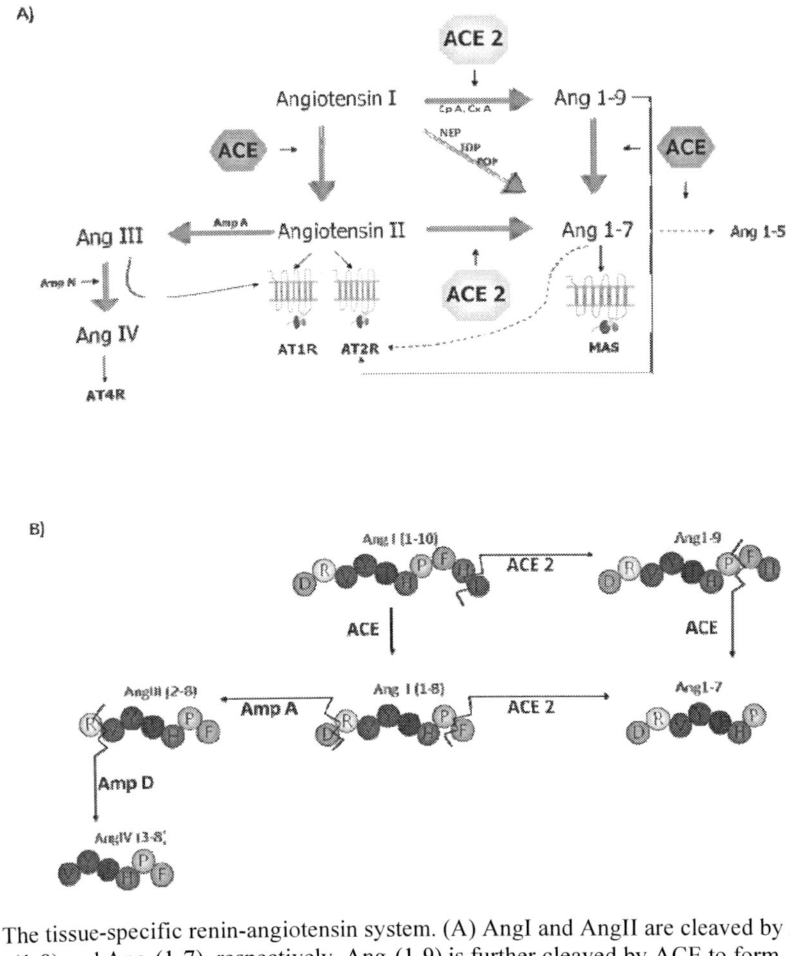

Figure 1. The tissue-specific renin-angiotensin system. (A) AngI and AngII are cleaved by ACE 2 to form Ang-(1-9) and Ang-(1-7), respectively. Ang-(1-9) is further cleaved by ACE to form Ang-(1-7). AngI can also be cleaved by cathepsin A (CpA) and carboxypeptidase A (Cx A) to form Ang-(1-9); or by prolyl endopeptidase (POP), neutral endopeptidase (NEP) and thimet oligopeptidase (TOP) to form Ang-(1-7). Ang-(1-7) is an active peptide that can antagonise AngII signalling whose effects are mediated by the Mas receptor. Ang-(1-7) is further cleaved by ACE to form the inactive peptide metabolite Ang-(1-5). AngII is also converted to AngIII through the cleavage of the N-terminus amino acid by Aminopeptidase A (Amp A). AngIII mediates actions through the AT_1R. AngIII is further cleaved by Aminopeptidase N and transformed into AngIV. AngIV binds to the insulin-regulated aminopeptidase (IRAP). (B) Schematic of angiotensin peptides and cleavage sites via action of different peptidases.

The Cardiac Counter-Regulatory RAS

In order to begin to elucidate the role of the counter-regulatory RAS, the heart has been a major focus of this research in pathophysiologies such as cardiac remodelling following experimental myocardial infarction, ischaemia reperfusion injury, cardiac hypertrophy in aortic banding and AngII infusion models and in heart failure. In these settings Ang-(1-7) and ACE 2 activity have been shown to have clear therapeutic benefit in reversing many of the phenotypes in these models. This chapter reviews the research in this area that has contributed to our current understanding of this counter regulatory RAS in the heart.

Angiotensin Converting Enzyme 2

ACE 2 is a zinc metalloproteinase that acts as a carboxypeptidase (Warner *et al.*, 2004). The gene maps to the X chromosome and has 42% homology with ACE in the catalytic site. ACE 2 is a membrane-bound enzyme expressed mainly in cardiac blood vessels and tubular epithelia of the kidney and testis (Tipnis *et al.*, 2000).

The main action of ACE 2 is the cleavage of the COO-H terminal amino acid from AngI and AngII generating the novel peptides Ang-(1-9) (from AngI) and Ang-(1-7) (from AngII) (Figure 1) (Donoghue *et al.*, 2000; Vickers *et al.*, 2002; Chappel and Ferrario, 2006; Trask *et al.*, 2007). ACE 2 also cleaves des-Arg(9)-bradykinin but not bradykinin and its activity is not affected by ACE inhibitors (Donoghue *et al.*, 2000).

ACE 2 knockout mice have been developed and have a phenotype of severe cardiac dysfunction characterized by decreased myocardial contractility, but however with no signs of cardiac hypertrophy or fibrosis (Crackower *et al.*, 2002). However, in another study in an independently generated strain of ACE 2 knockout mice no effect on cardiac function or size was observed (Gurley *et al.*, 2006). Furthermore, inhibition of ACE 2 in hypertensive rats promoted increased cardiac levels of AngII as well as left ventricular hypertrophy with increased interstitial deposition of collagen (Trask *et al.*, 2010). It has been demonstrated that in a rat model of myocardial infarction the loss of ACE 2 promotes fibroblast proliferation by activating extracellular signal-regulated kinases (ERK) 1/2 and c-Jun kinases (JNK) 1/2, as well as inflammation by increasing neutrophil infiltration to the infarct zone (Kassiri *et al.*, 2009). This in turn leads to an increase in inflammatory components such as cytokines including interleukin (IL) 6, and a deficiency in matrix metalloproteinase (MMP) 2 activity which leads to disruption of the extracellular matrix (Kassiri *et al.*, 2009). It was also found that in these mice the lack of ACE 2 induced the upregulation of hypoxic genes and levels of AngII were increased. In a rat model of myocardial infarction, lentiviral vector-mediated overexpression of ACE 2 also had a protective role by rescuing cardiac function through improved cardiac output, ejection fraction and contractility, as well as reducing left ventricular wall thinning (Der Sarkissian *et al.*, 2008). Furthermore, transfection of fibroblasts with an ACE 2 expression plasmid attenuated collagen and cytokine production (Grobe *et al.*, 2007a). Adenoviral overexpression of ACE 2 in rat heart prior to induction of myocardial infarction reduced myocardial fibrosis with decreased expression of collagen I (Zhao *et al.*, 2010). In similarity to these findings, ACE 2 knockout mice have also been reported to develop defects in conduction and contraction (Crackower *et al.*, 2002) as well as eccentric remodelling and pathological systolic parameters (Bodiga *et al.*, 2011). Furthermore, Zhong *et al.* demonstrated that ACE 2 knockout mice infused with AngII via osmotic minipumps developed more severe fibrosis and cardiac hypertrophy when compared to wild type mice (Zhong *et al.*, 2010). In this model it was also demonstrated that replacement of ACE 2 with osmotic minipump-mediated infusion of recombinant human ACE 2 blocked AngII-induced cardiac fibrosis and expression of collagen I and III. In addition, ACE 2 was able to block phosphorylation of protein kinase C (PKC), ERK1/2 and Janus kinase 2 (Zhong *et al.*, 2010). These studies suggest a protective role for ACE 2 in heart failure. However, other studies have also shown a negative role for ACE 2 activity. For example, Donoghue *et al.* showed that cardiac specific overexpression of ACE 2 in transgenic mice caused severe and progressive malfunction of rhythm and conduction leading to ventricular tachycardia and sudden death (Donoghue *et al.*, 2003). It was also demonstrated that ACE 2 overexpressing transgenic mice had mild interstitial fibrosis. Masson *et al.* also reported induction of severe cardiac fibrosis and deficits in ejection fraction and fractional shortening in stroke prone spontaneously hypertensive rats (SHRSP) overexpressing ACE 2 which was mediated by adeno-associated virus serotype 6 delivery (Masson *et al.*, 2009). In this study ACE 2 increased the expression of collagen type IIIα1, fibronectin and lysyl oxidase genes, suggesting a profibrotic action of ACE 2. In accordance expression of genes involved in cardiac maintenance (apelin, myosin heavy chain II and GATA6) were diminished. Therefore further research is still required to address the true role of ACE 2 in cardiovascular physiology and pathophysiology.

Angiotensin 1-7

Ang-(1-7) is the main effector peptide of the counter-regulatory RAS and its generation is the result of the activity of several different pathways (Figure 1). Ang-(1-7) is a seven amino acid peptide first described to be generated in the endothelium (Santos *et al.*, 1992). Ang-(1-7) is mainly formed by the cleavage of the terminal amino acid of AngII (phenylalanine) by ACE 2 (Garabelli *et al.*, 2008). Alternatively, AngI can be converted into Ang-(1-7), via either cleavage by ACE 2, to form Ang-(1-9) which is then hydrolyzed by ACE transforming it into Ang-(1-7), or by a direct conversion by the action of prolyl endopeptidase, neutral endopeptidase or thimet oligopeptidase (Welches *et al.*, 1993; Keidar *et al.*, 2007; Trask *et al.*, 2007) (Figure 1-3). The half life of Ang-(1-7) in the circulation has been reported to be approximately 10 seconds before it is further cleaved by ACE to form the inactive metabolite Ang-(1-5) (Chappell *et al.*, 1998; Yamada *et al.*, 1998). In normal conditions the circulating levels of Ang-(1-7) are much lower than AngII (20.1 pg/mL versus 47 pg/mL, respectively) (Yamada *et al.*, 1998; Vilas-Boas *et al.*, 2009). Ang-(1-7) mediates most of its effects through engaging the orphan Mas proto-oncogene (Santos *et al.*, 2003). The interest in Ang-(1-7) comes from the fact that it is able to antagonize many of the effects of AngII. Roks *et al.* demonstrated for the first time that in human blood vessels Ang-(1-7) inhibited AngII-induced vasoconstriction (Roks *et al.*, 1999). Ang-(1-7) has also been shown to mediate vasodilatation, as well as a producing antiproliferative, anti-inflammatory and cardioprotective effects.

Ang-(1-7) was originally proposed to mediate its effects via the classical AngII receptors in peripheral arterioles (Kono *et al.*, 1986). However, Santos *et al.* generated Mas-knockout mice and showed through a radioligand binding assay in rat kidneys a lack of Ang-(1-7) binding (Santos *et al.*, 2003). In addition chinese hamster ovary (CHO) cells were transfected with Mas cDNA and fluorescent labelled Ang-(1-7) was shown to bind to the receptor, confirming that Ang-(1-7) bound to this orphan G-protein coupled receptor (Santos *et al.*, 2003). The gene encoding the Mas receptor has been mapped to the distal half of chromosome 6q and encodes for a 325 amino acid protein (Alenina *et al.*, 2008). Its distribution is tissue-specific and it is expressed largely in the brain, but is also found in the testis, heart and kidney (Metzger *et al.*, 1995). Many studies have been carried out to demonstrate that the effects of Ang-(1-7) are mediated via Mas and much of this work has been produced via the use of the peptide antagonist of the Mas receptor, A779 (Santos *et al.*, 1994).

Although the role of Mas in Ang-(1-7) function is well established the existence of crosstalk between Mas and other angiotensin and bradykinin receptors has also been reported (Soares de Moura *et al.*, 2004; Castro *et al.*, 2005; Kostenis *et al.*, 2005). Castro *et al.* showed differences in perfusion pressure when stimulating Mas with Ang-(1-7) in the presence or absence of AT_1R and AT_2R antagonists, suggesting crosstalk between the three receptors (Castro *et al.*, 2005). In $Mas^{-/-}$ mice the changes in perfusion pressure were not seen. In CHO-K1 cells overexpression of Mas and AT_1R demonstrated an interaction between the two receptors (Kostenis *et al.*, 2005). In the presence of both receptors the initial AngII-induced production of inositol phosphate and intracellular calcium (Ca^{2+}) mobilization decreased approximately 50%, suggesting that Mas acted as an antagonist of the AT_1R. However, it has also been suggested that Mas expression upregulates AT_1R expression and activates PKC (Canals *et al.*, 2006). Furthermore, an interaction between Mas and the bradykinin B_2 receptor has also been shown as relaxation of mesenteric arteries in $Mas^{-/-}$ mice is abolished both basally and when stimulated with bradykinin (Peiro *et al.*, 2007). Soares de Moura *et al.* demonstrated that both Mas and the AT_2R enhanced the vasodilator effect of the bradykinin B_2 receptor (Soares de Moura *et al.*, 2004).

Ang-(1-7) has also been reported to be produced in the heart via either AngI or AngII (Wei *et al.*, 2002; Zisman *et al.*, 2003). Several authors have described Ang-(1-7) as a regulator of the cardiac conduction system (Ferreira *et al.*, 2001; De Mello *et al.*, 2007; Castro-Chaves *et al.*, 2009; Stewart *et al.*, 2009). For example, it has been described that in induced ischaemia in rat hearts Ang-(1-7) reduces the incidence of arrhythmias after reperfusion compared to AngII perfused hearts (Ferreira *et al.*, 2001), as well as inducing vasodilatation in postural tachycardia syndrome (Stewart *et al.*, 2009). De Mello *et al.* showed that in cardiomyocytes exposed to Ang-(1-7) the cardiac action potential was reduced and there was an increase in conduction velocity due to the activation of the sodium pump, assigning Ang-(1-7) antiarrhythmic properties (De Mello *et al.*, 2007). Interestingly, when cardiomyocytes were exposed to higher doses of Ang-(1-7) (10^{-7}M) the action potential was not decreased, but in fact augmented, as well as producing early-after depolarisations, leading to promotion of arrhythmias. In rabbit papillary muscle Ang-(1-7) has been shown to reduce muscle contraction (Castro-Chaves *et al.*, 2009). Relaxation was related to the integrity of endocardial endothelium, suggesting that Ang-(1-7) has negative inotropic effects mediated through endothelium. However, the effects of Ang-(1-7) were completely abolished when cardiac papillary muscle was incubated with the Mas antagonist A779. Using a long-term atrial tachycardia model in dogs, Liu *et al.* showed that infusion of Ang-(1-7) prevented increased ERK1/2 expression and activity and interstitial fibrosis in canine hearts, as well as reducing the inducibility and duration of atrial tachycardia (Liu *et al.*, 2010) (Figure 2).

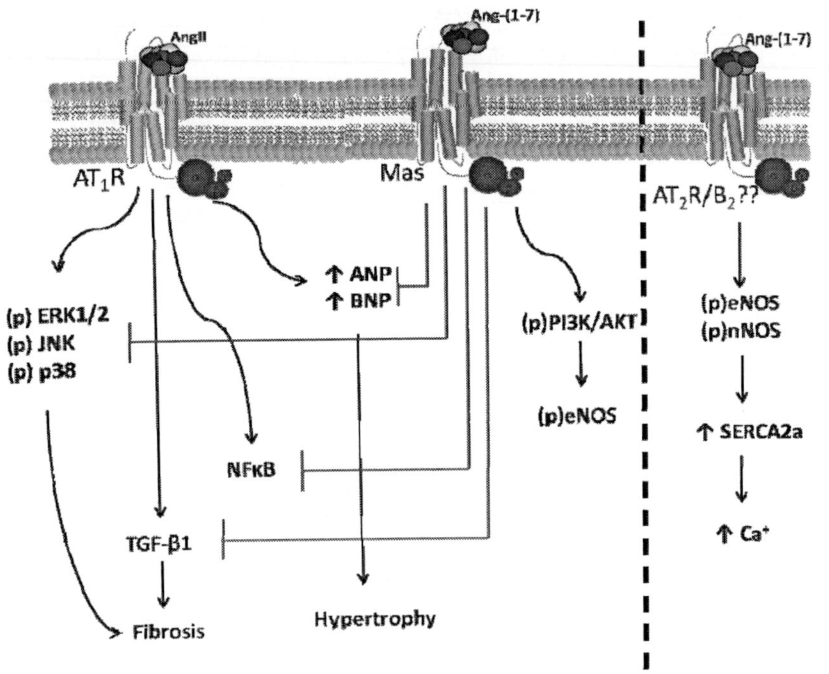

Figure 2. Ang-(1-7) actions in cardiac remodelling. Ang-(1-7) through coupling to the Mas receptor blocks the AngII-induced cardiac phosphorylation of ERK1/2, JNK and p38. Ang-(1-7) also decreases the levels of NF-κB, reduces TGF-β levels and blocks the increase in ANP and BNP resulting in reduced myocyte hypertrophy and cardiac interstitial fibrosis. Ang-(1-7) also increases endothelial nitric oxide synthase (eNOS) phosphorylation due to mediated activation of the phosphoinositide 3 kinase (PI3K)/Akt signalling pathway. Ang-(1-7) can also modulate Ca^{2+} handling by increasing nitric oxide and eNOS activity leading to activation of the sarcoplasmic endoreticulum calcium ATPase (SERCA2a) through an AT_2R/bradykinin B_2 receptor-dependent mechanism.

In the heart it has been shown that Ang-(1-7) can regulate many growth cell signalling pathways (Ferreira and Santos, 2005) (Figure 2). In Sprague-Dawley rats co-infusion of AngII and Ang-(1-7) blocked the cardiac phosphorylation of ERK1/2 and Rho kinases induced by AngII alone and furthermore the effects of Ang-(1-7) were abolished in the presence of the Mas antagonist A779 (Giani *et al.*, 2007). Interestingly, Ang-(1-7) also activated signal transducer and activator of transcription (STAT) 3 and STAT5a/b in the heart in this study. However this effect was not abolished by A779, but, however, was by an AT_1R antagonist suggesting its involvement in this setting. Ang-(1-7) has also been shown to have a role in recovery following ischaemia/reperfusion injury (Castro *et al.*, 2006; Zhang *et al.*, 2008; Al-Maghrebi *et al.*, 2009). In rat models of myocardial infarction (left coronary artery ligation), infusion of Ang-(1-7) has been demonstrated to prevent left ventricular deterioration (Loot *et al.*, 2002). In this same study endothelium-dependent relaxation in isolated aortic rings of rats infused with Ang-(1-7) was improved demonstrating a preservation of the endothelial function. Ang-(1-7) blocked the deterioration in aortic relaxation by preserving endothelial function when compared to rats subjected to myocardial infarction alone. Al-Maghrebi *et al* treated diabetic rats with Ang-(1-7) before inducing ischemia and demonstrated recovery of left ventricular function after ischemia, an effect that was abolished by the co-infusion of A779 (Al-Maghrebi *et al.*, 2009). At the molecular level Ang-(1-7) decreased the levels of nuclear factor κB (NF-κB) (Figure 2) and the expression of genes required for activation of NF-κB; including toll-like receptor 2, IL-1 receptor associated kinase 1 and inhibitor of kappa B kinase (Al-Maghrebi *et al.*, 2009). Furthermore, an inhibitory effect for Ang-(1-7) in inflammatory pathways was demonstrated as it reduced expression of complement component C3, IL-1β, IL-6 and caspase 1.

Many authors have confirmed that Ang-(1-7) has some effect on at least one of the components of cardiac remodelling. Grobe *et al.* demonstrated reduced myocyte hypertrophy, interstitial fibrosis and transforming growth factor beta (TGF-β) levels in response to Ang-(1-7) in an Ang II-induced rat model of hypertension and cardiac remodeling (Grobe *et al.*, 2007b). These effects of Ang-(1-7) were also blocked in the presence of A779, and were independent of effects on blood pressure. Studies with transgenic mice overexpressing Ang-(1-7) in the heart have shown that in the presence of AngII hypertrophy and fibrosis of the left ventricle is reduced, as well as expression of the hypertrophy markers atrial natriuretic peptide (ANP) and brain natriuretic peptide (BNP), and TGF-β1 (Mercure *et al.*, 2008) (Figure 2). In these mice Ang-(1-7) had no effect on AngII-induced ERK1/2 phosphorylation but reduced AngII-induced phosphorylation of c-Src and p38 kinases. One important finding was the fact that Ang-(1-7), both in the presence or absence of AngII, increased the levels of Src homology 2 domain containing phosphatase 1 (SHP-1) protein (Mercure *et al.*, 2008). However, Giani *et al.* showed decreased phosphorylation levels of ERK1/2, JNK1/2 and p38 in heart of high fructose-fed rats when infused chronically with Ang-(1-7) (Giani *et al.*, 2010). Dias-Peixoto *et al.* investigated the molecular mechanisms of the actions of Ang-(1-7) in cardiac hypertrophy (Dias-Peixoto *et al.*, 2008). An increase in nitric oxide (NO) phosphorylation due to Ang-(1-7)-mediated activation of the phosphoinositide 3 kinase (PI3K)/Akt signalling pathway was observed and these actions were blocked by co-treatment with A779, confirming the importance of Mas. Ang-(1-7) also promoted the phosphorylation of endothelial nitric oxide synthase (eNOS) at Ser177 which augmented enzyme activity (Figure 2). Furthermore, this study showed that in cardiomyocytes of Mas knockout ($Mas^{-/-}$) mice a lack of NO production due to decreased Akt activity, led to decreased phosphorylation of eNOS at Ser177 and therefore decreased activation (Dias-Peixoto *et al.*, 2008). Caveolin-3 expression, which inhibits basal activity of eNOS, was also increased; and heat shock protein 90 (Hsp90) (a scaffold protein which recruits Akt) was also decreased. Furthermore in normal cardiomyocytes Ang-(1-7) was not able to produce changes in Ca^{2+} transient parameters but curiously in $Mas^{-/-}$ cardiomyocytes Ang-(1-7) showed a smaller peak in the intracellular Ca^{2+} transient and slower Ca^{2+} kinetics, which was explained by a decreased expression of the sarcoplasmic reticulum Ca^{2+} ATPase (SERCA2a) (Dias-Peixoto *et al.*, 2008). This suggests that Ang-(1-7) modulates Ca^{2+} handling by increasing eNOS activity and NO production, leading to activation of SERCA2a (Figure 2). In accordance with this Costa *et al.* showed that infusion of Ang-(1-7) in hypertensive rats increased NOS activity and eNOS and neuronal nitric oxide synthase (nNOS) phosphorylation in the ventricle. Interestingly, this effect was mediated by an AT_2R/bradykinin B_2 receptor-dependent mechanism and not by Mas (Costa *et al.*, 2010) (Figure 2).

Models of transgenic rats overexpressing Ang-(1-7) either systemically or in the heart have also been utilised to dissect the function of Ang-(1-7). In 2004 Santos *et al.*, created a transgenic rat model expressing an Ang-(1-7)-producing protein. This resulted in high levels of circulating Ang-(1-7) (Santos et al, 2004). This protein was able to over-express Ang-(1-7) due to the unique design of its conformation consisting of a signal peptide from human prorenin linked to a portion of the mouse heavy chain constant region immunoglobulin (Ig)G, a design originally reported for the transgenic overexpression of AngII (van Kats *et al.*, 2001). This is followed by a portion of the human prorenin prosegment containing a cleavage site for furin protease and finally the biologically active Ang-(1-7). Finally this fusion protein was put under the control of the cytomegalovirus (CMV) promoter/enhancer (Santos *et al.*, 2004). By using transgenic rats that overexpressed Ang-(1-7) systemically in a deoxycorticosterone acetate-salt hypertension model, Santiago *et al.* showed a block in the development of cardiac hypertrophy and a decrease in expression of collagen I and III in these transgenic rats (Santiago *et al.*, 2010). Using the same fusion protein but this time under the control of the α-myosin heavy chain promoter/enhancer, Ferreira *et al.*, overexpressed Ang-(1-7) specifically in the heart of rats (Ferreira *et al.*, 2010). Using these transgenic rats in a isoproterenol infusion model of hypertrophy and fibrosis, Ang-(1-7) reduced deposition of collagen III and fibronectin without affecting blood pressure (Ferreira *et al.*, 2010).

Similar approaches have also been used to deliver Ang-(1-7) via somatic gene transfer through the use of viral gene transfer vectors. For example, direct lentiviral vector-mediated delivery of Ang-(1-7) into the left ventricle of a rat model of myocardial infarction led to improved cardiac function and remodelling as well as increased expression of ACE 2 and bradykinin B_2 receptors and decreased expression of tumor necrosis factor alpha (TNF-α) and IL-6 (Qi *et al.*, 2011).

Although in general Ang-(1-7) has been shown to be protective Velkoska *et al.* reported similar effects of Ang-(1-7) to those observed following AngII infusion, including increased blood pressure, cardiac hypertrophy and fibrosis in nephrectomised rats infused via osmotic minipumps with Ang-(1-7) (Velkoska *et al.*, 2011). However, to date this is the only study to demonstrate these adverse findings.

In cardiac fibrosis, exposure of AngII-stimulated cardiac fibroblasts to Ang-(1-7) inhibited collagen synthesis and expression of the growth factors endothelin-1 and leukaemia inhibitory factor (Iwata *et al.*, 2005). It was also described that Ang-(1-7) normalises the decreased levels of MMPs in AngII-stimulated cardiac fibroblasts and myocytes (Pan *et al.*, 2008). In human cardiac fibroblasts, Ang-(1-7) has been reported to increase expression of ACE 2 through Mas signalling (Lin *et al.*, 2010). In addition, Grobe *et al.* showed that Ang-(1-7) was able to prevent interstitial fibrosis by decreasing collagen deposition in the deoxycorticosterone acetate (DOCA) salt hypertensive rat model (Grobe *et al.*, 2006). In this model Ang-(1-7) did not prevent the increase in ventricular mass or myocyte diameter, or have any effect on blood pressure. In nephrectomised mice Ang-(1-7) infusion prevented left ventricular remodelling and preserved cardiac function, and also diminished interstitial fibrosis by reducing the levels of TGF-β and increasing MMP2 and 9 (Li *et al.*, 2009). Ang-(1-7) also decreased the expression levels of inflammatory cytokines and suppressed oxidative damage (Li *et al.*, 2009).

$Mas^{-/-}$ mice have been generated and have contributed to the knowledge of the actions of Ang-(1-7) in the heart (Lemos *et al.*, 2005). For example, Santos *et al.* characterized the phenotype of $Mas^{-/-}$ mice and showed lower global ventricular function (Santos *et al.*, 2006). Lack of Mas caused a decrease in systolic tension and heart rate, as well as left ventricular posterior wall thickness and decreased fractional shortening. At a molecular level, $Mas^{-/-}$ mice demonstrate increased expression of type I and III collagen and fibronectin, while type IV collagen expression was decreased. In accordance with these findings, Castro et al showed a decrease in cardiac contractility in Mas$^{-/-}$ mice (Castro *et al.*, 2006).

Angiotensin 1-9

Ang-(1-9) is a 9 amino acid peptide that results from the metabolism of AngI by ACE 2 as ACE 2 cleaves the terminal amino acid leucine of AngI and transforms it into Ang-(1-9) (Donoghue *et al.*, 2000; Li *et al.*, 2005) (Figure 1). Although ACE 2 is the main enzyme to form Ang-(1-9), it has also been reported that following incubation of AngI with human heart homogenates Ang-(1-9) is generated. Kokkonen *et al.* showed that incubation of AngI with heart homogenates generated AngII through cardiac chymase and ACE and Ang-(1-9) through the activity of carboxypeptidase A (Kokkonen *et al.*, 1997) (Figure 1). In addition, the same study reported a strong inhibition of AngII formation due to the generation of Ang-(1-9). Formation of Ang-(1-9) was also confirmed in ACE$^{-/-}$ and ACE 2$^{-/-}$ null mice where Ang-(1-9) was the main product of AngI following its cleavage by carboxypeptidase A (Garabelli *et al.*, 2008). These reports showed that formation of Ang-(1-9) from AngI is the main pathway in cardiomyocytes as well as suggesting for the first time that Ang-(1-9) was an active peptide and could mediate effects as an endogenous inhibitor of AngII generation (Kokkonen *et al.*, 1997; Garabelli *et al.*, 2008). Furthermore, Jackman *et al.* showed that the conversion of AngI to Ang-(1-9) can also occur through the action of cathepsin A in human heart extracts (Jackman *et al.*, 2002). Once Ang-(1-9) is formed ACE cleaves the 2 N-terminal amino acids (phenylalanine and histidine) generating Ang-(1-7) (Figure 1). Little is currently known about Ang-(1-9). Ang-(1-9) has also been reported to be a competitive inhibitor of ACE because it is an ACE substrate at the same catalytic site as AngI (Snyder and Wintroub, 1986). Ang-(1-9) has also been reported to potentiate bradykinin B_2 receptor activity 3-fold, by enhancing the release of arachidonic acid in human atria and ventricles induced by a B_2 agonist (Erdos *et al.*, 2002). Ang-(1-9) also enhances intracellular Ca^{2+} concentration and NO synthesis triggered by exposure of endothelial cells to bradykinin by 2.4-fold (Erdos *et al.*, 2002). Importantly, these studies also showed that Ang-(1-9) was an active peptide and that it was a more potent in potentiating the effects of bradykinin than Ang-(1-7) (Erdos *et al.*, 2002; Jackman *et al.*, 2002).

Recent work investigating Ang-(1-9) function has revealed it may also play a role in the counter-regulatory RAS. For example, Ang-(1-9) was demonstrated to block cardiac hypertrophy in a rat myocardial infarction model (Ocaranza *et al.*, 2010). Ocaranza *et al.* delivered Ang-(1-9) via osmotic minipumps and showed attenuation of cardiac hypertrophy when compared to control rats. Furthermore, this effect was maintained when co-infused with the Mas blocker A779, suggesting no transformation to Ang-(1-7) was needed for Ang-(1-9) to block hypertrophy.

Additionally, these authors reported an increase in Ang-(1-9) plasma levels when rats which had undergone myocardial infarction were infused with AT_1R blockers or ACE inhibitors, suggesting that Ang-(1-9) may be an endogenous component of the counter-regulatory RAS. Flores-Muñoz *et al.* have also demonstrated anti-hypertrophic effects in cardiomyocytes with Ang1-9 (Flores-Muñoz, 2011). Incubation of rat neonatal and adult rabbit cardiomyocytes with Ang-(1-9) blocked AngII and arg-vasopressin-induced hypertrophy. Moreover, incubation with the ACE inhibitor captopril or A779 had no effect over the anti-hypertrophic effect of Ang-(1-9) (Flores-Muñoz *et al.*, 2011). Importantly, using adenoviral over-expression of the AT_2R in HeLa cells, Flores-Muñoz *et al.* have shown that Ang-(1-9) is able to displace radiolabeled AngII from binding at the AT_2R (Flores-Muñoz *et al.*, 2011) and that the anti-hypertrophic effects of Ang-(1-9) were inhibited only in the presence of the selective AT_2R antagonist PD123,319, indicating that Ang-(1-9) may be an endogenous functional AT_2R ligand. Both these studies have shown Ang-(1-9) having direct effects and distinguishable from Ang-(1-7). Furthermore, Ocaranza *et al.* have also reported that inhibition of Rho kinase in deoxycorticosterone acetate-salt hypertensive rats significantly increased Ang-(1-9) plasma levels, suggesting that inhibition of the prohypertrophic Rho signalling pathway may be implicated in the effects of Ang-(1-9) (Ocaranza *et al.*, 2011).

This is the first study to elucidate potential downstream signalling partners of Ang-(1-9), which will be an important area for future research.

Angiotensin 1-12

Ang-(1-12) is one of the most recent novel RAS peptides to be described. The structure of Ang-(1-12) contains 2 extra amino acids (leucine and tyrosine) at the C-terminal compared to Ang I (12 amino acids in total). Therefore, Ang-(1-12) is thought to be derived from angiotensinogen since their structure is similar (Nagata *et al.*, 2006). Ang-(1-12) was found to be ubiquitously present in different tissues including heart, aorta, brain and kidneys.

Interestingly, levels of Ang-(1-12) in plasma were lower than the levels in tissue, suggesting Ang-(1-12) may be part of a local RAS and produced directly in tissues. Furthermore, when incubating rat aortic rings with Ang-(1-12), Nagata *et al.* reported dose dependent vasoconstriction, an effect that was abolished in the presence of ACE inhibitors or AT_1R blockers, suggesting Ang-(1-12) may be a tissue substrate to form AngII (Nagata *et al.*, 2006; Jessup *et al.*, 2008). Furthermore, it has also been reported that Ang-(1-12) is present at significantly higher levels in the hearts of hypertensive rats than normotensive rats (Jessup *et al.*, 2008) and that this peptide is rapidly metabolized into AngI, AngII and Ang-(1-7) by ACE and neprilysin (Trask *et al.*, 2008). All these data contribute to initial definition of Ang-(1-12) as a new member of the counter-regulatory RAS system, however it still remains poorly characterised.

Other Angiotensin Peptide Metabolites

Angiotensin III (2-8)

Angiotensin III (AngIII) is generated via the cleavage of the N-terminal amino acid of AngII (aspartic acid) by aminopeptidase A (Zini *et al.*, 1996) (Figure 1). AngIII has been reported to signal through the AT_1R, however, its affinity for the AT_1R is 10 times lower than AngII and to have similar actions to AngII in the brain (Pendleton *et al.*, 1989). For example, infusion of AngIII to rat brains stimulated release of vasopressin (Yamaguchi *et al.*, 1979;

Hohle *et al.*, 1995; Reaux *et al.*, 2001), suggesting that AngIII may be an active metabolite of the RAS in the brain.

Angiotensin IV (3-8)

Angiotensin IV (AngIV) is formed from the cleavage of AngIII at the N-terminus amino acid by aminopeptidase N and was originally considered to be an inactive peptide. However, it has been shown that this peptide binds with high affinity to the insulin-regulated aminopeptidase (IRAP) (Swanson *et al.*, 1992; Albiston *et al.*, 2001) (Figure 1). The distribution of IRAP is tissue-specific, being mainly expressed in different areas of the brain (Chai *et al.*, 2000), in the heart, adrenal cortex, kidney and vascular smooth muscle cells (de Gasparo *et al.*, 2000). AngIV has been shown to have a role in the cognitive and sensory functions of the brain such as memory and locomotor behaviour (Braszko *et al.*, 1988; Wright *et al.*, 1993).

Conclusion

The RAS is integral to the normal physiology of the cardiovascular system and furthermore its dysregulation is important in the development of many cardiovascular diseases. A clear role for AngII acting via the AT_1R to activate downstream cell signalling pathways has been established. These downstream effects are pleiotropic and occur in many different cells and tissues including smooth muscle cells, endothelial cells, fibroblasts and cardiomyocytes. However, there still remain many unanswered questions regarding the integrated function of the RAS. The ACE 2/Ang-(1-7)/ Mas axis is well established as being central to the counter-regulatory RAS and its function in the heart is able to inhibit many of the pathophysiological effects of cardiovascular disease. Other peptide metabolites of the RAS such as Ang-(1-9) and Ang-(1-12) may also play a role in cardiovascular disease development and also be effectors of the counter-regulatory RAS. However, there still remains a great deal to investigate to increase our understanding in this important area of research. Although cell signalling mechanisms for Ang-(1-7) via Mas are beginning to be reported, there is still a lack of knowledge of the molecular mechanisms of action and very little known about the effects of other peptides. Translational data is also lacking and detailed knowledge of the levels of different counter regulatory RAS components and how they change in clinical cardiovascular disease will be key to fully defining this important research area as an avenue for future research in the development of next generation cardiovascular therapeutic interventions.

References

Al-Maghrebi M, Benter IF and Diz DI. (2009). Endogenous angiotensin-(1-7) reduces cardiac ischemia-induced dysfunction in diabetic hypertensive rats. *Pharmacol. Res* 59, 263-268.

Albiston AL, McDowall SG, Matsacos D, Sim P, Clune E, Mustafa T, Lee J, Mendelsohn FA, Simpson RJ, Connolly LM and Chai SY. (2001). Evidence that the angiotensin IV (AT(4)) receptor is the enzyme insulin-regulated aminopeptidase. *J. Biol. Chem.* 276, 48623-48626.

Alenina N, Xu P, Rentzsch B, Patkin EL and Bader M. (2008). Genetically altered animal models for Mas and angiotensin-(1-7). *Exp. Physiol.* 93, 528-537.

Bodiga S, Zhong JC, Wang W, Basu R, Lo J, Liu GC, Guo D, Holland SM, Scholey JW, Penninger JM, Kassiri Z and Oudit GY. (2011). Enhanced susceptibility to biomechanical stress in ACE2 null mice is prevented by loss of the p47phox NADPH oxidase subunit. *Cardiovasc. Res.* 91, 151-161.

Booz GW and Baker KM. (1996). Role of type 1 and type 2 angiotensin receptors in angiotensin II-induced cardiomyocyte hypertrophy. *Hypertension* 28, 635-640.

Braszko JJ, Kupryszewski G, Witczuk B and Wisniewski K. (1988). Angiotensin II-(3-8)-hexapeptide affects motor activity, performance of passive avoidance and a conditioned avoidance response in rats. *Neuroscience* 27, 777-783.

Burrell LM, Risvanis J, Kubota E, Dean RG, MacDonald PS, Lu S, Tikellis C, Grant SL, Lew RA, Smith AI, Cooper ME and Johnston CI. (2005). Myocardial infarction increases ACE2 expression in rat and humans. *Eur Heart J* 26, 369-375; discussion 322-364.

Canals M, Jenkins L, Kellett E and Milligan G. (2006). Up-regulation of the angiotensin II type 1 receptor by the MAS proto-oncogene is due to constitutive activation of Gq/G11 by MAS. *J. Biol. Chem.* 281, 16757-16767.

Castro-Chaves P, Pintalhao M, Fontes-Carvalho R, Cerqueira R and Leite-Moreira AF. (2009). Acute modulation of myocardial function by angiotensin 1-7. *Peptides* 30, 1714-1719.

Castro CH, Santos RA, Ferreira AJ, Bader M, Alenina N and Almeida AP. (2005). Evidence for a functional interaction of the angiotensin-(1-7) receptor Mas with AT1 and AT2 receptors in the mouse heart. *Hypertension* 46, 937-942.

Castro CH, Santos RA, Ferreira AJ, Bader M, Alenina N and Almeida AP. (2006). Effects of genetic deletion of angiotensin-(1-7) receptor Mas on cardiac function during ischemia/reperfusion in the isolated perfused mouse heart. *Life Sci.* 80, 264-268.

Chai SY, Bastias MA, Clune EF, Matsacos DJ, Mustafa T, Lee JH, McDowall SG, Paxinos G, Mendelsohn FA and Albiston AL. (2000). Distribution of angiotensin IV binding sites (AT4 receptor) in the human forebrain, midbrain and pons as visualised by in vitro receptor autoradiography. *J Chem. Neuroanat* 20, 339-348.

Chappel MC and Ferrario CM. (2006). ACE and ACE2: their role to balance the expression of angiotensin II and angiotensin-(1-7). *Kidney Int.* 70, 8-10.

Chappell MC, Pirro NT, Sykes A and Ferrario CM. (1998). Metabolism of angiotensin-(1-7) by angiotensin-converting enzyme. *Hypertension* 31, 362-367.

Costa MA, Lopez Verrilli MA, Gomez KA, Nakagawa P, Pena C, Arranz C and Gironacci MM. (2010). Angiotensin-(1-7) upregulates cardiac nitric oxide synthase in spontaneously hypertensive rats. *Am. J. Physiol. Heart Circ. Physiol.* 299, H1205-1211.

Crackower MA, Sarao R, Oudit GY, Yagil C, Kozieradzki I, Scanga SE, Oliveira-dos-Santos AJ, da Costa J, Zhang L, Pei Y, Scholey J, Ferrario CM, Manoukian AS, Chappell MC, Backx PH, Yagil Y and Penninger JM. (2002). Angiotensin-converting enzyme 2 is an essential regulator of heart function. *Nature* 417, 822-828.

de Gasparo M, Catt KJ, Inagami T, Wright JW and Unger T. (2000). International union of pharmacology. XXIII. The angiotensin II receptors. *Pharmacol. Rev.* 52, 415-472.

De Mello WC, Ferrario CM and Jessup JA. (2007). Beneficial versus harmful effects of Angiotensin (1-7) on impulse propagation and cardiac arrhythmias in the failing heart. *J. Renin Angiotensin Aldosterone Syst* 8, 74-80.

Der Sarkissian S, Grobe JL, Yuan L, Narielwala DR, Walter GA, Katovich MJ and Raizada MK. (2008). Cardiac overexpression of angiotensin converting enzyme 2 protects the heart from ischemia-induced pathophysiology. *Hypertension* 51, 712-718.

Dias-Peixoto MF, Santos RA, Gomes ER, Alves MN, Almeida PW, Greco L, Rosa M, Fauler B, Bader M, Alenina N and Guatimosim S. (2008). Molecular mechanisms involved in the angiotensin-(1-7)/Mas signaling pathway in cardiomyocytes. *Hypertension* 52, 542-548.

Donoghue M, Hsieh F, Baronas E, Godbout K, Gosselin M, Stagliano N, Donovan M, Woolf B, Robison K, Jeyaseelan R, Breitbart RE and Acton S. (2000). A novel angiotensin-converting enzyme-related carboxypeptidase (ACE2) converts angiotensin I to angiotensin 1-9. *Circ. Res.* 87, E1-9.

Donoghue M, Wakimoto H, Maguire CT, Acton S, Hales P, Stagliano N, Fairchild-Huntress V, Xu J, Lorenz JN, Kadambi V, Berul CI and Breitbart RE. (2003). Heart block, ventricular tachycardia, and sudden death in ACE2 transgenic mice with downregulated connexins. *J. Mol Cell Cardiol* 35, 1043-1053.

Erdos EG, Jackman HL, Brovkovych V, Tan F and Deddish PA. (2002). Products of angiotensin I hydrolysis by human cardiac enzymes potentiate bradykinin. *J. Mol. Cell Cardiol.* 34, 1569-1576.

Ferreira AJ and Santos RA. (2005). Cardiovascular actions of angiotensin-(1-7). *Braz J. Med. Biol. Res.* 38, 499-507.

Ferreira AJ, Santos RA and Almeida AP. (2001). Angiotensin-(1-7): cardioprotective effect in myocardial ischemia/reperfusion. *Hypertension* 38, 665-668.

Ferreira AJ, Shenoy V, Qi Y, Fraga-Silva RA, Santos RA, Katovich MJ and Raizada MK. (2010). Angiotensin-converting enzyme 2 activation protects against hypertension-induced cardiac fibrosis involving extracellular signal-regulated kinases. *Exp. Physiol.* 96, 287-294.

Flores-Muñoz M, Smith NJ, Haggerty C, Milligan G and Nicklin SA. (2011). Angiotensin1-9 antagonises pro-hypertrophic signalling in cardiomyocytes via the angiotensin type 2 receptor. *J. Physiol.* 589, 939-951.

Garabelli PJ, Modrall JG, Penninger JM, Ferrario CM and Chappell MC. (2008). Distinct roles for angiotensin-converting enzyme 2 and carboxypeptidase A in the processing of angiotensins within the murine heart. *Exp. Physiol.* 93, 613-621.

Giani JF, Gironacci MM, Munoz MC, Pena C, Turyn D and Dominici FP. (2007). Angiotensin-(1 7) stimulates the phosphorylation of JAK2, IRS-1 and Akt in rat heart in vivo: role of the AT1 and Mas receptors. *Am. J. Physiol. Heart Circ. Physiol.* 293, H1154-1163.

Giani JF, Munoz MC, Mayer MA, Veiras LC, Arranz C, Taira CA, Turyn D, Toblli JE and Dominici FP. (2010). Angiotensin-(1-7) improves cardiac remodeling and inhibits growth-promoting pathways in the heart of fructose-fed rats. *Am. J. Physiol Heart Circ. Physiol.* 298, H1003-1013.

Grobe JL, Der Sarkissian S, Stewart JM, Meszaros JG, Raizada MK and Katovich MJ. (2007a). ACE2 overexpression inhibits hypoxia-induced collagen production by cardiac fibroblasts. *Clin. Sci .(Lond)* 113, 357-364.

Grobe JL, Mecca AP, Lingis M, Shenoy V, Bolton TA, Machado JM, Speth RC, Raizada MK and Katovich MJ. (2007b). Prevention of angiotensin II-induced cardiac remodeling by angiotensin-(1-7). *Am. J. Physiol. Heart Circ. Physiol.* 292, H736-742.

Grobe JL, Mecca AP, Mao H and Katovich MJ. (2006). Chronic angiotensin-(1-7) prevents cardiac fibrosis in DOCA-salt model of hypertension. *Am. J. Physiol. Heart Circ. Physiol* 290, H2417-2423.

Gurley SB, Allred A, Le TH, Griffiths R, Mao L, Philip N, Haystead TA, Donoghue M, Breitbart RE, Acton SL, Rockman HA and Coffman TM. (2006). Altered blood pressure responses and normal cardiac phenotype in ACE2-null mice. *J. Clin. Invest* 116, 2218-2225.

Hirsch AT, Talsness CE, Schunkert H, Paul M and Dzau VJ. (1991). Tissue-specific activation of cardiac angiotensin converting enzyme in experimental heart failure. *Circ. Res.* 69, 475-482.

Hohle S, Spitznagel H, Rascher W, Culman J and Unger T. (1995). Angiotensin AT1 receptor-mediated vasopressin release and drinking are potentiated by an AT2 receptor antagonist. *Eur. J. Pharmacol* 275, 277-282.

Iwata M, Cowling RT, Gurantz D, Moore C, Zhang S, Yuan JX and Greenberg BH. (2005). Angiotensin-(1-7) binds to specific receptors on cardiac fibroblasts to initiate antifibrotic and antitrophic effects. *Am. J. Physiol. Heart Circ. Physiol.* 289, H2356-2363.

Jackman HL, Massad MG, Sekosan M, Tan F, Brovkovych V, Marcic BM and Erdos EG. (2002). Angiotensin 1-9 and 1-7 release in human heart: role of cathepsin A. *Hypertension* 39, 976-981.

Jessup JA, Trask AJ, Chappell MC, Nagata S, Kato J, Kitamura K and Ferrario CM. (2008). Localization of the novel angiotensin peptide, angiotensin-(1-12), in heart and kidney of hypertensive and normotensive rats. *Am. J. Physiol. Heart Circ. Physiol.* 294, H2614-2618.

Kassiri Z, Zhong J, Guo D, Basu R, Wang X, Liu PP, Scholey JW, Penninger JM and Oudit GY. (2009). Loss of angiotensin-converting enzyme 2 accelerates maladaptive left ventricular remodeling in response to myocardial infarction. *Circ. Heart Fail* 2, 446-455.

Keidar S, Kaplan M and Gamliel-Lazarovich A. (2007). ACE2 of the heart: From angiotensin I to angiotensin (1-7). *Cardiovasc. Res.* 73, 463-469.

Kokkonen JO, Saarinen J and Kovanen PT. (1997). Regulation of local angiotensin II formation in the human heart in the presence of interstitial fluid. Inhibition of chymase by protease inhibitors of interstitial fluid and of angiotensin-converting enzyme by Ang-(1-9) formed by heart carboxypeptidase A-like activity. *Circulation* 95, 1455-1463.

Kono T, Taniguchi A, Imura H, Oseko F and Khosla MC. (1986). Biological activities of angiotensin II-(1-6)-hexapeptide and angiotensin II-(1-7)-heptapeptide in man. *Life Sci.* 38, 1515-1519.

Kostenis E, Milligan G, Christopoulos A, Sanchez-Ferrer CF, Heringer-Walther S, Sexton PM, Gembardt F, Kellett E, Martini L, Vanderheyden P, Schultheiss HP and Walther T. (2005). G-protein-coupled receptor Mas is a physiological antagonist of the angiotensin II type 1 receptor. *Circulation* 111, 1806-1813.

Lemos VS, Silva DM, Walther T, Alenina N, Bader M and Santos RA. (2005). The endothelium-dependent vasodilator effect of the nonpeptide Ang(1-7) mimic AVE 0991 is abolished in the aorta of mas-knockout mice. *J. Cardiovasc. Pharmacol.* 46, 274-279.

Li N, Zimpelmann J, Cheng K, Wilkins JA and Burns KD. (2005). The role of angiotensin converting enzyme 2 in the generation of angiotensin 1-7 by rat proximal tubules. *Am. J. Physiol. Renal. Physiol.* 288, F353-362.

Li Y, Wu J, He Q, Shou Z, Zhang P, Pen W, Zhu Y and Chen J. (2009). Angiotensin (1-7) prevent heart dysfunction and left ventricular remodeling caused by renal dysfunction in 5/6 nephrectomy mice. *Hypertens Res.* 32, 369-374.

Lin CS, Pan CH, Wen CH, Yang TH and Kuan TC. (2010). Regulation of angiotensin converting enzyme II by angiotensin peptides in human cardiofibroblasts. *Peptides* 31, 1334-1340.

Liu E, Yang S, Xu Z, Li J, Yang W and Li G. (2010). Angiotensin-(1-7) prevents atrial fibrosis and atrial fibrillation in long-term atrial tachycardia dogs. *Regul. Pept.* 162, 73-78.

Loot AE, Roks AJ, Henning RH, Tio RA, Suurmeijer AJ, Boomsma F and van Gilst WH. (2002). Angiotensin-(1-7) attenuates the development of heart failure after myocardial infarction in rats. *Circulation* 105, 1548-1550.

Masson R, Nicklin SA, Craig MA, McBride M, Gilday K, Gregorevic P, Allen JM, Chamberlain JS, Smith G, Graham D, Dominiczak AF, Napoli C and Baker AH. (2009). Onset of experimental severe cardiac fibrosis is mediated by overexpression of Angiotensin-converting enzyme 2. *Hypertension* 53, 694-700.

Mercure C, Yogi A, Callera GE, Aranha AB, Bader M, Ferreira AJ, Santos RA, Walther T, Touyz RM and Reudelhuber TL. (2008). Angiotensin(1-7) blunts hypertensive cardiac remodeling by a direct effect on the heart. *Circ. Res.* 103, 1319-1326.

Metzger R, Bader M, Ludwig T, Berberich C, Bunnemann B and Ganten D. (1995). Expression of the mouse and rat mas proto-oncogene in the brain and peripheral tissues. *FEBS Lett.* 357, 27-32.

Nagata S, Kato J, Sasaki K, Minamino N, Eto T and Kitamura K. (2006). Isolation and identification of proangiotensin-12, a possible component of the renin-angiotensin system. *Biochem. Biophys. Res. Commun.* 350, 1026-1031.

Ocaranza MP, Lavandero S, Jalil JE, Moya J, Pinto M, Novoa U, Apablaza F, Gonzalez L, Hernandez C, Varas M, Lopez R, Godoy I, Verdejo H and Chiong M. (2010). Angiotensin-(1-9) regulates cardiac hypertrophy in vivo and in vitro. *J. Hypertens* 28, 1054-1064.

Ocaranza MP, Rivera P, Novoa U, Pinto M, Gonzalez L, Chiong M, Lavandero S and Jalil JE. (2011). Rho kinase inhibition activates the homologous angiotensin-converting enzyme-angiotensin-(1-9) axis in experimental hypertension. *J. Hypertens* 29, 706-715.

Pan CH, Wen CH and Lin CS. (2008). Interplay of angiotensin II and angiotensin(1-7) in the regulation of matrix metalloproteinases of human cardiocytes. *Exp. Physiol.* 93, 599-612.

Paul M, Wagner J and Dzau VJ. (1993). Gene expression of the renin-angiotensin system in human tissues. Quantitative analysis by the polymerase chain reaction. *J. Clin. Invest* 91, 2058-2064.

Peiro C, Vallejo S, Gembardt F, Azcutia V, Heringer-Walther S, Rodriguez-Manas L, Schultheiss HP, Sanchez-Ferrer CF and Walther T. (2007). Endothelial dysfunction through genetic deletion or inhibition of the G protein-coupled receptor Mas: a new target to improve endothelial function. *J. Hypertens* 25, 2421-2425.

Pendleton RG, Gessner G and Horner E. (1989). Studies defining minimal receptor domains for angiotensin II. *J. Pharmacol. Exp. Ther* 250, 31-36.

Qi Y, Shenoy V, Wong F, Li H, Afzal A, Mocco J, Sumners C, Raizada MK and Katovich MJ. (2011). Lentiviral mediated overexpression of Angiotensin-(1-7) attenuated ischemia-induced cardiac pathophysiology. *Exp. Physiol.*

Reaux A, Fournie-Zaluski MC and Llorens-Cortes C. (2001). Angiotensin III: a central regulator of vasopressin release and blood pressure. *Trends Endocrinol. Metab.* 12, 157-162.

Roks AJ, van Geel PP, Pinto YM, Buikema H, Henning RH, de Zeeuw D and van Gilst WH. (1999). Angiotensin-(1-7) is a modulator of the human renin-angiotensin system. *Hypertension* 34, 296-301.

Santiago NM, Guimaraes PS, Sirvente RA, Oliveira LA, Irigoyen MC, Santos RA and Campagnole-Santos MJ. (2010). Lifetime overproduction of circulating Angiotensin-(1-7) attenuates deoxycorticosterone acetate-salt hypertension-induced cardiac dysfunction and remodeling. *Hypertension* 55, 889-896.

Santos RA, Brosnihan KB, Jacobsen DW, DiCorleto PE and Ferrario CM. (1992). Production of angiotensin-(1-7) by human vascular endothelium. *Hypertension* 19, II56-61.

Santos RA, Campagnole-Santos MJ, Baracho NC, Fontes MA, Silva LC, Neves LA, Oliveira DR, Caligiorne SM, Rodrigues AR, Gropen Junior C and et al. (1994). Characterization of a new angiotensin antagonist selective for angiotensin-(1-7): evidence that the actions of angiotensin-(1-7) are mediated by specific angiotensin receptors. *Brain Res. Bull* 35, 293-298.

Santos RA, Castro CH, Gava E, Pinheiro SV, Almeida AP, Paula RD, Cruz JS, Ramos AS, Rosa KT, Irigoyen MC, Bader M, Alenina N, Kitten GT and Ferreira AJ. (2006). Impairment of in vitro and in vivo heart function in angiotensin-(1-7) receptor MAS knockout mice. *Hypertension* 47, 996-1002.

Santos RA, Ferreira AJ, Nadu AP, Braga AN, de Almeida AP, Campagnole-Santos MJ, Baltatu O, Iliescu R, Reudelhuber TL and Bader M. (2004). Expression of an angiotensin-(1-7)-producing fusion protein produces cardioprotective effects in rats. *Physiol. Genomics* 17, 292-299.

Santos RA, Simoes e Silva AC, Maric C, Silva DM, Machado RP, de Buhr I, Heringer-Walther S, Pinheiro SV, Lopes MT, Bader M, Mendes EP, Lemos VS, Campagnole-Santos MJ, Schultheiss HP, Speth R and Walther T. (2003). Angiotensin-(1-7) is an endogenous ligand for the G protein-coupled receptor Mas. *Proc. Natl. Acad. Sci. USA* 100, 8258-8263.

Snyder RA and Wintroub BU. (1986). Inhibition of angiotensin-converting enzyme by des-Leu10-angiotensin I: a potential mechanism of endogenous angiotensin-converting enzyme regulation. *Biochim. Biophys. Acta* 871, 1-5.

Soares de Moura R, Resende AC, Emiliano AF, Tano T, Mendes-Ribeiro AC, Correia ML and de Carvalho LC. (2004). The role of bradykinin, AT2 and angiotensin 1-7 receptors in the EDRF-dependent vasodilator effect of angiotensin II on the isolated mesenteric vascular bed of the rat. *Br. J. Pharmacol.* 141, 860-866.

Stewart JM, Ocon AJ, Clarke D, Taneja I and Medow MS. (2009). Defects in cutaneous angiotensin-converting enzyme 2 and angiotensin-(1-7) production in postural tachycardia syndrome. *Hypertension* 53, 767-774.

Swanson GN, Hanesworth JM, Sardinia MF, Coleman JK, Wright JW, Hall KL, Miller-Wing AV, Stobb JW, Cook VI, Harding EC and et al. (1992). Discovery of a distinct binding site for angiotensin II (3-8), a putative angiotensin IV receptor. *Regul. Pept* 40, 409-419.

Tipnis SR, Hooper NM, Hyde R, Karran E, Christie G and Turner AJ. (2000). A human homolog of angiotensin-converting enzyme. Cloning and functional expression as a captopril-insensitive carboxypeptidase. *J. Biol. Chem* 275, 33238-33243.

Trask AJ, Averill DB, Ganten D, Chappell MC and Ferrario CM. (2007). Primary role of angiotensin-converting enzyme-2 in cardiac production of angiotensin-(1-7) in transgenic Ren-2 hypertensive rats. *Am. J. Physiol. Heart Circ. Physiol.* 292, H3019-3024.

Trask AJ, Groban L, Westwood BM, Varagic J, Ganten D, Gallagher PE, Chappell MC and Ferrario CM. (2010). Inhibition of angiotensin-converting enzyme 2 exacerbates cardiac hypertrophy and fibrosis in Ren-2 hypertensive rats. *Am. J. Hypertens* 23, 687-693.

Trask AJ, Jessup JA, Chappell MC and Ferrario CM. (2008). Angiotensin-(1-12) is an alternate substrate for angiotensin peptide production in the heart. *Am. J. Physiol. Heart Circ. Physiol.* 294, H2242-2247.

van Kats JP, Danser AH, van Meegen JR, Sassen LM, Verdouw PD and Schalekamp MA. (1998). Angiotensin production by the heart: a quantitative study in pigs with the use of radiolabeled angiotensin infusions. *Circulation* 98, 73-81.

van Kats JP, Methot D, Paradis P, Silversides DW and Reudelhuber TL. (2001). Use of a biological peptide pump to study chronic peptide hormone action in transgenic mice. Direct and indirect effects of angiotensin II on the heart. *J. Biol. Chem.* 276, 44012-44017.

Velkoska E, Dean RG, Griggs K, Burchill L and Burrell LM. (2011). Angiotensin-(1-7) infusion is associated with increased blood pressure and adverse cardiac remodelling in rats with subtotal nephrectomy. *Clin. Sci. (Lond)* 120, 335-345.

Vickers C, Hales P, Kaushik V, Dick L, Gavin J, Tang J, Godbout K, Parsons T, Baronas E, Hsieh F, Acton S, Patane M, Nichols A and Tummino P. (2002). Hydrolysis of biological peptides by human angiotensin-converting enzyme-related carboxypeptidase. *J. Biol. Chem.* 277, 14838-14843.

Vilas-Boas WW, Ribeiro-Oliveira A, Jr., Pereira RM, Ribeiro Rda C, Almeida J, Nadu AP, Simoes e Silva AC and dos Santos RA. (2009). Relationship between angiotensin-(1-7) and angiotensin II correlates with hemodynamic changes in human liver cirrhosis. *World J. Gastroenterol* 15, 2512-2519.

Warner FJ, Smith AI, Hooper NM and Turner AJ. (2004). Angiotensin-converting enzyme-2: a molecular and cellular perspective. *Cell Mol. Life Sci* 61, 2704-2713.

Wei CC, Ferrario CM, Brosnihan KB, Farrell DM, Bradley WE, Jaffa AA and Dell'Italia LJ. (2002). Angiotensin peptides modulate bradykinin levels in the interstitium of the dog heart in vivo. *J. Pharmacol Exp. Ther.* 300, 324-329.

Welches WR, Brosnihan KB and Ferrario CM. (1993). A comparison of the properties and enzymatic activities of three angiotensin processing enzymes: angiotensin converting enzyme, prolyl endopeptidase and neutral endopeptidase 24.11. *Life Sci.* 52, 1461-1480.

Wright JW, Miller-Wing AV, Shaffer MJ, Higginson C, Wright DE, Hanesworth JM and Harding JW. (1993). Angiotensin II(3-8) (ANG IV) hippocampal binding: potential role in the facilitation of memory. *Brain Res. Bull* 32, 497-502.

Yamada K, Iyer SN, Chappell MC, Ganten D and Ferrario CM. (1998). Converting enzyme determines plasma clearance of angiotensin-(1-7). *Hypertension* 32, 496-502.

Yamaguchi K, Negoro H, Hama H, Kamoi K and Sakaguchi T. (1979). [A comparison between the effects of angiotensin II and angiotensin III injected into the third cerebral ventricle on vasopressin secretion in conscious rats (author's transl)]. *Nippon Naibunpi Gakkai Zasshi* 55, 1286-1295.

Zhang Y, Lu J, Shi J, Lin X, Dong J, Zhang S, Liu Y and Tong Q. (2008). Central administration of angiotensin-(1-7) stimulates nitric oxide release and upregulates the endothelial nitric oxide synthase expression following focal cerebral ischemia/reperfusion in rats. *Neuropeptides* 42, 593-600.

Zhao YX, Yin HQ, Yu QT, Qiao Y, Dai HY, Zhang MX, Zhang L, Liu YF, Wang LC, Liu de S, Deng BP, Zhang YH, Pan CM, Song HD, Qu X, Jiang H, Liu CX, Lu XT, Liu B, Gao F and Dong B. (2010). ACE2 overexpression ameliorates left ventricular remodeling and dysfunction in a rat model of myocardial infarction. *Hum. Gene Ther* 21, 1545-1554.

Zhong J, Basu R, Guo D, Chow FL, Byrns S, Schuster M, Loibner H, Wang XH, Penninger JM, Kassiri Z and Oudit GY. (2010). Angiotensin-converting enzyme 2 suppresses pathological hypertrophy, myocardial fibrosis, and cardiac dysfunction. *Circulation* 122, 717-728, 718 p following 728.

Zini S, Fournie-Zaluski MC, Chauvel E, Roques BP, Corvol P and Llorens-Cortes C. (1996). Identification of metabolic pathways of brain angiotensin II and III using specific aminopeptidase inhibitors: predominant role of angiotensin III in the control of vasopressin release. *Proc. Natl. Acad. Sci. USA* 93, 11968-11973.

Zisman LS, Meixell GE, Bristow MR and Canver CC. (2003). Angiotensin-(1-7) formation in the intact human heart: in vivo dependence on angiotensin II as substrate. *Circulation* 108, 1679-1681.

In: Angiotensin: New Research
Editors: S. Harada, I. Moi, pp. 113-129
ISBN: 978-1-62100-773-9

Chapter 4

NEW ROLES FOR THE NEUROPEPTIDE ANGIOTENSIN II: STRESS AND DRUG ABUSE

Claudia Bregonzio[1], Brenda Casarsa[2], Natalia A. Marchese[1] and Gustavo Baiardi[2]

[1] Departamento de Farmacología, Facultad de Ciencias Químicas, Universidad Nacional de Córdoba, IFEC-CONICET, Córdoba, Argentina.
[2] Laboratorio de Neurofarmacología, Facultad de Ciencias Químicas, Universidad Católica de Córdoba, IIBYT-CONICET, Córdoba, Argentina.

ABSTRACT

Angiotensin II (Ang II) is known as a peripheral hormone involved in the control of blood pressure and fluid homeostasis. The study and characterization of Ang II and its receptors in the brain has opened a new vision of its physiological role and also offers a variety of research fields. Ang II is involved in the response to stress, which stimulates the brain and the peripheral (hormonal) Ang II systems. Activation of brain angiotensin II AT_1 receptors is required for stress-induced hormone secretion, including CRH, ACTH, corticoids and vasopressin, and for stimulation of central sympathetic activity. The blockade of peripheral but also brain AT_1 receptors prevents the hormonal and sympathoadrenal response to isolation stress and prevents the formation of stress-induced gastric ulcers, through ischemia and inflammation. The AT_1 receptor antagonists prevent inflammation (neutrophil infiltration and increase in ICAM-1 and TNF-α) in the gastric mucosa and partially inhibit sympathoadrenal stimulation, without affecting the protective effect of glucocorticoid release during stress. The coordination of behavioral and autonomic responses to stress is partially under the control of extrahypothalamic, including cortical, CRF neurons expressing CRF_1 receptors. AT_1 receptor activation is thus also involved in the cortical decrease of CRF_1 binding induced by stress.

A large number of studies have been conducted on the effect of drugs of abuse on hypothalamic and extrahypothalamic CRF systems in the brain and on the role of CRF in mediating the behavioral and physiological effects of drugs of abuse. It is also known that dopaminergic neurotransmission in the nucleus accumbens and caudate-putamen plays a critical role in the locomotor and stereotypic effects of psychostimulant drugs. Ang II receptors are found on the soma and terminals of dopaminergic neurons and it has been shown that Ang II, acting through its AT_1 receptors, facilitates the release of dopamine in the rat striatum in vitro and in vivo. Repeated exposure to amphetamine, as with most addictive drugs, results in progressive and lasting enhancement of their psychomotor and positive reinforcing effects. Neuroadaptive changes in mesotelencephalic dopaminergic projections play a key role in the induction and expression of amphetamine sensitization. Recently, we found evidence showing that brain AT_1 receptor activation is involved in the neuroadaptive changes induced by amphetamine.

The results of studies on the physiological role of brain Ang II offer new pharmacological tools for the treatment of some stress-related disorders such as drug abuse.

INTRODUCTION

Angiotensin II was discovered in 1940 and described as a peripheral hormone. Later its synthesis and metabolism were characterized, currently known as the renin angiotensin system (RAS) [1]. The precursor molecule is the angiotensinogen synthesized in the liver and cleaved by a renal protease, giving an inactive decapeptide, angiotensin I. This is converted into the active octapeptide Angiotensin II (ANG II), by action of a circulating enzyme called angiotensin converting enzyme (ACE), which is also responsible for inactivating bradykinin. The principal actions related to Ang II are vasoconstriction, aldosterone release, sodium retention and a key role in blood pressure control and fluid homeostasis.

All the components of the RAS, including the receptors, have been found in brain tissue, indicating a role as a hormone or neuromodulator in the central nervous system [2, 3]. Ang II exerts its principal known actions at the AT_1 receptor. Its functions related to AT_2 receptors are controversial and associated with AT_1 opposite effects, although there is evidence showing cross-talk between both receptors. The metabolism of Ang II generates other active peptides, such as Angiotensin 1-7 and Angiotensin IV, which will not be discussed in this chapter.

The role of Ang II at the periphery and in the central nervous system is vast and complex; for this reason, in this chapter we will focus in the role of brain RAS in stress responses and related pathologies from many other important aspects of Ang II research.

Brain Ang II

Ang II from the periphery does not cross the blood-brain barrier (BBB) but stimulates the AT_1 receptors located in the circumventricular organ outside the BBB [4]. This stimulation increases the intake of fluids and salt. The brain RAS generates the Ang II which stimulates receptors inside the BBB [5]. The neuroanatomical localization of Ang II, AT_1 and AT_2 receptors has been precisely described in different brain areas [4], placed on neurons, astrocytes and oligodendrocytes. The presence of components of RAS in glial cells suggests a more important role for these than was previously postulated [6].

Both subtypes of receptors were found with a similar, but not identical, distribution in all the mammalian species studied, including humans [4]. While AT_1 receptors predominate in adult animals, AT_2 are expressed in the developing brain [4]. AT_1 receptors are located in brain areas related with the control of neuroendocrine functions and the autonomic regulation of limbic and cardiovascular systems [7], while AT_2 receptors are involved in organogenesis and in the functions of motor and sensorial systems.

The role of brain Ang II is complex and is related with control of the autonomic, hormonal system, and sensorial and cognitive processes including regulation of cerebral blood flow [4].

Ang II is Involved in Stress Response

There is a large body of evidence, at pharmacological, neuroanatomical and physiological level, supporting a key role for Ang II in the stress response, including regulation of the sympathetic and neuroendocrine systems [8-10]. The presence of AT_1 receptors has been shown at all levels of the hypothalamus-pituitary-adrenal (HPA) axis, with a higher concentration in key areas for the control of stress response, such as the paraventricular nucleus (PVN) [11], median eminence, anterior pituitary, zona glomerulosa and adrenal medulla [12]. Exposure to stress induces an increase in circulating and brain Ang II levels [13, 14]. Brain Ang II stimulates local receptors in the PVN and locus coeruleus, among other nuclei, while circulating Ang II also stimulates the AT_1 receptors in the subfornical organ, to which it is connected through the median eminence and PVN [12, 15].

It has been found that exposure to acute stress induced an increase in AT_1 receptor density in the anterior pituitary, although exposure to repeated stress sessions increased AT_1 receptor density in the PVN [16], expressed in the cellular body of neurons that synthesize corticotrophin releasing hormone (CRH) [12, 15]. In agreement with this, it has been found that AT_1 receptor stimulation by Ang II induced an increase in the production of CRH [17, 18]. This hormone is released to the circulation and increases ACTH release from the pituitary. In the same way, high levels of adrenal glucocorticoids, due to stress, induced an increase in the expression of AT_1 receptors in the PVN [17]. Moreover, there is local production of Ang II in the anterior pituitary which, acting together with circulating Ang II, induces an increase in ACTH secretion [19].

The PVN is an important area in the processing and integration of many different stress signals [20]. This nucleus receives noradrenergic input from the locus coeruleus and serotoninergic input from the dorsal raphe nucleus, and there are reciprocal interactions between these two regions and the PVN [21, 22]. In addition, there are reciprocal neural connections between CRH neurons from the PVN and noradrenergic neurons from the locus coeruleus. It has been shown that both adrenergic receptor subtypes regulate the ACTH secretion, and CRH controls central noradrenergic activity. Most of the available evidence suggests that CRH acts as a neurotransmitter in the locus coeruleus modulating the noradrenergic activation in response to stress [23].

The evidence obtained using AT_1 antagonists gives support for a key role for Ang II in the stress response. It is important to highlight that the results obtained using AT_1 blockers as a pre-treatment in animals exposed to different stress conditions, such as isolation, cold restraint or novelty, suggest that their actions may not be limited to the HPA axis only.

Exposure to one session of social isolation for 24 hs or 2hs of cold restraint induced an increase in the enzyme tirosine hydroxilase (TH) mRNA in the locus coeruleus and, in both cases, this increase was prevented by previous administration of an AT_1 blocker [24, 25]. This suggests that AT_1 receptors are involved in the control of central sympathetic activity through the regulation of TH transcription. The influence of AT_2 receptor activation in the locus coeruleus cannot be discarded. This is based on results showing dual control by AT_1 and AT_2 receptors in TH transcription and in the synthesis of catecholamines at the adrenal medulla [26].

In addition, pretreatment with candesartan, an AT_1 blocker, prevents isolation-induced decrease in CRH_1 receptors and the $GABA_A$ complex in the brain cortex [24]. When animals were tested in the plus maze they exhibited an increase in the parameters associated with anxiolytic effects. All together, these strongly suggest a role for AT_1 receptors not only in autonomic and hormonal, but also in behavioral response to stress [24, 27].

AT1 Antagonists Attenuate Central Responses to Stress and Have Anxiolytic Effects

Despite the major role of the HPA axis in stress response being mediated by CRH, the behavioral stress response mediated by CRH occurs in a manner independent of the HPA axis. This is based, among other evidence, on the fact that hypophysectomy and the blockade of the HPA axis response with dexametaxone do not alter the stress response induced by brain CRH administration. This strongly suggests a central action responsible for the coordination of stress-related behaviors [28].

It has been found that isolation stress [24], electric shock [29] and chronic unpredictable stress [30] produce, among others, a decrease in brain CRH_1 density. This can be reproduced in the prefrontal cortex by intracerebral CRH administration, and a decrease in mRNA levels of CRH_1 receptors has been shown *in vitro* in a cell line derived from CRH neurons incubated with CRH.

These results support the idea of down-regulation induced by the CRH increase [31]. An AT_1 blocker that crosses the BBB was found to prevent a decrease in brain cortex CRH_1 induced by isolation stress [24], indicating that cortical CRH activation is positively regulated by AT_1 receptors, similar to what occurs at hypothalamic level. Even so, the presence of AT_1 receptors has been determined in the piriform and entorhinal cortex [32] but only of the mRNA of AT_1 receptors in the neocortex [33]. This suggests that AT_1 receptor blockade could reduce the decrease in cortical CRH_1 receptors [24]. There is a reciprocity between CRH and noradrenergic systems during stress: the locus coeruleus is activated by CRH [34] and stress induces an increase in CRH in this brain area [35].

In addition, CRH injected in the locus coeruleus induces behavioral activation, and prefrontal cortex noradrenaline release can be blocked by a CRH receptor antagonist [36]. AT_1 receptors seem to modulate only the CRH_1 receptors because there is no evidence showing any action on the CRH_2 receptors [24]. The CRH is also related with the GABA system, since $GABA_A$ receptors are located in CRH neurons.

In response to different kinds of stressors, there is a decrease in benzodiazepine binding in the frontal cortex, increasing anxiety behavior [37, 38]. AT_1 antagonists decrease CRH release, and this could explain the prevention of the $GABA_A$ binding decrease in animals exposed to isolation stress [24]. Moreover, the anxiolytic effect of AT_1 receptor antagonists has also been described [39-41].

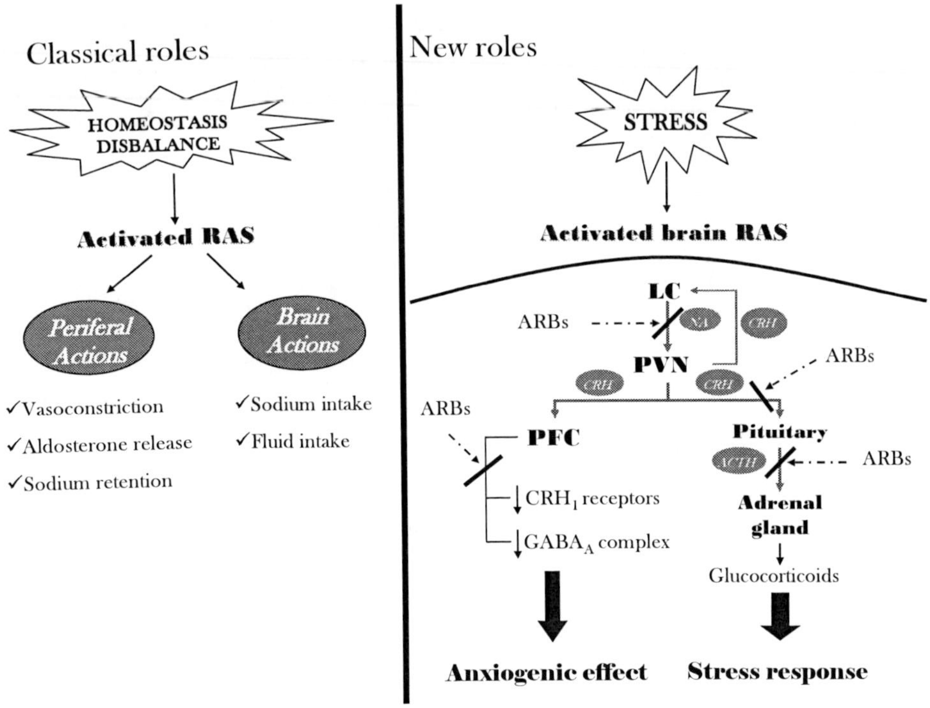

Figure 1. New roles of brain RAS versus classical. Brain RAS has a key role in the stress response in dependant and independent manner of HPA axis level. LC (locus coeruleus), PVN (paraventricular nucleus), ARBs (angiotensin receptor blockers), PFC (prefrontal cortex).

Ang II and stress-related disorders

Gastric Lesions Induced by Stress

When an organism is subjected to stress, gastric ulcers or ulcerations are commonly developed [42] as a result of complex psychological factors influencing individual vulnerability, the stimulation of brain specific pathways regulating autonomic function, decreased blood flow to the mucosa, increase in muscular contractility, mast cell degranulation, leukocyte activation, and increased free radical generation, resulting in increased lipid peroxidation [42-45].

The events associated with ulcer formation are sudden blood flow reduction to the gastric mucosa and increased free radical formation [44]. For this reason, the maintenance of gastric blood flow is important to protect the mucosa from endogenous and exogenous damage factors. Ang II levels increase during stress in plasma and tissues, including the stomach [13]. The role of Ang II in the stomach is the regulation of gastric vascular tone through AT_1 receptor stimulation [46]. It is known that Ang II generates reactive oxygen species, with cellular damage and inflammation [47]. The mucosal vasoconstriction and proinflammatory effects of Ang II could contribute to the production of stress-induced gastric ulcers.

An experimental model commonly used to induce acute gastric damage is cold-restraint stress, which is also clinically relevant [48]. Using this stress model in male spontaneously hypertensive rats (SHR), it was found that AT_1 receptor inhibition prevented gastric lesions by combined local and systemic mechanisms, including gastric blood flow maintenance, inhibition of proinflammatory cascade activation, preventing the gastric ischemia and inflammation characteristic of a major stress response, and resulting in the protection of the gastric mucosa from stress-induced ulcerations [49]. The experiment was carried out in SHR which have an increased expression of the brain RAS components and have been described as stress-prone animals. More specifically it was found that blood flow to the stomach was significantly increased in animals treated with the AT_1 receptor antagonist compared with vehicle-treated controls [49]. Interestingly, the maintenance of a normal pituitary- adrenal response to stress parallels protection from gastric injury, with the results supporting the hypothesis that, although large doses of exogenously administered corticosteroids are ulcerogenic, endogenous corticoids actually contribute to protecting the gastric mucosa from ulceration during stress, probably by contributing to an increase in blood flow and secretion of bicarbonate [50].

The presence and density of Ang II receptors in the stomach analyzed by autoradiography showed AT_1 receptors and a lower number of AT_2 receptors, in all layers of the stomach [49]. The AT_1 antagonist treatment decreased AT_1 receptor binding [49]. This could be the result of receptor occupancy with the insurmountable antagonist candesartan or of receptor downregulation [51]. So the decreased number of gastric AT_1 receptors after stress may be related to receptor occupancy by the increased Ang II levels or to a receptor compensatory mechanism due to Ang II increased stimulation [8].

It was also confirmed that cold restraint drastically increases the expression of the adhesion molecule ICAM-1 and the proinflammatory cytokine TNF-α and the number of infiltrating neutrophils in the gastric mucosa [49]. These components play crucial roles in the progression of gastric injury [52]. It is known that activated neutrophils release inflammatory mediators, capable of damaging endothelial cells, and inhibition of neutrophil infiltration prevents the stress-induced reduction of mucosal blood flow and the production of gastric lesions [53]. Likewise, it has been described that Ang II promotes tissue inflammation through AT_1 receptor stimulation, enhancing neutrophil infiltration [54, 55], increasing the expression of TNF-α [54, 56, 57] and ICAM-1 [58]. It was reported that TNF-α down-regulated AT_1 receptors [59, 60], and that TNF-α, acting with other proinflammatory cytokines, upregulated AT_1 receptors and increased the profibrotic effects induced by Ang II [61, 62]. The increase of TNF-α and neutrophil infiltration in the gastric mucosa induced by cold restraint was prevented by the AT_1 receptor blockade [49].

The increased ICAM-1 expression induced by cold restraint exposure in the endothelium of arteries of the gastric mucosa and submucosa, and in venules of the submucosa (where AT_1 receptors are located), was also prevented by the AT_1 receptor blockade. The anti-inflammatory effects of AT_1 receptor blockade could thus be important for protection against stress-induced gastric ulcers.

Stress Is Related to Drug Abuse

The hormonal changes, involving increased peripheral glucocorticoid levels and CRF release in different brain sites, initiate a cascade of biological responses to counteract the altered homeostatic balance of the organism in response to stress. The modification in the brain physiology induced by stress triggers the release of neuroactive hormones, such as biogenic amines and adrenal steroids, which activate the same neuronal circuit as the psychostimulant drugs, cocaine or amphetamine. Many years ago, clinical studies on methadone-treated heroin addicts [63] showed atypical stress responsivity in both active and long-term abstinent heroin addicts, similar to the atypical stress response of the HPA axis that has been found in abstinent cocaine addicts [64]. Thus, it has been hypothesized that an atypical response to stressors may contribute to compulsive drug use [65]. Moreover, in a series of studies, Piazza et al. [66] have demonstrated that rats with higher levels of behavioral and neuroendocrine response to stress develop psychostimulant drug self-administration more rapidly than low responders [66]. Together with other evidence, this supports a major role for stress in individual vulnerability to self-administer drugs of abuse. In addition, corticosterone, the major glucocorticoid end-product of HPA axis activation in rodents, is self-administered by rats [67], and pharmacological manipulation of the circulating corticosterone levels altered cocaine self-administration behavior [68]. These results and many others suggest that the activity of the HPA axis may play a role in different phases of drug addiction.

Brain Ang II Is Involved in Psychostimulant Sensitization

One of the principal systems involved in drug abuse is the dopaminergic mesolimbic system, a critical component in the brain reward circuit [69]. Ang II belongs to the group of peptides known to stimulate dopamine release [70-72]. Moreover, the Ang II receptors are located in dopamine-rich brain areas [72, 73], such as the nucleus accumbens (NAC) and caudate putamen, strongly related with self-administration and sensitization to drugs of abuse [74].

Sensitization to drugs, such as amphetamine, is associated with alterations in the morphology of neurons in the NAC, a brain region critical to motivation and reward. It is known that Ang II is involved in the control of salt appetite, and it has been shown that sodium depletion that promotes salt appetite also leads to alterations in neurons in NAC. Medium spiny neurons in the shell of the NAC of rats that had experienced sodium depletion had significantly more dendritic branches and spines than controls [75]. In addition, a history of sodium depletion was found to have cross-sensitization effects, leading to enhanced psychostimulant responses to amphetamine [76]. Thus, neuronal alterations common to salt and drug sensitization may provide a general mechanism for enhanced behavioral responses to subsequent exposures to these challenges.

Recently, behavioral cross-sensitization between sodium depletion and cocaine has also been described. In rats, repeated administration of the mineralocorticoid agonist deoxycorticosterone acetate (DOCA) initially induced incremental increases in daily hypertonic saline consumption (i.e., sensitization of sodium appetite) in spite of the retention of sodium [77]. This study investigated whether sodium appetite sensitization induced by DOCA shares mechanisms similar to those of psychomotor stimulant-induced sensitization, and whether there is evidence for reciprocal cross-sensitization. They found that animals pretreated with DOCA without access to saline showed greater locomotor responses to cocaine than animals receiving vehicle treatments. The results of these experiments indicate that treatments generating a sustained salt appetite and producing cocaine-induced psychomotor responses show reciprocal behavioral cross-sensitization [77]. The underlying mechanisms accounting for this relationship may be the fact that psychostimulants and an unresolved craving for sodium can act as potent stressors.

The extent to which sensitization is induced by drug pre-exposure is highly dependent on the nature of the pretreatment regimen. Thus repeated intermittent treatment with moderate doses of drugs is far more effective in inducing sensitization than chronic exposure to high or escalating drug doses. Remarkably, studies in mouse and rats show that a single exposure to psychostimulants (amphetamine or cocaine) induces behavioral sensitization [69, 78].

Ang II AT_1 receptors have recently been found to be involved in the neuroadaptative changes induced by a single exposure to amphetamine, and such changes are related to the development of behavioral and neurochemical sensitization. The study examined the expression of amphetamine-enhanced (0.5 mg/kg i.p.) locomotor activity in animals pretreated with candesartan, an AT_1 blocker, (3 mg/kg p.o. x 5 days), 3 weeks after an amphetamine injection (5 mg/kg i.p.).

The dopaminergic hyperreactivity associated with sensitization was tested by measuring 3H-DA release *in vitro* from NAC slices, induced by K+ stimulus. Behavioral sensitization to amphetamine was confirmed in the two-injection protocol, and pretreatment with an AT_1 receptor blocker, candesartan, attenuated this response [79] (Figure 2). In respect to the neurochemical sensitization tested, using ex vivo 3H-DA release experiments, it was found that candesartan pretreatment blunted the enhanced response induced by K+ stimulus [79] (Figure 3).

Similarly, the involvement of brain Ang II AT_1 receptors was studied in the development of neuronal changes in the activity of the immediate early gene, c-fos, as a function of exposure to amphetamine in a two-injection protocol, and it was found that amphetamine-induced neuronal plasticity was blunted by previous AT_1 receptor blockade (unpublish data) (Figure 4). These three experiments support a role for brain AT_1 receptors in the development of neuroadaptive changes in response to amphetamine exposure.

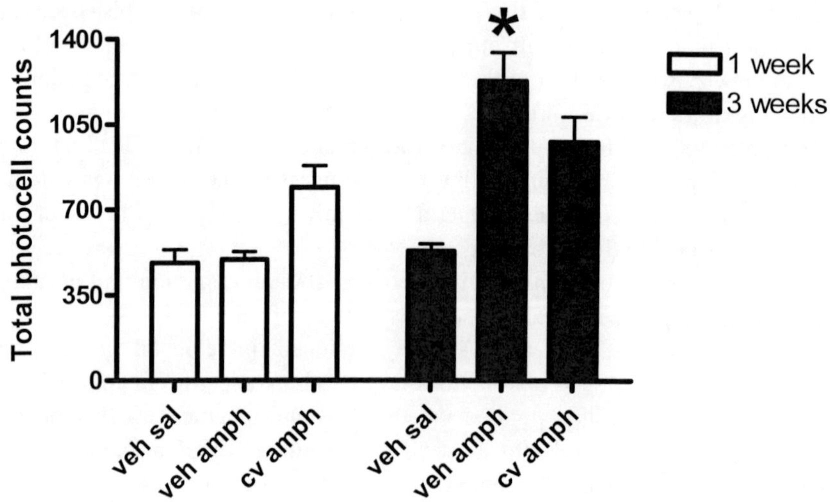

Figure 2. AT_1 receptor blockade attenuated behavioral sensitization to amphetamine. Sensitized locomotor responses to amphetamine challenge (0.5 mg/ kg, i.p.) in rats pretreated with candesartan (cv) 3 mg/kg, p.o or vehicle (veh) 1ml/kg, p.o.; and amphetamine (amph) 5 mg/kg, i.p. or saline (sal) 1 ml/kg, i.p. (n=8); 1 week vs. 3 weeks after treatment. Data are expressed as mean ± SEM of total photocell counts per 120 min after amphetamine challenge. *$p < 0.01$ (Two-way ANOVA, Bonferroni post hoc test).

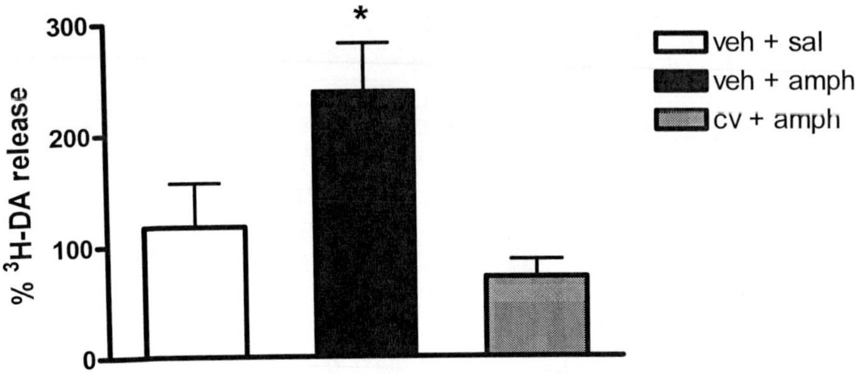

Figure 3. AT_1 receptor blockade attenuated neurochemical sensitization to amphetamine K^+ 28mM-evoked ^{3}H-DA release from superfused nucleus accumbens slices of rats pretreated with candesartan (cv) 3 mg/kg, p.o. or vehicle (veh) 1ml/kg, p.o.; and amphetamine (amph) 5 mg/ kg, i.p. ; or saline (sal) 1 ml/kg, i.p. (n= 6); three weeks after pretreatment. Data are expressed as percent increase above their basal ^{3}H-DA release (mean ± SEM). *p<0.01 vs. all treatments (One-way ANOVA, Student Newman-Keuls).

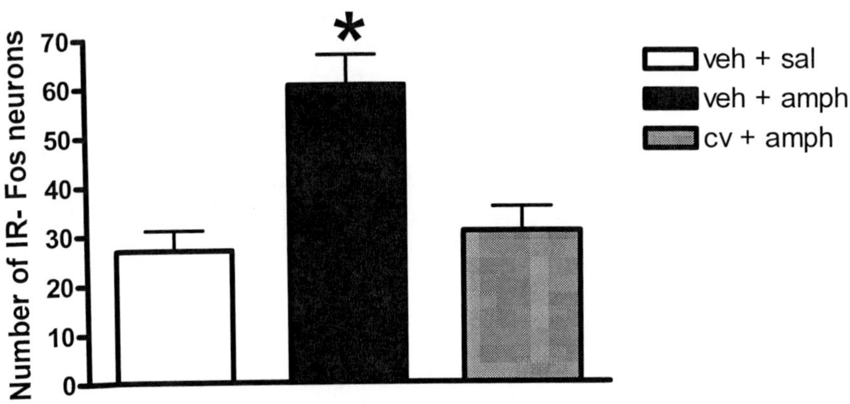

Figure 4. AT_1 receptor blockade attenuated neuronal plasticity induced by amphetamine. Average number of Fos-ir neurons in the NAC Core induced by amphetamine challenge from rats pretreated with candesartan (cv) 3 mg/kg, p.o. or vehicle (veh) 1ml/kg, p.o.; and amphetamine (amph) 5 mg/ kg, i.p. ; or saline (sal) 1 ml/kg, i.p. three weeks after pretreatment. Values are mean ± SEM; n= 6. *p<0.01 vs. all treatments (One-way ANOVA, Student Newman-Keuls).

Brain RAS and Alcohol Abuse

The involvement of the RAS in ethanol consumption behavior has been studied and long debated [80-82]. It has become evident that neuroadaptations in the amygdala CRH system are responsible for alcohol dependence and are a major target for its treatment [83]. As described above, there is a role of brain RAS in the regulation of extrahypothalamic (cortical, subcortical) and hypothalamic (PVN) responses to stress. The activation of the RAS is integrated with stimulatory CRH, arginine vasopressin and catecholamine, and with inhibitory $GABA_A$ and natriuretic (atrial natriuretic factor) systems, influencing both the hypothalamic and extrahypothalamic regulatory centers. Blockade of CRH and Ang II receptors may improve adaptation mechanisms, restore the balance, and promote the return to homeostasis [84].

The clinical defining features of alcoholism are uncontrolled heavy drinking and chronic relapsing. Experimentally, it has been shown, in animals trained to respond to ethanol, in an operant self-administration paradigm followed by an extinction period, that ethanol-seeking can be reinstated after presentation of the conditioned cue, a small dose of ethanol (interpreted as a *model of reward craving*) [84]. Alternatively, stress (e.g., foot shock) can reinstate responding (*relief craving model).* Interestingly, AT_1 receptor blockade could be helpful in models both of reward craving and relief craving, because AT_1 receptors, independently of the RAS–CRH system interaction, may also affect dopamine release [84].

Recent studies in animals with genetic modifications in various components of the RAS demonstrate that Ang II, via AT_1 action, is a positive modulator of spontaneous ethanol consumption in rodents [85]. Furthermore, increased expression of Angiotensinogen was found in microarray studies of brains from different rodent lines selectively bred for high ethanol preference (HAP mice, P and AA rats), compared to their respective controls [84].

Supporting the idea that angiotensin-mediated dopamine release plays an essential role in Ang II-triggered regulation of alcohol intake, altered dopamine concentrations were found in relevant brain areas of TGR(ASrAOGEN)680 animals in which angiotensin generation is drastically reduced in the CNS. Indeed, concentrations of dopamine as well as DOPAC were found to be strongly reduced in a region covering the ventral tegmental area of TGR(ASrAOGEN)680 rats [85]. Moreover, these rats consumed markedly less alcohol in comparison to their wild-type controls. An inhibitor of the angiotensin-converting enzyme (ACE), which passes the blood-brain barrier, did not influence alcohol consumption in TGR(ASrAOGEN)680, but it did significantly reduce alcohol intake in wild-type rats [85]. These results clearly support the hypothesis that pharmacological manipulations of the central RAS, e.g., after oral application of ACE inhibitors reaching the CNS, alter alcohol intake via AT_1-mediated dopamine modulation. This report suggests that drugs interfering with the RAS could be of particular advantage, because the available compounds (such as ACE inhibitors and AT_1 antagonists) are nearly free of severe side effects and are widely used in the treatment of hypertension and in cardioprotection [85].

Interestingly, in a double-blind, placebo-controlled clinical study, 15 alcoholics who met DSM-IV criteria were randomized to receive captopril 100 mg/day or placebo for 12 weeks. Captopril did not alter alcohol consumption in alcoholics when compared with placebo but it did reduce craving [86]. More epidemiological studies are needed to reveal how effective long-term treatment with modern ACE inhibitors or AT_1 blockers can be in the treatment of alcohol addiction.

Brain Ang II and Morphine Reward

Recently, evidence has been found that brain Ang II could be related with the rewarding effects of morphine. An experiment using the conditioning place preference (CPP) test in rats showed that an injection of captopril before testing significantly decreased the time difference spent in compartment A between pre- and post-conditioning compared to the morphine group.

In the same way, the self- administration experiment showed that the number of active lever presses was significantly greater than the inactive in the morphine group. In the captopril group the number of active lever presses was significantly lower than in the morphine group, but there was no significant difference between the number of active and inactive lever presses. The results showed that captopril significantly decreased morphine-induced conditional place preference and morphine self-administration [87].

Another experiment designed to investigate the effect of captopril injection into the NAC on morphine self-administration in rats showed a significantly higher number of active than inactive lever presses during all 5 days of testing and was also significantly higher than in the saline group. In the captopril group, there were no significant differences between the number of active and inactive lever presses. However, the number of active lever presses was significantly lower than in the morphine group [88].

These results highlight the interaction between RAS and the opioid system in NAC. All this strongly indicates that RAS may have a role in the rewarding properties associated with the opioid system.

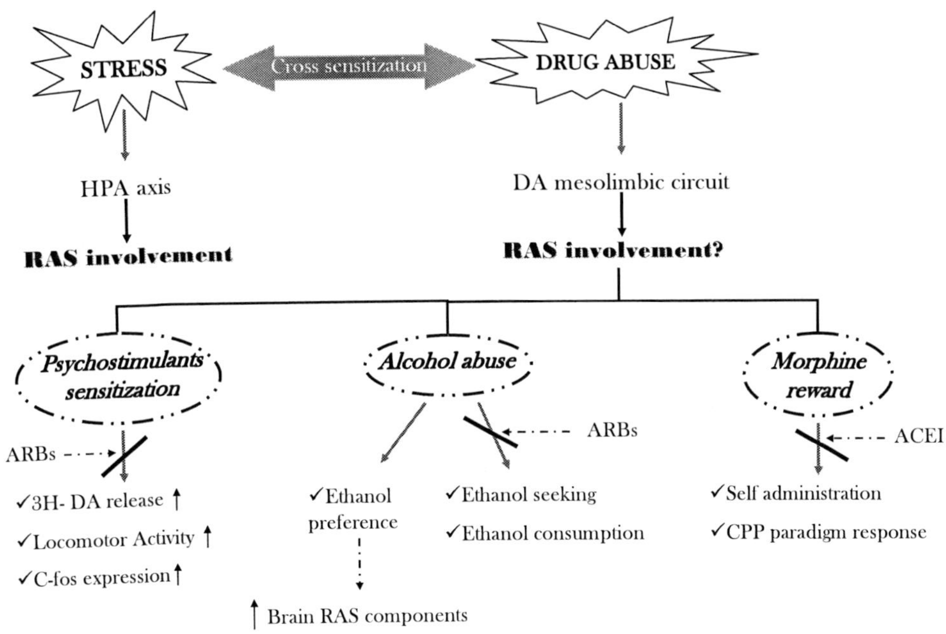

Figure 5. Brain RAS actions related to drug abuse. Brain RAS seems to be involved in the neuroadaptative changes induced by different kinds of drugs of abuse. ARBs (angiotensin receptor blockers), CPP (conditioned place preference).

CONCLUSION

The results from studies on the physiological role of brain Ang II presented here aim to encourage the study of this system in the context of the search for new pharmacological tools in the treatment of stress-related disorders (Figure 5). Moreover, the advantage of the available compounds that interfere with the RAS, ACE inhibitors and AT_1 receptor blockers, is that they are very well tolerated and widely used in the treatment of hypertension.

REFERENCES

[1] Braun-Menéndez E, Fasciolo JC, Leloir LF, Muñoz JM. The substance causing renal hypertension. *J. Physiol.* 1940;98:283-98.

[2] Lavoie JL, Sigmund CD. Minireview: overview of the renin-angiotensin system- an endocrine and paracrine system. *Endocrinology.* 2003;144:2179-83.

[3] Danser AH. Local renin-angiotensin systems: the unanswered questions. *Int. J. Biochem Cell Biol.* 2003;35:759-68.

[4] Saavedra JM. Brain and pituitary angiotensin. *Endocr. Rev.* 1992;13(2):329-80.

[5] Mendelsohn FAO, Quirion R, Saavedra JM, Aguilera G, Catt KJ. Autoradiographic localization of angiotensin II receptors in rat brain. *Proc. Natl. Acad Sci. USA.* 1984;81:1575-9.

[6] Fogarty DJ, Matute C. Angiotensin receptor-like immunoreactivity in adult brain white matter astrocytes and oligodendrocytes. *Glia.* 2001;35(2):131-46.

[7] Phillips MI, Sumners C. Angiotensin II in the central nervous system physiology. *Regul. Pept.* 1998;78:1-11.

[8] Armando I, Carranza A, Nishimura Y, Hoe KL, Barontini M, Terrón JA, et al. Peripheral administration of an angiotensin II AT1 receptor decreases the hypothalamic-pituitary-adrenal response to stress. *Endocrinology.* 2001;142:3880-9.

[9] Aguilera G, Young WS, Kiss A, Bathia A. Direct regulation of hypothalamic corticotropin -releasing hormone neurons by angiotensin II. *Neuroendocrinology.* 1995;61:437-44.

[10] Baiardi G, Bregonzio C, Jezova M, Armando I, Saavedra JM. Angiotensin II AT1 receptor blockade prolongs the lifespan and reduces stress-induced release of catecholamines, glucocorticoids and vasopressin. *Ann. NY Acad Sci.* 2004;1018:131-6.

[11] Armando I, Volpi S, Aguilera G, Saavedra JM. Angiotensin II AT1 receptor blockade prevents the hypothalamic corticotropin-releasing factor response to isolation stress. *Brain Res.* 2007;1142:92-9.

[12] Tsutsumi K, Saavedra JM. Angiotensin II receptor subtypes in median eminence and basal forebrain areas involved in the regulation of pituitary function. *Endocrinology.* 1991;129:3001-8.

[13] Xang G, Xi ZX, Wan Y, Wang H, Bi G. Changes in circulating and tissue angiotensin II during acute and chronic stress. *Biol. Signals.* 1993;2:166-72.

[14] Yang G, Wan Y, Zhu Y. Angiotensin II an important stress hormone. *Biol. Signals.* 1996;5:1-8.

[15] Shigematsu K, Saavedra JM, Plunkett LM, Correa FMA. Angiotensin II binding site in the anteroventral-third ventricle (AV3V) area and related structures of the rat brain. *Neurosci. Lett.* 1986;67:37-41.

[16] Castrén E, Saavedra JM. Repeated stress increase the density of angiotensin II binding sites in the rat paraventricular nucleus and subfornical organ. *Endocrinology.* 1988;122:370-2.

[17] Aguilera G, Kiss A, Luo X. Increased expression of type 1 of angiotensin II receptors in the hypothalamic paraventricular nucleus following stress and glucocorticoid administration. *J. Neuroendocrinol.* 1995;7:775-83.

[18] Jezova D, Ochedalski T, Kiss A, Aguilera G. Brain angiotensin II modulates sympathoadrenal and hypothalamic pituitary adrenocortical activation during stress. *J. Neuroendocrinol.* 1998;10:67-72.

[19] Ganong WF, Murakami K. The role of angiotensin II in the regulation of ACTH secretion. *Ann. NY Acad Sci.* 1987;512:176-86.

[20] Makara GB, Antoni FA, Stark E, Karteszi M. Hypothalamic organization of corticotropin releasing factor (CRF) producing structures. In: Muller E, Macleod RM, editors. *Endocrine Perspective.* Amsterdam: Elsevier; 1984. p. 71-120.

[21] Cedarbaum JM, Aghajanian GK. Afferent projections to the rat locus coeruleus as determined by retrograde tracing technique. *J. Comp. Neurol.* 1978;178:1-14.

[22] Thiboliet E, Dreifuss JJ. Localization of neurons projecting to the hipothalamic paraventricular nucleus area of the rat : a horseradish peroxidase study. *Neuroscience.* 1981;6:1315-28.

[23] Koob GF. Corticotropin-releasing factor, norepinephrine, and stress. *Biol. Psychiatry.* 1999;46:1167-80.

[24] Saavedra JM, Armando I, Bregonzio C, Juorio A, Macova M, Pavel J, et al. A centrally acting, anxiolytic angiotensin II AT1 receptor antagonist prevents the isolation stress-induced decrease in cortical CRF1 receptor and benzodiazepine binding. *Neuropsychopharmacology.* 2006;31:1123-34.

[25] Bregonzio C, Seltzer A, Armando I, Pavel J, Saavedra JM. Angiotensin II AT(1) receptor blockade selectively enhances brain AT(2) receptor expression, and abolishes the cold-restraint stress-induced increase in tyrosine hydroxylase mRNA in the locus coeruleus of spontaneously hypertensive rats. *Stress.* 2008;11(6):457-66.

[26] Jezova M, Armando I, Bregonzio C, Yu Z-X, Quian S, Ferrans VJ, et al. Angiotensin II AT1 and AT2 receptors contribute to maintain basal adrenomedullary norepinephrine synthesis and tyrosine hydroxilase transcription. *Endocrinology.* 2003;144:2092-101.

[27] Shekhar A, Sajdyk TJ, Gehlert DR, Rainnie DG. The amygdala, panic disorder, and cardiovascular responses. *Ann. NY Acad. Sci.* 2003 Apr;985:308-25.

[28] Valdez GR, Koob GF. Allostasis and dysregulation of corticotropin-releasing factor and neuropeptide Y systems: implications for the development of alcoholism. *Pharmacol. Biochem. Behav.* 2004;79:671-89.

[29] Anderson SM, Kant JG, De Souza EB. Effect of chronic stress on anterior pituitary and brain corticotropin-releasing factor receptors. *Pharmacol. Biochem. Behav.* 1993;44:755-61.

[30] Iredale PA, Terwilliger R, Widnell KL, Nestler EJ, Duman RS. Differential regulation of corticotrophin-releasing factor receptor 1 expression by stress and agonist treatments in brain and cultured cells. *Mol. Pharmacol.* 1996;50:1103-10.

[31] Brunson KL, Grigoriadis DE, Lorang MT, Baram TZ. Corticotropin-releasing hormone (CRH) downregulates the function of its receptor (CRF1) and induces CRF1 expression in hippocampal and cortical regions of inmature rat brain. *Exp. Neurol.* 2002;176:75-86.

[32] Tsutsumi K, Saavedra JM. Characterization and development of angiotensin II receptor subtypes (AT1 and AT2) in rat brain. *Am. J. Phisiol.* 1991;261:R209-16.

[33] Lenkei Z, Palkovits M, Corvol P, Llorens-Cortes C. Distribution of angiotensin type 1 receptor messenger RNA expression in the adult rat brain. *Neuroscience.* 1998;82:827-41.

[34] Berridge CW, Waterhouse BD. The locus coeruleus-noradrenergic system: modulation of behavioral state and state-dependent cognitive processes. *Brain Res. Rev.* 2003;42:33-84.

[35] Chappell PB, Smith MA, Kilts CD, Bissette G, Ritchie J, Anderson C. Alterations in corticotropin-releasing factor like immunoreactivity in discrete rat brain regions after acute and chronic stress. *J. Neurosci.* 1986;6:2908-14.

[36] Shimizu N, Nakane H, Hori T, Hayashi Y. CRF receptor antagonist attenuates stress-induced noradreanline release in the medial prefrontal cortex of rats. *Brain Res.* 1994;654:145-8.

[37] Biggio G, Concas A, Corda MG, Giorgi O, Sanna E, Serra M. Gabaergic and dopaminergic transmission in the rat cerebral cortex: effects of stress, anxiolytic and anxiogenis drugs. *Pharmacol. Ther.* 1990;48:121-42.

[38] Nutt DJ, Malizia AL. New insights into the role of the GABA (A)-benzodiazepine receptor in psychiatric disorder. *Br. J. Psychiatry.* 2001;179:390-94.

[39] Barnes NM, Costall B, Kelly ME, Murphy DA, Naylor RJ. Anxiolityc-like action by DuP753 , a non-peptide angiotensin II receptor antagonist. *Neuroreport.* 1990;1:20-1.

[40] Kaiser FC, Palmer GC, Wallace AV, Carr RD, Fraser-Rae L, Hallam C. Antiaxiety properties of the angiotensin II antagonist, Dup753, in the rat using the elevated plus-maze. *Neuroreport.* 1992;3:922-24.

[41] Saavedra JM, Ando H, Armando I, Baiardi G, Bregonzio C, Juorio A, et al. Anti-stress and anti-anxiety effects of centrally acting angiotensin II AT1 receptor antagonists. *Regul. Pept.* 2005;128:237-38.

[42] Overmier JB, Murison R. Anxiety and helplessness in the face of stress predisposes, precipitates, and sustains gastric ulceration. *Behav. Brain Res.* 2000;110:161-74.

[43] Andrade TG, Graeff FG. Effect of electrolytic and neurotoxic lesions of the median raphe nucleus on anxiety and stress. *Pharmacol. Biochem. Behav.* 2001 Sep;70(1):1-14.

[44] Tuncel N, Erkasap N, Sahinturk V, Ak DD, Tuncel M. The protective effect of vasoactive intestinal peptide (VIP) on stress-induced gastric ulceration in rats. *Ann. NY Acad. Sci.* 1998 Dec 11;865:309-22.

[45] Yelken B, Dorman T, Erkasap S, Dundar E, Tanriverdi B. Clonidine pretreatment inhibits stress-induced gastric ulcer in rats. *Anesth. Analg.* 1999 Jul;89(1):159-62.

[46] Heinemann A, Sattler V, Jocic M, Wienen W, Holzer P. Effect of angiotensin II and telmisartan, an angiotensin1 receptor antagonist, on rat gastric mucosal blood flow. *Aliment Pharmacol. Ther.* 1999 Mar;13(3):347-55.

[47] Rajagopalan S, Kurz S, Munzel T, Tarpey M, Freeman BA, Griendling KK, et al. Angiotensin II-mediated hypertension in the rat increases vascular superoxide production via membrane NADH/NADPH oxidase activation. Contribution to alterations of vasomotor tone. *J. Clin. Invest.* 1996 Apr 15;97(8):1916-23.

[48] Senay CE, Levine RJ. Synergism between cold and restraint for rapid production of stress ulcer in rats. *Proc. Soc. Exp. Biol. Med.* 1967;124:1221-3.

[49] Bregonzio C, Armando I, Ando H, Jezova M, Baiardi G, Saavedra JM. Anti-inflammatory effects of angiotensin II AT1 receptor antagonism prevent stress-induced gastric injury. *Am. J. Phisiol.* 2003;285:G414-23.

[50] Filaterova LP, Filaretov AA, Makara GB. Corticosterone increase inhibits stress-induced gastric erosions in rats. *Am. J. Phisiol.* 1998;274:G1024-30.

[51] Nishimura Y, Ito T, Hoe K, Saavedra JM. Chronic peripheral administration of the angiotensin II AT(1) receptor antagonist candesartan blocks brain AT(1) receptors. *Brain Res.* 2000 Jul 14;871(1):29-38.

[52] Hamaguchi M, Watanabe T, Higuchi K, Tominaga K, Fujiwara Y, Arakawa T. Mechanisms and roles of neutrophil infiltration in stress-induced gastric injury in rats. *Dig. Dis. Sci.* 2001 Dec;46(12):2708-15.

[53] Liu W, Okajima K, Murakami K, Harada N, Isobe H, Irie T. Role of neutrophil elastase in stress-induced gastric mucosal injury in rats. *J. Lab Clin. Med.* 1998 Nov;132(5):432-9.

[54] Ruiz-Ortega M, Ruperez M, Lorenzo O, Esteban V, Blanco J, Mezzano S, et al. Angiotensin II regulates the synthesis of proinflammatory cytokines and chemokines in the kidney. *Kidney Int. Suppl.* 2002 Dec(82):S12-22.

[55] Tamarat R, Silvestre JS, Durie M, Levy BI. Angiotensin II angiogenic effect in vivo involves vascular endothelial growth factor- and inflammation-related pathways. *Lab Invest.* 2002 Jun;82(6):747-56.

[56] Kalra D, Sivasubramanian N, Mann DL. Angiotensin II induces tumor necrosis factor biosynthesis in the adult mammalian heart through a protein kinase C-dependent pathway. *Circulation.* 2002 May 7;105(18):2198-205.

[57] Nakamura A, Johns EJ, Imaizumi A, Niimi R, Yanagawa Y, Kohsaka T. Role of angiotensin II-induced cAMP in mesangial TNF-alpha production. *Cytokine.* 2002 Jul 7;19(1):47-51.

[58] Strawn WB, Dean RH, Ferrario CM. Novel mechanisms linking angiotensin II and early atherogenesis. *J. Renin Angiotensin Aldosterone Syst.* 2000 Mar;1(1):11-7.

[59] Bucher M, Ittner KP, Hobbhahn J, Taeger K, Kurtz A. Downregulation of angiotensin II type 1 receptors during sepsis. *Hypertension.* 2001 Aug;38(2):177-82.

[60] Sasamura H, Nakazato Y, Hayashida T, Kitamura Y, Hayashi M, Saruta T. Regulation of vascular type 1 angiotensin receptors by cytokines. *Hypertension.* 1997 Jul;30(1 Pt 1):35-41.

[61] Cowling RT, Gurantz D, Peng J, Dillmann WH, Greenberg BH. Transcription factor NF-kappa B is necessary for up-regulation of type 1 angiotensin II receptor mRNA in rat cardiac fibroblasts treated with tumor necrosis factor-alpha or interleukin-1 beta. *J. Biol. Chem.* 2002 Feb 22;277(8):5719-24.

[62] Peng J, Gurantz D, Tran V, Cowling RT, Greenberg BH. Tumor necrosis factor-alpha-induced AT1 receptor upregulation enhances angiotensin II-mediated cardiac fibroblast responses that favor fibrosis. *Circ. Res.* 2002 Dec 13;91(12):1119-26.

[63] Dole VP, Nyswander ME. Rehabilitation of heroin addicts after blockade with methadone. *NY State J. Med.* 1966 Aug 1;66(15):2011-7.

[64] Kreek MJ. Effects of opiates, opioid antagonists and cocaine on the endogenous opioid system: clinical and laboratory studies. *NIDA Res. Monogr.* 1992;119:44-8.

[65] Kreek MJ, Koob GF. Drug dependence: stress and dysregulation of brain reward pathways. Drug Alcohol Depend. 1998 Jun-Jul;51(1-2):23-47.

[66] Piazza PV, Le Moal M. The role of stress in drug-self administration. *Trends Pharmacol. Sci.* 1998;19:67-74.

[67] Piazza PV, Deroche V, Deminiere JM, Maccari S, Le Moal M, Simon H. Corticosterone in the range of stress-induced levels possesses reinforcing properties: implications for sensation-seeking behaviors. *Proc. Natl. Acad. Sci. USA*. 1993 Dec 15;90(24):11738-42.

[68] Goeders NE. Stress, the hypothalamic-pituitary-adrenal axis, and vulnerability to drug abuse. *NIDA Res. Monogr*. 1998 Mar;169:83-104.

[69] Vanderschuren LJ, Schmidt ED, De Vries TJ, Van Moorsel CA, Tilders FJ, Schoffelmeer AN. A single exposure to amphetamine is sufficient to induce long-term behavioral, neuroendocrine, and neurochemical sensitization in rats. *J. Neurosci*. 1999;19(21):9579-86.

[70] Brown DC, Steward LJ, Ge J, Barnes NM. Ability of angiotensin II to modulate striatal dopamine release via the AT1 receptor in vitro and in vivo. *Br. J. Pharmacol*. 1996 May;118(2):414-20.

[71] Tchekalarova J, Sotiriou E, Georgiev V, Kostopoulos G, Angelatou F. Up-regulation of adenosine A1 receptor binding in pentylenetetrazol kindling in mice: effects of angiotensin IV. *Brain Res*. 2005 Jan 25;1032(1-2):94-103.

[72] Tchekalarova J, Georgiev V. Angiotensin peptides modulatory system: how is it implicated in the control of seizure susceptibility? *Life Sci*. 2005;76:955-70.

[73] Daubert DL, Meadows GG, Wang JH, Sanchez PJ, Speth RC. Changes in angiotensin II receptors in dopamine-rich regions of the mouse brain with age and ethanol consumption. *Brain Res*. 1999;816:8-16.

[74] White F, Kalivas PW. Neuroadaptations involved in amphetamine and cocaine addiction. *Drug and Alcohol dependence*. 1998;51:141-53.

[75] Roitman MF, Na E, Anderson G, Jones TA, Bernstein IL. Induction of a salt appetite alters dendritic morphology in nucleus accumbens and sensitizes rats to amphetamine. *J. Neurosci*. 2002 Jun 1;22(11):RC225.

[76] Clark JJ, Bernstein IL. Reciprocal cross-sensitization between amphetamine and salt appetite. *Pharmacol. Biochem. Behav*. 2004 Aug;78(4):691-8.

[77] Acerbo MJ, Johnson AK. Behavioral cross-sensitization between DOCA-induced sodium appetite and cocaine-induced locomotor behavior. *Pharmacol. Biochem. Behav*. 2011 May;98(3):440-8.

[78] Valjent E, Bertran-Gonzalez J, Aubier B, Greengard P, Herve D, Girault JA. Mechanisms of locomotor sensitization to drugs of abuse in a two-injection protocol. *Neuropsychopharmacology*. 2010;35(2):401-15.

[79] Paz MC, Assis MA, Cabrera RJ, Cancela LM, Bregonzio C. The AT angiotensin II receptor blockade attenuates the development of amphetamine-induced behavioral sensitization in a two-injection protocol. *Synapse*. 2011 Jun;65(6):505-12.

[80] Fitts DA. Angiotensin and captopril increase alcohol intake. *Pharmacol. Biochem. Behav*. 1993 May;45(1):35-43.

[81] Fitts DA, Hoon RG. Ethanol-induced changes in plasma proteins, angiotensin II, and salt appetite in rats. *Behav. Neurosci*. 1993 Apr;107(2):339-45.

[82] Weisinger RS, Blair-West JR, Burns P, Denton DA. Intracerebroventricular infusion of angiotensin II increases water and ethanol intake in rats. *Am. J. Physiol*. 1999 Jul;277(1 Pt 2):R162-72.

[83] Heilig M, Koob GF. A key role for corticotropin-releasing factor in alcohol dependence. *Trends Neurosci*. 2007 Aug;30(8):399-406.

[84] Sommer WH, Saavedra JM. Targeting brain angiotensin and corticotrophin-releasing hormone systems interaction for the treatment of mood and alcohol use disorders. *J. Mol. Med.* 2008 Jun;86(6):723-8.

[85] Maul B, Krause W, Pankow K, Becker M, Gembardt F, Alenina N, et al. Central angiotensin II controls alcohol consumption via its AT1 receptor. *Faseb J.* 2005;19:1474-81.

[86] Guivernau M, Pallavicini J. [Effect of angiotensin II synthesis inhibition on alcohol consumption]. *Rev. Med. Chil.* 2008 Aug;136(8):968-75.

[87] Hosseini M, Sharifi MR, Alaei H, Shafei MN, Karimooy HA. Effects of angiotensin II and captopril on rewarding properties of morphine. Indian *J. Exp. Biol.* 2007 Sep;45(9):770-7.

[88] Hosseini M, Alaei HA, Headari R, Eslamizadeh MJ. Effects of microinjection of angiotensin II and captopril into nucleus accumbens on morphine self-administration in rats. *Indian J. Exp. Biol.* 2009 May;47(5):361-7.

In: Angiotensin: New Research
Editors: S. Harada, I. Moi, pp. 131-148

ISBN: 978-1-62100-773-9

Chapter 5

ANGIOTENSIN I-CONVERTING ENZYME INHIBITORY ACTIVITY IN LIMA BEAN (*PHASEOLUS LUNATUS*) PROTEIN HYDROLYSATES PRODUCED WITH ALCALASE OR PEPSIN-PANCREATIN

***L. Chel-Guerrero*[1], *M. Domínguez-Magaña*[2], *G.Dávila-Ortiz*[2], *and D. Betancur-Ancona*[1*]**

[1] Facultad de Ingeniería Química, Universidad Autónoma de Yucatán, Periférico Norte Km. 33.5, Tablaje Catastral 13615, Colonia Chuburná de Hidalgo Inn, C.P. 97203, Mérida Yucatán, México.

[2] Escuela Nacional de Ciencias Biológicas, Instituto Politécnico Nacional, Casco de Santo Tomás, Prolongación Manuel M. Carpio S/N Esquina Plan de Ayala, Delegación Miguel Hidalgo.

ABSTRACT

Protein concentrates from ungerminated and germinated lima bean *Phaseolus lunatus* seed flours were hydrolyzed with alcalase 2.4L or pepsin-pancreatin sequential hydrolysis, and ACE inhibitory activity measured in the different hydrolysis treatments. A 2^3 factorial design with four replicates of the central trial was used. Evaluated factors were protein concentrate source (ungerminated seeds, PC_1; germinated seeds, PC_2), enzyme/substrate ratio E/S (1/50 or 1/10) and hydrolysis time (0.5 or 2.0 h for alcalase; 1 or 3 h for pepsin-pancreatin). Degree of hydrolysis (DH) was high for the alcalase hydrolysates (24.12 - 58.94%), but the pepsin-pancreatin hydrolysates exhibited the highest ACE inhibitory activity (IC_{50} = 0.250 - 0.692 mg/mL). Under the tested conditions, the hydrolysates with the highest ACE inhibitory activity were produced with sequential pepsin-pancreatin using either PC_1 at 1 h hydrolysis time and a 1/10 E/S ratio or PC_2 at 1 h hydrolysis time and a 1/50 E/S ratio. Lima bean protein hydrolysates

* Telephone (52) 999 9460989, Fax (52) 999 9460994. E-mail:bancona@uady.mx.

prepared with alcalase or pepsin-pancreatin are a potential ingredient in the production of physiologically functional foods with antihypertensive activity.

Keywords: Lima bean, Protein hydrolysates, Degree of hydrolysis, ACE inhibition, IC_{50}

INTRODUCTION

Hypertension is a major risk factor for stroke and other cardiovascular diseases. Among other strategies, angiotensin I-converting enzyme (ACE-I) inhibitors are used in the prevention of hypertension and congestive heart failure [1]. Studies have also been done of ACE-I inhibitors in the treatment of chronic heart failure and myocardial infarction [2], as well as cancer [3, 4]. ACE-I (peptidyldipeptide hydrolase, EC 3.4.15.1) catalyzes various reactions, two of which play key physiological roles in regulating blood pressure: conversion of inactive decapeptide angiotensin I into angiotensin II, a powerful vasoconstrictor and salt-retaining octapeptide; and inactivation of the vasodilator nonapeptide bradykinin, which is conducive to lowering blood pressure [5]. ACE-I inhibitors have been shown to exhibit antihypertensive activity in spontaneously hypertensive rats and hypertensive patients [6].

Recent research has focused on ACE-I inhibitory hydrolysates and peptides from animal and vegetal sources. The primary animal sources are proteins from casein, whey protein, fish protein, pig and chicken muscle, hemoglobin, blood plasma protein, gelatin [7] and egg yolks [8, 9]. The primary plant sources are proteins from legume seeds such as mung bean [10], soybean [11, 12], pea [13], and chickpea [14]; oilseeds such as rapeseed [15, 16]; and cereal crop derivatives such as maize gluten, wheat germ and buckwheat [7]. These studies involve hydrolysate and peptide extraction with commercial enzymes (alcalase, flavourzyme, pepsin, pancreatin, trypsin, chymotrypsin, neutrace, etc.) at different hydrolysis times and enzyme/substrate ratios. An important variable in these studies is the concentration (mg protein/mL) of hydrolysate or peptide required to inhibit 50% of ACE-I activity under assayed conditions (IC_{50}); most enzymatic hydrolysates and peptides have values between 0.20 and 246.7 mg/mL [10]. Protein hydrolysis can be done chemically using acids or alkalines, although this oxidizes, destroys or modifies some amino acids, thus reducing protein quality [17]. Enzymatic hydrolysis is therefore preferred since it can improve the physicochemical, functional and sensory properties of native proteins without affecting their nutritional value [18]. In addition to modifying technological functionality, enzymatic hydrolysates have also been used to reduce allergenicity, and formulate pharmaceutical products and substances for clinical applications [19, 20].

Legume seeds have higher nutritional protein content (200-400 g/kg) than other seeds, such as cereals (70-140 g/kg) [21]. The high protein content of legume protein isolates or concentrates are making them increasingly important in the food industry, where they represent a promising alternative ingredient for preparing and developing new foods [22]. Germinated legumes currently account for an increasingly larger proportion of total worldwide food legume consumption because germination produces beneficial modifications in their chemical components; among other applications, they are used to produce high nutritional value flours [23]. Lima bean (*Phaseolus lunatus*) is grown in tropical regions such as Mexico. Its seeds have high protein (210-260g/kg) and high carbohydrate contents (550-640 g/kg), low fat (10-23 g/kg) and fiber levels (32-68 g/kg), high levels of minerals such as

K, Zn, Ca and Fe, and low levels of Na and P [24]. Use of plant products as functional ingredients in foods is rising rapidly, due both to their cost-effectiveness and the improvements they provide in product nutritional quality [25]. *Phaseolus lunatus* is a promising source of protein hydrolysates with antihypertensive properties. The present study aim was to obtain hydrolysates from protein concentrates produced from ungerminated and germinated *Phaseolus lunatus* seeds using alcalase or pepsin-pancreatin sequential hydrolysis, and evaluate hydrolysate ACE-I inhibitory activity.

MATERIALS AND METHODS

Seeds and Chemicals

Phaseolus lunatus L. seeds were purchased at a local market in Merida, Yucatan, Mexico. Any impurities were manually removed from the seeds. Flours from ungerminated and germinated seeds were prepared by cleaning the seeds, milling them in a Mycros impact mill, and screening through a 20 mesh screen (0.85 mm pore opening). Angiotensin I-converting enzyme (ACE-I), Hippuryl-L-histidyl-L-leucine (HHL), 2,4,6-trichloro-s-triazine (TT), o-phthaldialdehyde (OPA), serine standard, gastric porcine pepsin, and porcine pancreatin were purchased from Sigma. Alcalase 2.4 L was obtained from Novo Nordisk, Bagsvaerd, Denmark. All other chemicals were analytical grade.

Seed Germination

Seeds were washed with water, soaked in distilled water and immersed for 1 min in 20 mL sodium hypochloride solution (0.2 w/v), and washed again three times in 25 mL distilled water. Following, germination was done for 48 h in a germination room in darkness at 16-18 °C and moisture levels maintained by spraying with distilled water every 8 h [26].

Protein Concentrates from Ungerminated and Germinated Seeds

Protein concentrates (PC) were extracted from the ungerminated and germinated seeds according to Chel-Guerrero et al., [21] method. Three, 1 Kg batches of flour were processed by preparing flour: water (1:6 w/v) suspension, and adjusting pH to 11 with 1 N NaOH. After soaking for 1 h, the suspensions were milled in a disk mill and passed through 80 and 100 mesh screens to separate the fiber-containing solid fraction from the liquid fraction, which contains the protein and starch. Residual solids were washed 5 times with distilled water at a 1:3 v/v ratio and then passed through 150 mesh screen to eliminate the finest fiber. Wash water was mixed with the supernatants from the initial suspension and this solution allowed to sediment for 30 min to recover the starch fraction and separate the solubilized protein. The pH of the solubilized proteins was adjusted to the isoelectric point (4.5) with 1 N HCl. The suspension was then centrifuged at 1317 x g for 12 min (Mistral 3000i, Curtin Matheson

Sci.), the supernatants discarded and the precipitates freeze-dried at -47 °C and 13 x 10-3 mbar.

Proximate Composition

Standard AOAC [27] methods were used to determine nitrogen (method 954.01); fat (920.39); ash (923.03); fiber (962.09); and moisture (925.09) contents of the flours and protein concentrates. Protein content was calculated as nitrogen (factor 6.25), and carbohydrate content was estimated as nitrogen-free extract (NFE).

Amino Acid Analysis of Protein Concentrates

Samples (2 mg) were hydrolyzed with 4 mL of 6 N HCl, the solutions sealed in tubes under nitrogen and incubated in an oven at 110 °C for 24 h. Amino acids were determined after derivatization with diethyl ethoxymethylenemalonate by high-performance liquid chromatography (HPLC) [28], using D,L-γ–aminobutyric acid as an internal standard. The HPLC system consisted of a Model 600E multi-system with a 484 UV–vis detector (Waters, Milford, MA) equipped with a 300x3.9 mm i.d. reversed-phase column (Novapack C18, 4 m; Waters). A binary gradient was used for elution with a flow of 0.9 mL/min. The solvents used were (A) sodium acetate (25 mM) containing sodium azide (0.02% w/v) at pH 6.0, and (B) acetonitrile. Elution was done as follows: time 0.0–3.0 min, linear gradient from A/B (91:9) to A/B (86/14); 3.0–13.0 min, elution with A/B (86/14); 13.0–30.0 min, linear gradient from A/B (86:14) to A/B (69/31); 30.0–35.0 min, elution with A/B (69:31). Eluted amino acids were detected at 280 nm and the column maintained at 18 °C.

Alcalase Protein Hydrolysis

Following the method of Li et al., [10], protein isolate suspensions (4 g protein in 100 ml water) were prepared from the ungerminated and germinated seed flours. Hydrolysis of these suspensions was done using Alcalase 2.4L, a commercial protease preparation with endopeptidase activity produced from *Bacillus licheniformis* [14]. Its specific activity is 2.4 Anson Units (AU) per gram, one AU being the amount of enzyme, which, under standard conditions, digests hemoglobin at an initial rate that generates an amount of trichloroacetic acid-soluble product which produces the same color with Folin reagent as one milliequivalent of tyrosine released per min. This enzyme is a microbial protease preparation used in the food industry to improve the functional and nutritional properties of protein preparations. A 2^3 factorial design was used to analyze DH and ACE-I inhibitory activity, with four replicates of the central trial. Factors and their corresponding levels were: Factor A, protein concentrate source (ungerminated, PC_1; germinated, PC_2); Factor B, enzyme/substrate ratio (E/S) (1/50 or 1/10); and Factor C: hydrolysis time (0.5 or 2.0 h). Hydrolysis was done in a pH stat, 50 mL vessel, by adding 0.3 AU/g alcalase. The reaction was run at 50 ºC, pH adjusted to 7.0 with 0.1 N NaOH and the suspension kept under constant agitation. Hydrolysis was finalized by inactivating the protease with heating to 85 °C for 10 min. The hydrolysates were freeze-dried (Labconco) for later analysis.

Pepsin-Pancreatin Protein Hydrolysis

Protein hydrolysis was done with a sequential pepsin-pancreatin system involving digestion with pepsin for half the hydrolysis time followed by incubation with pancreatin for the other half [29]. A 2^3 factorial design was again used to analyze DH and ACE-I inhibitory activity, with four replicates of the central trial. Factors and their corresponding levels were: Factor A, PC source (PC_1, PC_2); Factor B, E/S ratio (1/50 or 1/10); and Factor C, hydrolysis time (1.0 or 3.0 h). Hydrolysis parameters were 4% (w/v) concentration for each enzyme; pH 2 for pepsin and 7.5 for pancreatin; and 37 °C temperature. Hydrolysis was done in a 50 mL reaction vessel equipped with a stirrer, thermometer and pH electrode. The hydrolysis reaction was stopped by heating at 80 °C for 20 min. Hydrolysates were lyophilized for later use. In both experiments, the response variables were DH and ACE-I inhibitory activity.

Degree of Hydrolysis

Degree of hydrolysis (DH) was calculated by determining free amino groups through reaction with OPA reagent [30], using a serine standard. Total number of amino groups was determined in a 100% hydrolyzed sample by treatment with 6 N HCl at 110 °C for 24 h in a vacuum oven.

ACE-I Inhibitory Activity

ACE-I inhibitory activity was determined according to Hayakari et al., [31] method, with some modifications. ACE-I hydrolyzes HHL, yielding hippuric acid and His-Leu. This method relies on the colorimetric reaction of hippuric acid with TT in a 0.5 mL incubation mixture containing 40 µmol potassium phosphate buffer, pH 8.3; 300 µmol NaCl; 1.5 µmol HHL; 20 µL ACE (100 mU); and different amounts of hydrolysate extracts. Incubation was run for 45 min at 37 °C, and the reaction stopped by adding 1.5 mL 3% TT in dioxane, followed by 3 mL 0.2 M phosphate buffer, pH 8.3. The resulting reaction mixtures were centrifuged at 10 000 x g for 10 min, and enzymatic activity determined in the supernatant by reading absorbance at 382 nm. The IC_{50} value was determined by regression analysis of ACE inhibition (%) vs. hydrolysate protein concentration.

Statistical Analysis

Statistical treatment of DH and ACE-I inhibitory activity results was done with an analysis of variance (ANOVA), a Duncan comparison of means and a 2^3 factorial design regression analysis. A Student *t* test (5% significance level) was applied to compare differences between means for the flour and PC chemical compositions (ungerminated and germinated seeds) [32]. All statistical analyses were done with the Statgraphics Plus version 5.0 statistical software.

RESULTS AND DISCUSSION

Proximate Composition

Germination for 48 h show significantly ($p<0.05$) effected in flour and PC composition (Table 1). This treatment reduced fat content by 16.5% (i.e. 1.76-1.47%), fiber by 15.6% (i.e. 5.64-4.76%) and NFE by 4.19% (i.e. 58.53-56.08%), but increased protein content by 11.5% (i.e. 30.18-33.65%) and ash by 3.9% (i.e. 3.89-4.04%). The increase in protein and ash content after germination of *P. lunatus* seeds coincides with Dibifori *et al.* [33], who showed a 2.4% increase in protein and 0.94% increase in ash after germination of *P. lunatus* seeds for 48 h in darkness. Rodríguez *et al.* [34] report a 0.5% increase in protein content in *P. vulgaris* cv. La Granja seeds after germination for 48 h, and Bau *et al.* [35] mentioned increases in soybean protein content after germination. Prolonging germination time can further increase protein contents. In a study of seeds from two *P. vulgaris* cultivars (black and white seeds), there was reported an increasing on protein content (4.1 and 2.9%, respectively) after five days of germination [36]

Table 1. Proximate composition of protein concentrates produced from ungerminated and germinated *P. lunatus* seed flours

Component (g/100 g)	F_1	F_2	PC_1	PC_2
Moisture	$(9.58)^b$	$(9.32)^a$	$(4.45)^A$	$(5.40)^B$
Protein (Nx6.25)	30.18^a	33.65^b	56.40^A	69.14^B
Fat	1.76^b	1.47^a	3.12^A	4.16^B
Fiber	5.64^b	4.76^a	1.83^B	0.96^A
Ash	3.89^a	4.04^b	3.32^A	3.68^B
NFE	58.53^b	56.08^a	35.33^B	22.06^A

$^{a-b, A-B}$ Different letter superscripts in the same row indicate significant difference ($P<0.05$). F_1: Flour from ungerminated seeds. F_1 : Flour from germinated seeds. PC_1: Protein concentrate from ungerminated seeds. PC_2: Protein concentrate from germinated seeds. NFE: Nitrogen-free extract.

Protein concentration levels were 56.40% in PC_1 and 69.14% in PC_2. Fat content increased in both PC_1 (3.12%) and PC_2 (4.16%), probably caused by concentration of fats at the alkaline pH (11). At this pH, fat saponifies with the alkali and these fats (mainly polar) precipitate together with the protein at the isoelectric point (pH 4.5), which has been reported in protein concentrates from *Cicer arietinum* L [25] and *Canavalia ensiformis* [21]. The extent of this saponification probably depends on legume seed fatty acid composition. Germination resulted in higher protein content, probably due to synthesis of enzyme proteins for seed dicotyledon development in the mother plant and degradation of reserve nutrients (lipids and carbohydrates), both vital to the purpose of providing the energy required for protein synthesis in plant growth [35]. Protein content in both flours and PCs was similar to previously showed levels in *P. lunatus* [21, 37, 38, 39]. The protein recovery percentages (i.e. process efficiency) for PC production were 34.30% for ungerminated seeds and 30.84% for germinated seeds, which are lower than mentioned for other seeds: 44% in faba beans [40]; 60% in lupine seeds [41]; and 46% in safflower seeds [42].

Amino Acids Composition

The PCs exhibited similar amino acid profiles (Table 2). Both contained high proportions of Asp (12.80 and 12.47% for PC_1 and PC_2, respectively); Glu (15.30 and 16.10%), Leu (9.19 and 9.01%), Pro (7.62 and 7.68%) and Ser (7.39 and 7.26%). Germination and the isoelectric point protein recovery process further increased levels of Glu (15.30-16.10%), Gly (4.67-4.84%), Ala (6.08-6.19%), Met (0.35-0.50%) and Phe (0.52-0.65%), but decreased Asp (12.80-12.47%), Ser (7.39-7.26%), His (3.24-3.17%), Tyr (3.54-3.09%), Ile (4.30-4.11%), Leu (9.19-9.01%) and Trp (0.98-0.79%). All other amino acids levels varied minimally between the PCs. Rodríguez *et al.* [34] reports similar decreases in Lys (6.64-6.16 g/16 g N) and Tyr (2.98-2.49 g/16 g N), but also observed an increase in His (2.92-3.04 g/16g N) in a study of germination in *P. vulgaris* cv. La Granja for 48 h in darkness. The PC amino acid profiles observed here are very similar to amino acid profiles reported for lima bean [39] and mung bean protein isolates [10].

Hydrolysis with Alcalase

Hydrolysis with the endoprotease alcalase increased DH with greater hydrolysis time in both PC_1 and PC_2, the highest DH being in PC_2 (DH = 58.94%) (Table 3). This greater alcalase activity in PC_2 may have resulted from partial elimination of lipids and carbohydrates during germination (Table 2). Another possibility is that denaturation during the concentration process produced a better molecular orientation in PC_2 than in PC_1, which would have enhanced the enzyme-substrate interaction, or that germination increased Ala, Met and Phe residues, upon which alcalase has broad specificity [19].

The variance analysis indicated that all factors and interactions influenced ($p<0.05$) DH (Figure 1, Eq. 1), and the regression analysis for this response variable indicated that the results fit ($p<0.05$) a first-order polynomial model. The mathematical model explaining the behavior of DH as a function of PC source (A); E/S ratio (B); hydrolysis time (C); PC source-E/S ratio (AB); PC source-hydrolysis time (AC); E/S ratio-hydrolysis time (BC); and PC source-E/S ratio-hydrolysis time (ABC) had a determination coefficient (R^2) of 0.998 (Figure 1). This model showed E/S ratio (B) and hydrolysis time (C) to have the most positive effects on DH ($p<0.05$), with coefficients of 4.11 and 9.94, respectively.

ACE-I inhibitory activity (IC_{50}) ranged from 0.61-2.40 mg/mL (Table 3). In the variance analysis, it was unaffected by the principal factors and double interactions, but was affected ($p<0.05$) by the triple interaction. The regression analysis showed it to fit a first-order polynomial model with an R^2=0.931. This explains the behavior of ACE-I inhibitory activity as a function of PC source-E/S ratio-hydrolysis time (ABC) (Figure 1, Eq. 2). From a cost standpoint, treatment 1 is optimum, although it did not have the best ACE-I inhibitory effect (0.94 mg/mL).

Table 2. Amino acid composition of protein concentrates produced from ungerminated (PC_1) and germinated (PC_2) *P. lunatus* seed flours

	Content (g/100 g of protein)	
Amino acid	PC_1	PC_2
Asp	12.80	12.47
Glu	15.30	16.10
Ser	7.39	7.26
His	3.24	3.17
Gly	4.67	4.84
Thr	4.4	4.41
Ala	6.08	6.19
Arg	4.96	5.02
Tyr	3.54	3.09
Cys	3.87	3.90
Val	4.79	4.88
Met	0.35	0.50
Phe	0.52	0.65
Ile	4.30	4.11
Leu	9.19	9.01
Lys	5.99	5.94
Pro	7.62	7.68
Trp	0.98	0.79
Amino Acid Distribution		
Hydrophobic	34.10	33.34
Neutral	20.90	21.06
Hydrophilic	45.00	45.60

Table 3. Degree of hydrolysis (DH) and ACE-I inhibition (IC_{50}) in alcalase hydrolysates of protein concentrates from a) ungerminated (PC_1) and b) germinated (PC_2) *P. lunatus* seeds

Treatment	Factor A Protein concentrate Source	Factor B E/S Ratio	Factor C Hydrolysis Time (h)	DH (%)	IC_{50} (mg/mL)
1	PC_1	1/50	0.5	24.12^a	0.94^d
2	PC_2	1/50	0.5	29.91^c	2.40^i
3	PC_1	1/10	0.5	33.40^b	2.05^g
4	PC_2	1/10	0.5	30.34^e	0.61^b
5	PC_1	1/50	2.0	40.39^d	2.11^h
6	PC_2	1/50	2.0	46.67^d	0.87^c
7	PC_1	1/10	2.0	51.28^g	0.56^a
8	PC_2	1/10	2.0	58.94^h	1.16^e
9A	PC_1-PC_2 (50/50 w/w)	1/30	1.25	39.56^f	1.00^f
9B	PC_1-PC_2 (50/50 w/w	1/30	1.25	40.07^f	1.02^f
9C	PC_1-PC_2 (50/50 w/w	1/30	1.25	39.76^f	1.01^f
9D	PC_1-PC_2 (50/50 w/w)	1/30	1.25	39.77^f	1.02^f

$^{a-i}$ Different letter superscripts in the same column indicate significant difference ($P<0.05$).
E/S = Enzyme/substrate ratio.
9A, 9B, 9C, 9D: central trial treatments.

Optimization of ACE-I inhibitory activity will require analysis of more than the three factors evaluated here. In a study of rice dreg hydrolysates with trypsin, [43] obtained a mathematical model with R^2=0.877, which explained ACE-I inhibitory activity based on five factors: pH; temperature; E/S ratio (B); water to rice dregs ratio (W/R); and hydrolysis time (C). In this study, pH and the water to rice dregs ratio (W/R) had an effect ($p<0.05$) on ACE-I inhibitory activity.

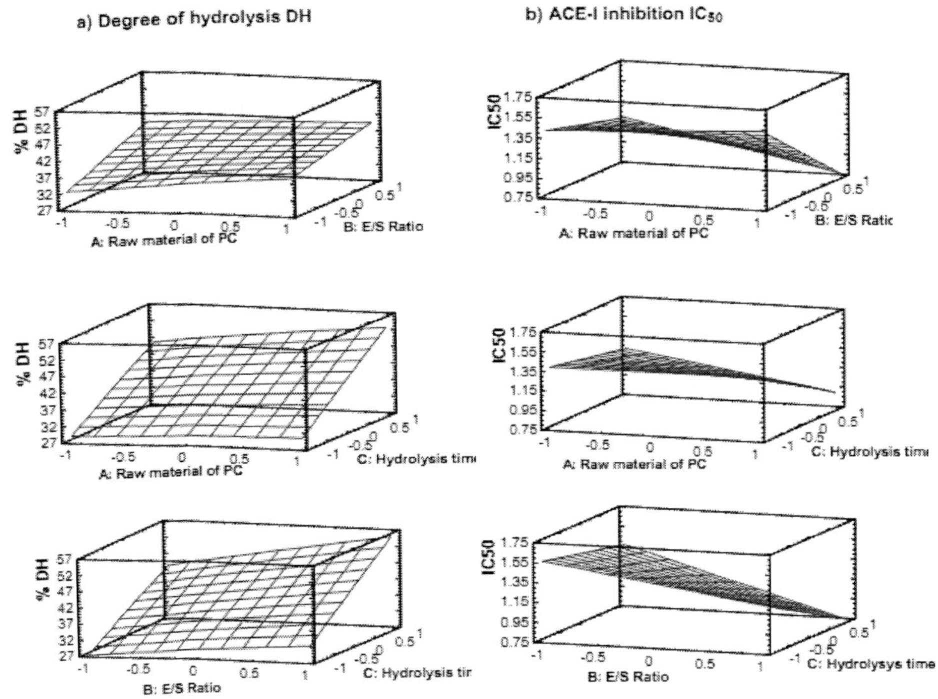

$$\% DH = 39.52+2.08A+4.11B+9.94C-0.93AB+01.40AC+1.68BC+1.28ABC \qquad R^2=0.998 \text{ (Eq. 1)}$$

$$IC_{50} = 1.23+0.59ABC \qquad R^2=0.931 \text{ (Eq. 2)}$$

Figure 1. Effect of significant factors in alcalase hydrolysis of protein concentrates from ungerminated (PC_1) and germinated (PC_2) *P. lunatus* seeds on a) Degree of hydrolysis (DH) and b) ACE-I inhibition (IC_{50}): Factor A, protein concentrate source (PC_1 and PC_2); Factor B, E/S ratio; Factor C, hydrolysis time.

At 0.5 h hydrolysis time and the 1/50 E/S (Table 3, Figure $2a_1$, $2b_1$), alcalase activity was highest in PC_2 (DH=29.91%), whereas ACE-I inhibitory activity was best in PC_1 (IC_{50}=0.94 mg/mL). This trend inverted when the E/S ratio increased to 1/10 (Table 3, Figure $2a_2$, $2b_2$), in that alcalase activity was highest in PC_1 (33.40%) and inhibitory activity was highest in PC_2 (IC_{50}=0.61 mg/mL). At 2 h hydrolysis time, PC_2 exhibited the highest enzymatic activity at both E/S levels (1/50: DH=46.67%, 1/10: DH=58.94%) (Table 3, Figure $2b_1$, $2b_2$). In contrast, inhibitory activity was independent of PC source and E/S ratio, with the best IC_{50} values in PC_1 at 1/10 (0.56 mg/mL) and PC_2 at 1/50 (0.87 mg/mL) (Table 3, Figure $2a_1$, $2b_1$). The inhibitory activity mathematical model and the fact that only the triple interaction (ABC) was significant, indicate that treatment 7 (PC_1, 1/10 E/S, 2 h hydrolysis time) produced the optimum ACE-I inhibitory activity (IC_{50}=0.56 mg/mL).

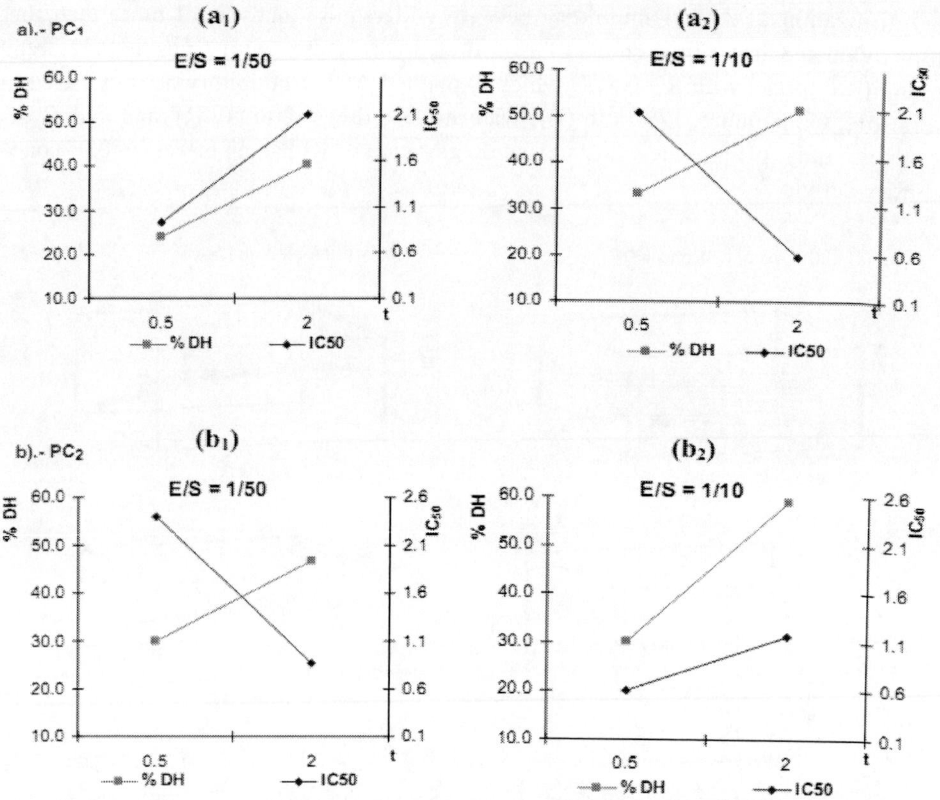

Figure 2. Degree of hydrolysis (% DH) and ACE-I inhibition (IC_{50}) produced by alcalase hydrolysis of protein concentrates from a) ungerminated (PC_1) and b) germinated (PC_2) *P. lunatus* seeds.

Inhibitory activity in treatments 2 (PC_2, 1/50 E/S) and 3 (PC_1, 1/10 E/S) improved with greater hydrolysis time (2.40-0.87 and 2.05-0.56 mg/mL, respectively), but declined in treatments 1 (PC_1, 1/50 E/S) and 4 (PC_2, 1/10 E/S) (0.93-2.11 and 0.61-1.16 mg/mL, respectively). This suggests that a peptide (or peptides) with good ACE-I inhibitory activity obtained at 0.5 h was hydrolyzed at 2 h hydrolysis time, consequently decreasing its antihypertensive effect. In other words, there is an optimal hydrolysis point or DH above which a larger amount of ACE-I inhibitory peptides are degraded than formed, lowering overall ACE-I inhibitory activity. Similar behavior has been reported for protein hydrolysates from sunflower [29], chickpea [14] and fish [44]. The central trial treatment had an average DH of 39.81% and an average IC_{50} of 1.01 mg/mL, meaning that PC_1-PC_2 mixtures are not recommended in terms of their inhibitory activity.

Overall, optimum ACE-I inhibitory activity among the alcalase hydrolysates was observed in PC_1 (IC_{50} between 0.56-2.11 mg/mL), although alcalase reacted better with PC_2. Both the DH and inhibitory activity values for the *P. lunatus* alcalase hydrolysates are similar to results reported for alcalase hydrolysates from other proteins: Alaska pollack skin (IC_{50}=0.63 mg/mL, 6 h hydrolysis time) [44]; chickpea protein isolate (IC_{50}=0.19 mg/mL, DH=18%, 0.5 h hydrolysis time) [45]; chickpea legumin (IC_{50}=0.18 mg/mL, DH=27%, 0.5 h hydrolysis time) [14]; and mung bean (IC_{50}=0.64 mg/mL, DH=17%, 2 h hydrolysis time) [10].

Hydrolysis with Pepsin-Pancreatin

Pepsin-pancreatin sequential hydrolysis did not hydrolyze the lima bean PCs as effectively as alcalase, producing comparatively lower DH values (15.35-37.07%), although ACE-I inhibitory activity was generally higher in these hydrolysates (Table 4, Figure 4). These differences in hydrolytic behavior may have originated in the hydrolysis method used (e.g. enzyme type and concentration) [46], or the low content of aromatic and cationic amino acid residues (5.04% and 10.95% in PC_1, respectively; 4.53% and 10.96% in PC_2, respectively), upon which pepsin and pancreatin have broad specificity (Table 2) [47]. The IC_{50} values for the pepsin-pancreatin hydrolysates ranged from 0.25-0.69 mg/mL with the generally best values in PC_2 (0.28-0.53 mg/mL). In the pepsin-pancreatin hydrolysates, DH improved with increasing hydrolysis time in both PC_1 and PC_2, as occurred in the alcalase hydrolysates, and inhibitory activity was independent of hydrolysis time.

The variance analysis showed that the E/S ratio, hydrolysis time, the PC source-E/S ratio interaction and the triple interaction (PC source-E/S ratio-hydrolysis time) influenced ($p<0.05$) DH (Figure 3, Eq. 3). The regression analysis indicated that the DH results fit ($p<0.05$) a first-order polynomial model. This mathematical model also explained DH behavior as a function of E/S ratio (B), hydrolysis time (C), the PC source-E/S ratio (AB) interaction and the PC source-E/S ratio-hydrolysis time (ABC) interaction, with a determination coefficient of $R^2=0.976$. The model indicated that E/S ratio (B) and hydrolysis time (C) had the greatest effect ($p<0.05$) on DH (coefficients = 3.88 and 3.86, respectively).

Table 4. Degree of hydrolysis (DH) and ACE-I inhibition (IC_{50}) in pepsin-pancreatin hydrolysates of protein concentrates from a) ungerminated (PC_1) and b) germinated (PC_2) *P. lunatus* seeds

Treatment	Factor A Protein concentrate source	Factor B E/S Ratio	Factor C Hydrolysis time (h)	DH (%)	IC_{50} (mg/mL)
10	PC_1	1/50	1.0	15.35^a	0.69^g
11	PC_2	1/50	1.0	27.04^c	0.29^b
12	PC_1	1/10	1.0	32.16^f	0.25^a
13	PC_2	1/10	1.0	25.68^b	0.38^d
14	PC_1	1/50	3.0	28.49^c	0.34^c
15	PC_2	1/50	3.0	29.28^d	0.28^b
16	PC_1	1/10	3.0	36.28^g	0.42^e
17	PC_2	1/10	3.0	37.07^h	0.53^f
18A	PC_1-PC_2 (50/50 w/w)	1/30	2.0	29.89^e	0.25^a
18B	PC_1-PC_2 (50/50 w/w)	1/30	2.0	30.84^e	0.26^a
18C	PC_1-PC_2 (50/50 w/w)	1/30	2.0	31.04^e	0.25^a
18D	PC_1-PC_2 (50/50 w/w)	1/30	2.0	30.59^e	0.26^a

[a-h] Different letter superscripts in the same column indicate significant difference ($P<0.05$).

E/S = Enzyme/substrate ratio.

18A, 18B, 18C, 18D: central trial treatments.

None of the factors or interactions had an effect ($p>0.05$) on ACE-I inhibitory activity, making it impossible to generate a regression analysis and produce a mathematical model for ACE-I inhibitory data in the pepsin-pancreatin hydrolysates. In other words, all of the pepsin-pancreatin treatments produced hydrolysates with ACE-I inhibitory properties. Further study is needed to identify factors that could optimize ACE-I inhibitory values in these hydrolysates [43].

Pepsin-pancreatin activity and ACE-I inhibitory activity were higher (DH=27.04%, IC_{50}=0.29 mg/mL) in Treatment 11 (PC_2, 1 h hydrolysis time, 1/50 E/S) than in Treatment 10 (PC_1, 1 h hydrolysis time, 1/50 E/S) (Table 4, Figure $4c_1$,$4d_1$). However, enzymatic and inhibitory activities in PC_1 increased (DH=32.16%, IC_{50}=0.25 mg/mL) at the 1/10 E/S (Figure $4c_2$, $4d_2$), suggesting that both enzymes may have limited the hydrolysis reaction in PC_1 at the 1/50 E/S. By contrast, DH and inhibitory activity in PC_2 decreased at the 1/10 E/S ratio (DH, 27.04-25.68%; IC_{50}=0.29-0.38 mg/mL) (Figure $4d_1$, $4d_2$). At 3 h hydrolysis time and the 1/50 E/S, DH was better in PC_2 (29.28%) than in PC_1 (28.49%), and PC_2 exhibited better inhibitory activity (IC_{50} = 0.28 mg/mL) (Figure $4c_1$, $4c_2$). At the 1/10 E/S, DH was again higher in PC_2 (37.07%) than in PC_1 (36.28%), but inhibitory activity was better in PC_1 (0.42 mg/mL) (Figure $4c_2$, $4d_2$).

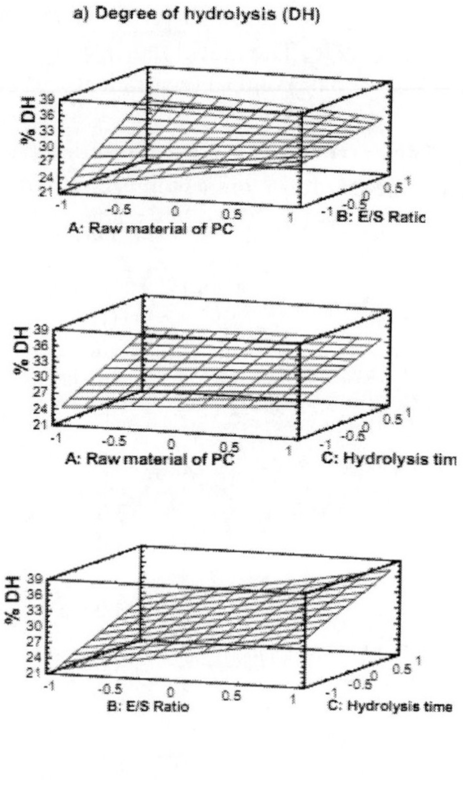

$$\% DH = 29.48 + 3.88B + 3.86C - 2.27AB + 2.27ABC \qquad R^2 = 0.976 \quad \text{(Eq. 3)}$$

Figure 3. Effect of significant factors in pepsin-pancreatin sequential hydrolysis of protein concentrates from ungerminated (PC_1) and germinated (PC_2) *P. lunatus* seeds on a) Degree of hydrolysis (DH): Factor A, protein concentrate source (PC_1 and PC_2); Factor B, E/S ratio; and Factor C, hydrolysis time.

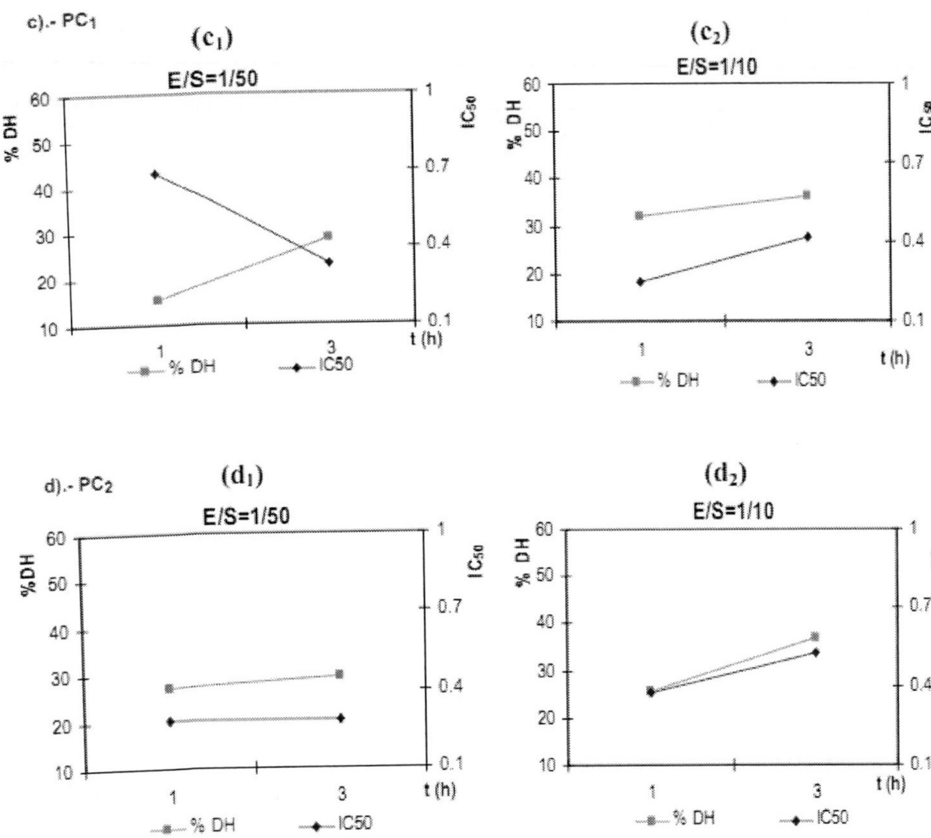

Figure 4. Degree of hydrolysis (% DH) and ACE-I inhibition (IC_{50}) produced by pepsin-pancreatin sequential hydrolysis of protein concentrates from a) ungerminated (PC_1) and b) germinated (PC_2) *P. lunatus* seeds.

The best overall ACE-I inhibitory activity with this hydrolysis method (0.25 mg/mL) was observed in Treatment 12 (PC_1, 1 h hydrolysis time, 1/10 E/S). The increase from 1 to 3 h hydrolysis time increased ACE-I inhibitory activity only in PC_1 at the 1/50 E/S (0.69-0.34 mg/mL), suggesting that this treatment generated peptides with good antihypertensive properties at 3 h hydrolysis time (Figure 4). Aside from a minor improvement in IC_{50} in PC_2 at 1/50 E/S with the increase from 1 to 3 h (0.29-0.28 mg/mL; $p>0.05$), increased hydrolysis time generally compromised ACE-I inhibitory activity, probably due to hydrolysis of some antihypertensive peptides as hydrolysis time increased. This coincides with Megías *et al* [29], who, in a study of sunflower protein hydrolysates produced with pepsin-pancreatin sequential hydrolysis, report that the best ACE-I inhibitory values were observed at DH 10-22% rather than at higher DHs of 30-35%.

All the *P. lunatus* protein concentrate hydrolysates, from alcalase or pepsin-pancreatin hydrolysis, had ACE-I inhibitory activity, with values ranging from 0.25 to 2.40 mg/mL. Under the study conditions, the best IC_{50} value was produced using protein concentrate from ungerminated seeds sequentially hydrolyzed with pepsin-pancreatin for 1 h at a 1/10 E/S ratio. The hydrolysates from ungerminated seed flour PCs had the highest IC_{50} values, although those from germinated seeds were also quite good. The IC_{50} value range observed in the present study encompasses protein hydrolysate IC_{50} values reported in the literature: 0.18 mg/mL for maize gluten [48]; 0.18 mg/mL for chickpea legumin [14]; 1.36 mg/mL for chickpea total protein [49]; 0.23 mg/mL for rapeseed cv. León [16]; 0.30-1.20 mg/mL for buckwheat protein [50]; and 0.64 mg/mL for mung bean protein [10].

Structure-activity correlations between different peptide ACE-I inhibitors indicate that ACE-I binding is strongly influenced by the substrate's C-terminal tripeptide sequence. The C-terminal tripeptide can interact with the three sub-sites at an active ACE-I site. This enzyme apparently prefers substrates or competitive inhibitors containing hydrophobic (aromatic or branched-side chain) amino acid residues at each of the three C-terminal positions. Many studies have shown that tripeptides or dipeptides with potent inhibitory activity have Trp, Tyr or Pro at their C-terminal, and branched aliphatic amino acids at the N-terminal [44]. A quantitative QSAR study of the structure-activity relationship of ACE-I inhibitory peptides has also confirmed that tripeptides composed of amino acids with strong hydrophobicity at their C- and N-terminals have potent ACE-I inhibitory activity [10]. Given that both the tested *P. lunatus* PCs contained high proportions (33.34-34.10%) of hydrophobic amino acids (Table 2), it is probable that this action mechanism contributed to their ACE-I inhibitory activity.

CONCLUSIONS

Protein concentrates from ungerminated and germinated *Phaseolus lunatus* seeds are good sources of ACE-I inhibitory peptides when hydrolyzed with the proteases alcalase or pepsin-pancreatin. The best ACE-I inhibitory activity was observed using sequential hydrolysis with pepsin-pancreatin, a potentially important fact since pepsin is the main proteolytic enzyme generated in the stomach during food digestion and pancreatin includes proteases such as trypsin, chymotrypsin and elastase, released by the pancreas into the small intestine. In other words, the pepsin-pancreatin protein hydrolysates produced in the present study represent a set of peptides resembling those generated during digestion of *P. lunatus* proteins in the human organism. Because they are resistant to pepsin and pancreatin, these peptides can be absorbed by digestive epithelial cells in the small intestine and then exert an antihypertensive effect within the organism. Lima bean protein hydrolysates produced with alcalase or pepsin-pancreatin are a potential ingredient in the production of physiologically functional foods with antihypertensive activity.

ACKNOWLEDGEMENTS

This research was partially funded by the Consejo Nacional de Ciencia y Tecnología (CONACYT), Project "Ciencia Básica 153012"and SIP-IPN (projects: 20060445, 20070800, and 20082532) and a scholarship from the Programa Institucional de Formación de Investigadores (PIFI).

REFERENCES

[1] Mark, K.S. and Davis, T.P. (2000). Stroke: development, prevention and treatment with peptidase inhibitors. *Peptides,* 21, 1965–1973.

[2] Varin, R. Mulder, P., Tamion, F., Richard, V., Henry, J.P., Lallemand, F., Lerebours, G. and Thuillez, C. (2000). Improvement of endothelial function by chronic angiotensin converting enzyme inhibition in heart failure: role of nitric oxide, prostanoids, oxidant stress, and bradykinin. *Circulation*, 102, 351–356.

[3] Lever, A.F., Hole, D.J., Gillis, C.R., McCallum, I.R., McInnes, G.T., McKinnon, P.L., Meredith, P.A., Murray, L.S., Reid, J.L. and Robertson, J.W. (1998). Do inhibitors of angiotensin-I-converting enzyme protect against risk of cancer? *The Lancet*, 352, 179-184.

[4] Lever, A.F., Hole, D.J., Gillis, C.R., McInnes, G.T., Meredith, P.A., Murray, L.S. and Reid, J.L. (1999). Is cancer related to hypertension or to its treatment? *Clinical Experimental Hypertension*, 21, 937–946.

[5] Gavras, H. and Gavras, I. (1999). Bioactive peptides in the treatment of hypertension and heart failure. *Biomedical and Health Research*, 22, 41-50.

[6] Li, G.H., Shi, Y.H., Liu, H. and Le, G.W. (2006). Antihypertensive effect of alcalase generated mung bean protein hydrolysates in spontaneously hypertensive rats. *European Food Research and Technology*, 222, 733-736.

[7] Li, G.H., Le, G.W., Shi, Y.H. and Shrestha, H. (2004). Angiotensin I-converting enzyme inhibitory peptides derived from food proteins and their physiological and pharmacological effects. *Nutrition Research*, 24, 469-486.

[8] Quirós, A., Chichón, R., Recio, I. and López-Fandiño, R. (2006). The use of high hydrostatic pressure to promote the proteolysis and release of bioactive peptides from ovalbumin. *Food Chemistry*, 54, 319-327.

[9] Miguel, M., Alonso, M.J., Salaices, M., Aleixandre, A. and López-Fandiño R. (2007). Antihypertensive, ACE-inhibitory and vasodilator properties of an egg white hydrolysate: Effect of a simulated intestinal digestion. *Food Chemistry*, 104,163-168.

[10] Li, G.H., Le, G.W., Liu, H. and Shi, Y.H. (2005). Mung-bean protein hydrolysates obtained with alcalase exhibit angiotensin I-converting enzyme inhibitory activity. *Food Science and Technology International,* 11 (4), 281-287.

[11] Shin, Z.I., Ahn, C.W., Nam, H.S., Lee, H.J. and Moon, T.H. (1995). Fractionation of angiotensin converting enzyme inhibitory peptide from soybean paste. *Korean Journal of Food Science and Technology*, 27, 230–234.

[12] Shin, Z.I., Yu, R., Park, S.A., Chung, D.K., Nam, H.S., Kim, K.S and Lee, H.J. (2001). His-His-Leu, an angiotensin I converting enzyme inhibitory peptide derived from Korean soybean paste, exerts antihypertensive activity in vivo. *Journal of Agricultural and Food Chemistry,* 49, 3004–3009.

[13] Vermeirssen, V., Van, C.P., Devos, L. and Verstraete, W. (2003). Release of angiotensin I converting enzyme (ACE). Inhibitory activity during in vitro gastrointestinal digestion: from batch experiment to semicontinuous model. *Journal of Agriculture and Food Chemistry*, 51, 5680-5687.

[14] Yust, M.M., Pedroche, J., Girón-Calle, J., Alaiz, M., Millán, F. and Vioque, J. (2003). Production of ACE inhibitory peptides by digestion of chickpea legumin with alcalase. *Food Chemistry*, 81, 363-369.

[15] Pedroche, J., Yust, M.M., Megías, C., Lqari, H., Alaiz, M., Girón-Calle, J., Millán, F. and Vioque, J. (2004). Utilisation of rapeseed proteína isolates for production of peptides with angiotensin I-converting enzyme (ACE)-inhibitory activity. *Grasas y Aceites*, 55, 354-358.

[16] Yoshie-Stark, Y., Wada, Y., Schott, M. and Wäshe, A. (2006). Functional and bioactive properties of rapeseed protein concentrates and sensory analysis of food application with rapeseed protein concentrates. *LWT-Food Science and Technology*, 39, 503-512.

[17] Manninen, A. (2004). Protein hydrolysates in sports and exercise: A brief review. *Journal of Sports Science and Medicine*, 3, 60-63.

[18] Kristinsson, H.G. and Rasco, B.A. (2000). Biochemical and functional properties of atlantic salmon (Salmo salar) muscle proteins hydrolyzed with various alkaline proteases. *Journal of Agricultural and Food Chemistry,* 48(3), 657-666.

[19] Doucet, D. Otter, D.E. Gauthier, S.F. and Foegeding, E.A. (2003). Enzyme-induced gelation of extensively hydrolyzed whey proteins by Alcalase: peptide identification and determination of enzyme specificity. *Journal of Agricultural and Food Chemistry*, 51(21), 6300-6308.

[20] Tardioli, P.W., Fernández-Lafuente. R., Guisán, J.M. and Giordano, R.L.C. (2003) Design of new immobilized-stabilized carboxypeptidase A derivative for production of aromatic free hydrolysates of proteins. *Biotechnology Progress*, 19(2), 565-574.

[21] Chel-Guerrero, L., Pérez-Flores, V., Betancur-Ancona, D. and Dávila-Ortíz, G. (2002). Functional properties of flours and protein isolates from Phaseolus lunatus and Canavalia ensiformis seeds. *Journal of Agricultural and Food Chemistry,* 50(3), 584-591.

[22] Lecomte, N., Zayas, J. and Kastner, C. (1993). Soy proteins functional and sensory characteristics improved in comminuted meals. *Journal of Food Science,* 58, 464–466, 472.

[23] Kuo, Y.H., Rosan, P., Lambein, F., Frias, J. and Vidal-Valverde C. (2004). Effects of different germination conditions on the contents of free protein and non-protein amino acids of commercial legumes. *Journal of Food Chemistry*, 86, 537-545.

[24] Oshodi, A.A. and Aletor, V.A. (1993). Functional Properties of haemagglutinins (lectins) extracted from some edible varieties of lima beans (Phaseolus lunatus L). *International Journal of Food Science and Nutrition,* 44:133-136.

[25] Sanchez-Vioque, R. Clemente, A. Vioque, J., Bautista, J. and Millan, F. (1999). Protein isolates from Chickpea (Cicer arietinum L.): Chemical composition, functional properties and protein characterization. *Food Chemistry,* 64, 237-143.

[26] Anon. (1999). *International Rules for Seeds Testing*. Published by The International Seed Testing Association (ISTA), Switzerland.

[27] A.O.A.C. (1995) *Official Methods of Analysis*. Association of Analytical Chemists, 15th Ed. Washington D.C.

[28] Alaiz, M., Navarro, J.L., Giron, J. and Vioque, E. (1992). Amino acid analysis by high performance liquid chromatography after derivatization with diethyletoxymethylenemalonate. *Journal of Chromatography*, 591, 181-186.

[29] Megías, C., Yust, M.M., Pedroche, J., Lquari, H. Girón-Calle, J., Alaiz, M., Millán, F. and Vioque, J. (2004). Purification of an ACE inhbitory peptide after hydrolysis of Sunflower (Helianthus annuus L.) protein isolates. *Journal of Agriculture and Food Chemistry*, 52,1928-1932.

[30] Nielsen, P.M., Petersen, D. and Dambmann, C. (2001). Improved method for determining food protein degree of hydrolysis. *Journal of Food Science,* 66 (5), 642-646.

[31] Hayakari, M., Kondo, Y. and Izumi, H. (1978). A rapid and simple spectrophotometric assay of angiotensin-converting enzyme. *Analytical Biochemistry,* 84, 361–369.

[32] Montgomery, D.C. (2004). *Diseño y análisis de experimentos*. Editorial Limusa-Wiley. Segunda Edición, México, pp. 228-241.

[33] Dibofori, A.N., Okoh, P.N. and Onigbinde, A.O. (1994). Effect of germination on the cyanide and oligosaccharide content of lima beans (Phaseolus lunatus). *Journal of Food Chemistry*, 51, 133-136.

[34] Rodríguez, C., Frias, J., Vidal-Valverde, C. and Hernández, A. (2008). Correlation between some nitrogen fractions, lysine, histidine, tyrosine, and ornithine contents during germination of peas, beans, and lentils. *Journal of Food Chemistry*, 108, 245-252.

[35] Bau, H., Villaume, C., Nicolas, J. and Méjean, L. (1997). Effect of germination on chemical composition, biochemical constituents and antinutritional factors of soya bean (Glycine max) seeds. *Journal of Science Food and Agriculture*, 73, 1-9.

[36] Sangronis, E., Rodríguez, M., Cava, R. and Torres, A. (2006). Protein quality of germinated Phaseolus vulgaris. *European Food Research and Technology,* 222, 144-148.

[37] Augustin, J. and Klein, P. (1989). Nutrient *composition of raw, cooked, canned and sprouted legumes*. In Legumes. Chap. 7, Ed. Matthews and Dekker, New York, pp. 187-204.

[38] Betancur-Ancona, D., Martinez-Rosado, R., Corona-Cruz, A., Castellanos-Ruelas, A., Jaramillo-Flores, M.E. and Chel-Guerrero, L. (2009). Functional properties of hydrolysates from Phaseolus lunatus seeds. *International Journal of Food Science and Technology*,. 44, 128-137.

[39] Betancur-Ancona, D., Gallegos-Tintoré, S. and Chel-Guerrero, L. (2004). Wet-fractionation of Phaseolus lunatus seeds: partial characterization of starch and protein. *Journal of Science Food and Agriculture*, 84, 1193-1201.

[40] Arntfield, S.D., Ismond, M.A.H. and Murray, E.D. (1985). The rate of antinutritional factors during the preparation of a faba bean protein isolate using a micellization technique. *Canadian Institute of Food Sciencie Technology Journal*, 18, 137-143.

[41] Rodríguez-Ambriz, S.L., Martínez-Ayala, A.L., Millán, F. and Dávila-Ortiz, G. (2005). Composition and functional properties of Lupinus campestris protein isolates. *Plant Foods for Human Nutrition*, 60, 99-107.

[42] Paredes-López, O. and Ondorica-Falomir, C. (1986). Production of safflower protein isolates: composition, yield and protein quality. *Journal of the Science and Food Agriculture*, 37, 1104-1109.

[43] He, G., Xuan, G. and Ruan, H. (2005). Optimization of angiotensin I-converting enzyme (ACE) inhibition by rice dregs hydrolysates using response surface methodology. *Journal of Zhejiang University Science,* 6B (6), 508-513.

[44] Byun, H.G. and Kim, S.K. (2001). Purification and characterization of angiotensin I converting enzyme (ACE) inhibitory peptides from Alaska pollack (Theragra chalcogramma) skin. *Journal of Process Biochemistry,* 36, 1155–1162.

[45] Pedroche, J., Yust, M.M., Girón-Calle, J., Alaiz, M., Millán, F. and Vioque, J. (2002). Utilization of chickpea protein isolates for production of peptides with angiotensin I-converting enzyme (ACE)-inhibitory activity. *Journal of the Science and Food Agriculture*, 82, 960-965.

[46] Mahmoud, I.M., Malone, T.W. and Cordle, T.C. (1992). Enzymatic hydrolysis of casein: effect of degree of hydrolysis on antigenicity and physical properties. *Journal of Food Science*, 57, 1223–1229.

[47] Adamson, N.J. and Reynolds, E.C. (1995). Characterization of multiply phosphorylated peptides selectively precipitated from pancreatin casein digest. *Journal of Dairy Science*, 78, 2653-2659.

[48] Kim, J.M., Whang, J.H. and Suh, H.J. (2004). Enhancement of angiotensin I convering enzyme inhibitory activity and improvement of the emulsifying and foaming properties of corn gluten hydrolysate using ultrafiltration membranes. *European Food Research and Technology*, 218, 133-138.

[49] Vermeirssen, V., Van Camp, J. and Verstraete, W. (2002). Optimization and validation of an angiotensin-converting enzyme inhibition assay for screening of bioactive peptides. *Journal of Biochemical and Biophysical Methods,* 51: 75–87.

[50] Li, C.H., Matsui, T., Matsumoto, K., Yamasaki, R. and Kawasaki, T. (2002). Latent production of angiotensin I-converting enzyme inhibitors from buckwheat protein. *Journal of Peptide Science*, 8, 267–274.

In: Angiotensin: New Research
Editors: S. Harada, I. Moi, pp. 149-163

ISBN: 978-1-62100-773-9

Chapter 6

PATHOPHYSIOLOGICAL ROLE OF ANGIOTENSIN-CONVERTING ENZYME IN THE CARDIOVASCULAR SYSTEM

***Maira Segura-Campos, Jorge Ruiz-Ruiz, Luis Chel-Guerrero, David Betancur-Ancona**[*]*

Facultad de Ingeniería Química, Universidad Autónoma de Yucatán, Periférico Nte. Km. 33.5, Tablaje Catastral 13615, Col. Chuburná de Hidalgo Inn, 97203 Mérida, Yucatán, México.

ABSTRACT

Angiotensin I-converting enzyme (ACE, EC 3.4.15.1) is a zinc metallopeptidase involved in release of angiotensin II (Ang II) and inactivation of bradykinin (BK), two peptide hormones which play key roles in regulation of blood pressure, renal and cardiovascular functions. Ang II is an end-product of the highly regulated renin-angiotensin-aldosterone system (RAAS) while bradykinin is an end-product of the kallikrein-kinin system (KKS). Ang II is produced by the RAAS system from the precursor angiotensinogen, cleaved by the enzyme renin to angiotensin I (Ang I), and then cleaved by ACE to Ang II. Ang II is considered the most active agonist of this system, and its physiological actions are implemented through stimulation of specific receptors distributed widely throughout the body. Ang II is known to bind to the AT1 and AT2 binding site subtypes. Stimulation of the AT1 receptor results in a signaling pathway cascade in several cell types, leading to processes such as vasoconstriction, inflammation and cell proliferation. These are extremely important in many cardiovascular diseases, including hypertension, atherosclerosis and ventricular hypertrophy. The AT2 receptor is mainly expressed during the fetal stage and is only minimally expressed in adults under normal circumstances. Its role in the adult cardiovascular system remains unclear, but it apparently produces oppositional effects to the AT1 receptor. The existence of two active sites for ACE has generated speculation about their functional significance. *In vitro* these two domains display relatively broad substrate specificity, including cleavage of Ang I and BK. However, some biochemical features differentiate these active sites. ACE-

[*] Tels. +52 (999) 9460956, 946-09-81 and 946-09-89; Fax. +52 (999) 946-09-94. E mail: bancona@uady.mx.

specific inhibitors are one of the most widely prescribed drug classes in cardiology and are used for treatment of hypertension and heart failure. This overview discusses the pathophysiological role of ACE and its enzymatic products, principally Ang II.

Keywords: ACE, Renin-Angiotensin-Aldosterone System, Ang II, Cardiovascular System

INTRODUCTION

Angiotensin I-converting enzyme (ACE) (peptidyl dipeptidase A, kininase II, EC 3.4.15.1) is a zinc dipeptidyl carboxypeptidase. This membrane-bound exopeptidase is found on the plasma membranes of various cell types, including vascular endothelial cells, microvillar brush border epithelial cells and neuroepithelial cells. It is thought to be physiologically important. A soluble form of ACE also exists in the plasma, but may simply reflect turnover and clearance of membrane-bound ACE. The primary activity of ACE is to cleave broad specificity free carboxyl group oligopeptides. Substrates containing Pro at the P1' position and Asp or Glu at P2' are resistant to ACE. However, on certain substrates ACE can also function as an endopeptidase or a tripeptidyl carboxypeptidase. With ACE, endopeptidase activity is observed on substrates having amidated carboxyl groups where the enzyme can cleave a C-terminal dipeptide amide and/or a C-terminal tripeptide amide [1].

ACE is responsible for converting angiotensin I (Ang I) to the powerful vasoconstrictor angiotensin II (Ang II) and inactivating the vasodilator peptide bradykinin (BK) by removal of C-terminal dipeptides [2]. In a functional sense, therefore, the enzymatic actions of ACE potentially cause increased vasoconstriction and decreased vasodilation [3]. ACE has attracted intense interest for development of orally-active ACE inhibitors to treat hypertension due to of its central role in vasoactive peptide metabolism, and because the ACE gene is a candidate gene in several cardiovascular diseases. An ACE homologue referred to as ACE2 was recently identified in humans and found to be an essential regulator of cardiac function. Unlike classic ACE, it is a carboxypeptidase which preferentially removes C-terminal hydrophobic or basic amino acids and is unaffected by ACE inhibitors [4].

ANGIOTENSIN-CONVERTING ENZYME DISTRIBUTION IN HUMAN TISSUES

Using high performance liquid chromatography (HPLC), Van Sande et al. [5] identified ACE in 27 human tissue homogenates and physiological fluids by measuring hydrolysis of the hippuryl-glycyl-glycine substrate. All the tissues studied contained measurable ACE activities inhibited by low captopril concentrations. High specific converting enzyme activities were found in several intestinal and urogenital tract tissues. Krassnigg et al. [6] observed ACE activity in male genital tract tissues (testis, epididymis and prostate), on the surface of endothelial cells in the lung, myocardium, liver, and intestine, as well as in epithelial cells of the kidney proximal tubules. Metzger et al. [7] described ACE distribution in human tissues by using a panel of anti-human ACE monoclonal antibodies and serial sections of the entire vascular tree. Endothelial cells (EC) of small muscular arteries and arterioles displayed high ACE immunoreactivity in all organs except the kidney, while EC in the large arteries and veins reacted poorly or were completely negative. On average, only 20% of capillary EC stained for ACE in each organ, including the heart; the remarkable exceptions were the lung and kidney. All capillary EC were intensively labeled for ACE in the lung, while in the kidney the entire vasculature was devoid of detectable ACE. This absence of ACE content in the renal vasculature may protect renal circulation against excess Ang II formation and kinin depletion, and maintain high renal blood flow.

Presence of ACE in some tissues may play a pathophysiological role in human cardiovascular disease. ACE expression has been immunohistochemically studied in non-atherosclerotic and diseased human coronary arteries. In non-atherosclerotic arteries, ACE immunoreactivity was found in luminal and adventitial vasa vasorum endothelium, while in early- and intermediate-stage atherosclerotic lesions high ACE immunoreactivity was detected in regions of fat-laden macrophages and in association with T lymphocytes. In advanced lesions, ACE immunoreactivity was localized to the microvasculature endothelium throughout the plaques. Immunoreactive Ang II was also detected in these areas. ACE accumulation within the plaque may contribute to increased production of local angiotensin which may participate in the pathobiology of coronary artery disease. Plaque ACE probably is an important target for drug action [8].

ANGIOTENSIN-CONVERTING ENZYME ISOFORMS

Two ACE isoforms are transcribed by the same gene [9] (Figure 1): a larger one referred to as somatic ACE (sACE), with 1277 amino acids and expressed in most tissues; and a smaller one referred to as testis ACE (tACE) with 701 amino acids and found in the adult testis[2]. Also known as kininase II, ACE is a single-chain protein with N- and C-domains (named according to their proximity to the N- or C-terminal). Somatic ACE is composed of two homologous catalytic domains (N- and C- domains), whereas tACE represents the C-domain with an additional N-terminal sequence. This difference originates in an alternate initiation site in intron 12 of the ACE gene. In both sACE and tACE, however, synthesis is directed by a single gene. Despite 89% homogeneity around the active centers, the two active sites cleave some substrates at different rates.

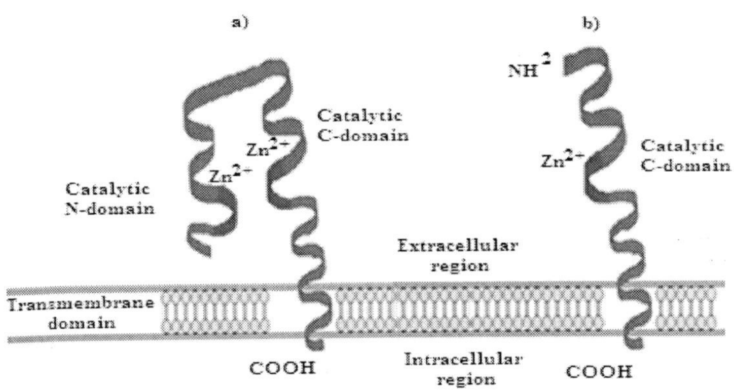

Figure 1. Angiotensin-converting enzyme isoforms: a) somatic ACE; b) testis ACE [9].

In addition to the active centers and substrate binding sites, the positions of all 7 cysteine residues in each domain are highly conserved (there are no cysteine residues in other regions of the molecule) indicating that both domains have some similarities in topological structure[10].

Catalytic activity of the N- and C- domains has been studied extensively. The most notable difference between them is their substrate specificity. Both are capable of hydrolyzing Ang I and BK, but other compounds are cleaved preferentially by one or the other, more frequently the N-domain. Among peptide hormones, for example, luteinizing hormone-releasing hormone (LHRH) is principally inactivated by release of <Glu^{1}-His^{2}-Trp^{3}, and the encephalin precursor Met^{5}-Enk-Arg^{6}-Phe^{7} is converted primarily to encephalin by the N-domain site [11]. Angiotensin (1-7) and the tetrapeptide AcSer-Asp-Lys-Pro (AcSDKP) are also cleaved by the N-domain [12]. Of note is that the vasodilator Ang (1-7) is cleaved at the N-domain catalytic site, but acts as an inhibitor at the C-domain [13].

Although the role of individual amino acids in the active center has been well studied, the function of the N-terminal sequence in preserving ACE N-domain integrity is not yet understood. The human intestinal brush border is quite rich in sACE, but ileal fluid contains only highly active intact ACE N-domain with no C-domain. This separate N-domain has an estimated sequence of 443 amino acids. The N-terminal preceding the N-domain active center would therefore lend stability to ACE in the intestine's protease-rich milieu. Integrity of the C-domain attached to the plasma membrane can be protected by the N-domain on one side and the ACE transmembrane anchor portion on the other [14]. The N- and C-domain sites differ in their sensitivity to ACE-inhibitor drugs; for instance, lisinopril more effectively inhibits the C-domain, and captopril more effectively inhibits the N-domain. The two sites also differ in their sensitivity to chloride activation. The N-domain exhibits maximum activity at low Cl^- concentrations, although it is still active in the total absence of Cl^-. The C-domain, in contrast, is highly dependent on Cl^- and is totally inactive in its absence [15].

Renin-Angiotensin-Aldosterone System

The renin-angiotensin aldosterone system (RAAS) plays an integral role in homeostatic control of arterial pressure, tissue perfusion and extracellular volume. It functions as an unusual endocrine axis in which the active hormone, Ang II, forms in the extracellular space by sequential proteolytic cleavage of its precursors. This pathway is initiated by the regulated secretion of renin, a rate-limiting processing enzyme (Figure 2). Although renin was discovered over a century ago, the importance of renin in the pathogenesis of cardiovascular and renal disorders has gained wide acceptance only during the last thirty years, largely due to development of specific pharmacologic agents aimed at blocking this system [16].

The RAAS hormonal cascade begins with renin biosynthesis by juxtaglomerular cells (JG) lining the afferent (and occasionally efferent) arteriole of the renal glomerulus. Renin is synthesized as a preprohormone, and mature (active) renin is formed by proteolytic removal of a 43-amino-acid prosegment peptide from the prorenin N-terminus, proenzyme or renin precursor. Mature renin is stored in JG cell granules and released into the kidney and then into systemic circulation by an exocytic process involving stimulus-secretion coupling. In addition to this regulated pathway, the kidney also apparently releases unprocessed prorenin via a constitutive pathway. In fact, prorenin accounts for about 70 to 90% of the immunoreactive renin in the human circulatory system.

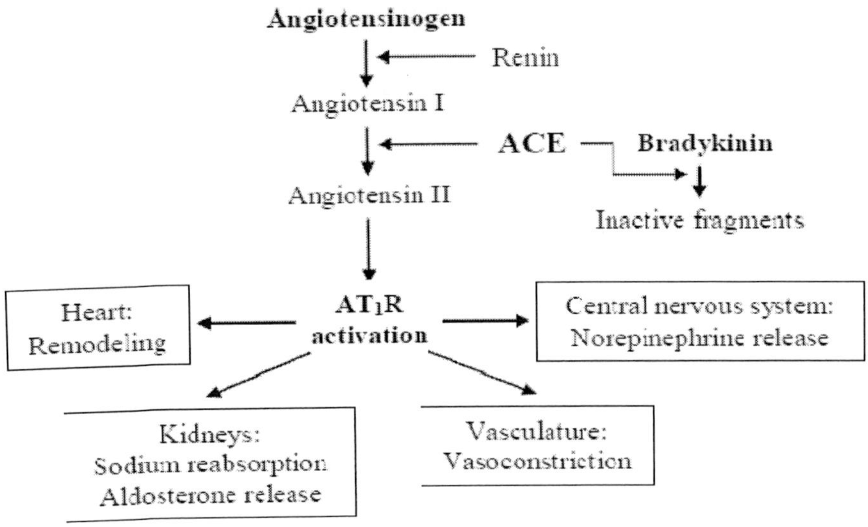

Figure 2. ACE activity in the renin-angiotensin-aldosterone and kallikrein-kinin systems.

Active renin secretion is regulated principally by four interdependent factors: (1) a renal baroreceptor mechanism in the afferent arteriole that senses changes in renal perfusion pressure; (2) changes in NaCl delivery (sensed as changes in Cl^- concentration) to the macula densa cells of the distal tubule (these are near the JG cells and conjointly form the "JG apparatus"); (3) sympathetic nerve stimulation via beta-1 adrenergic receptors; and (4) negative feedback by direct Ang II action on the JG cells. Renin secretion is stimulated by a fall in perfusion pressure or NaCl delivery, and an increase in sympathetic activity [17]. Control of renin secretion is a key determinant of RAAS activity. Renin regulates the RAAS's initial, rate-limiting step by cleaving the N-terminal portion of the high molecular weight globulin angiotensinogen to form the biologically inert Ang I or Ang (1-10) decapeptides. The primary source of systemic circulating angiotensinogen is the liver, but angiotensinogen mRNA expression has also been detected in many other tissues, including kidney, brain, heart, vascular, adrenal gland, ovary, placenta, and adipose tissues. Angiotensinogen is secreted constitutively by the liver, so plasma levels are generally stable and do not change acutely. However, both hepatic and extra-hepatic synthesis have been shown to increase in response to glucocorticoids, estrogens and other sexual steroids; thyroid hormone; inflammatory cytokines (e.g. interleukin-1 and tumor necrosis factor); and Ang II [18].

The inactive decapeptide Ang I is hydrolyzed by ACE, removing the C-terminal dipeptide to form the octapeptide Ang II or Ang (1-8), a potent, biologically-active vasoconstrictor. Although Ang II is the primary active product of the RAAS, there is evidence that other Ang I and II metabolites may have significant biological activity, particularly in tissues. Ang III and IV are formed by sequential removal of amino acids from the Ang II N-terminus by aminopeptidase action (Figure 3) [19]. They are probably produced in tissues with high levels of aminopeptidases A and N, such as brain and kidney tissue. Ang III or Ang

(2-8), a heptapeptide formed by removal of the first N-terminal amino acid, is present in the central nervous system (CNS), where it is thought to play an important role in tonic blood pressure maintenance and hypertension. Ang IV or Ang (3-8) is a hexapeptide formed by further enzymatic degradation of Ang III. Preclinical studies have suggested a cooperative effect of Ang IV in Ang II signaling. For instance, Ang IV apparently increases blood pressure in the brain by cooperating with Ang II [20].

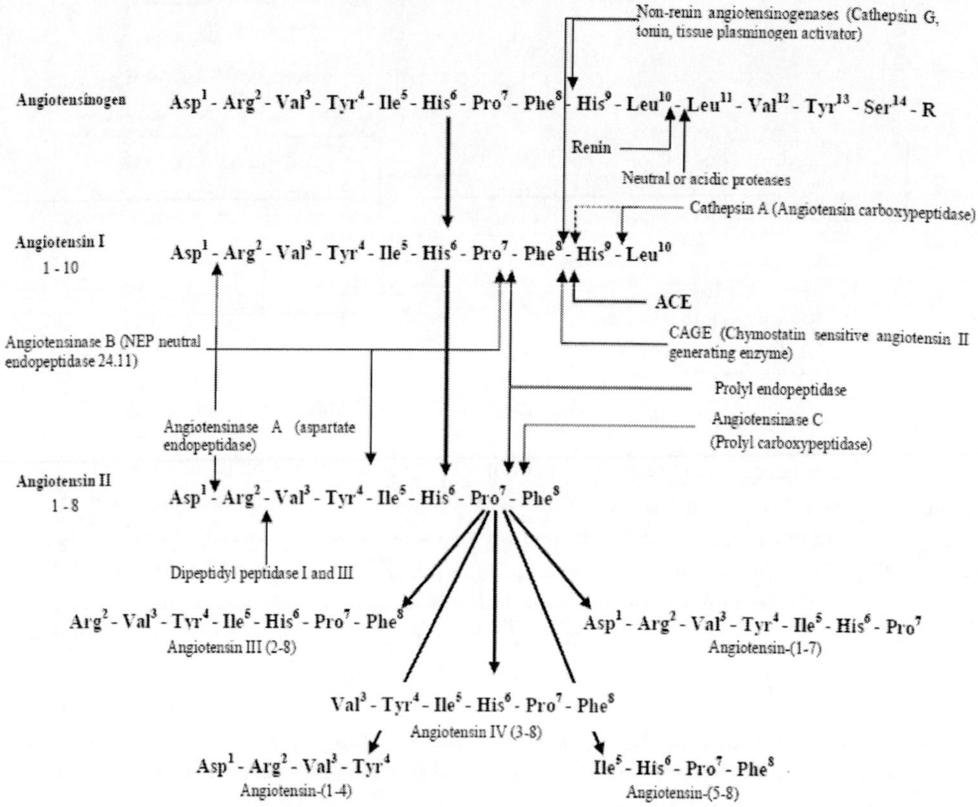

Figure 3. Metabolic pathways for angiotensin II formation and degradation [19].

ANGIOTENSIN II RECEPTORS IN CARDIOVASCULAR PATHOPHYSIOLOGY

The Ang II receptors mediate the effects of the RAAS, which plays an important role in cardiovascular physiology. Four types of angiotensin receptors are known, of which the AT1 and AT2 receptors are the most important. Stimulation of the AT1 receptor produces a signaling pathway cascade in several cell types. This eventually leads to processes such as vasoconstriction, inflammation and proliferation (Figure 4) [21], all important in cardiovascular diseases, including hypertension, atherosclerosis and ventricular hypertrophy [22]. The AT2 receptor is mainly expressed in the fetal stage. In adults, it expresses minimally under normal circumstances. What role it plays in the adult cardiovascular system is not well established, but it appears to have opposing effects to the AT1 receptor [23] (Figure 5) [21].

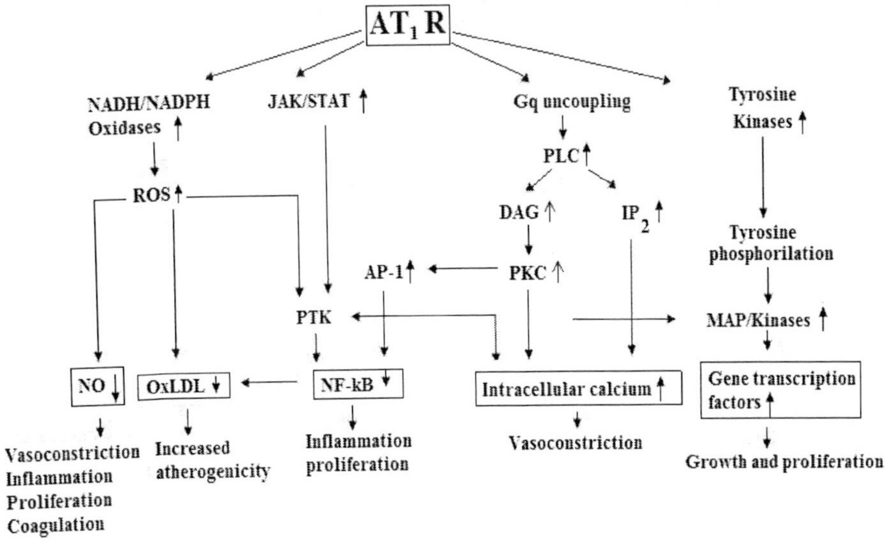

Figure 4. Schematic overview of AT1 receptor signal transduction [21]. (AP-1: Activator protein-1;AT1R: Angiotensin II type 1 receptor; DAG: Diacylglycerol; IP_3: 1,4,5-inositoltriphosphate; JAK: Janus kinase; MAP: Mitogen-activated protein; NADH: Nicotinamide-adenine dinucleotide; NADPH: Nicotinamide-adenine dinucleotide phosphate; NF-κB: Nuclear factor kappa-B; NO: Nitric oxide; OxLDL: Oxidized low-density lipoprotein; ROS: Reactive oxygen species; STAT: Signal transducer and activator transcription factor; PKC: Protein kinase C; PLC: Phospholipase C; PTK: Phosphotyrosine kinase).

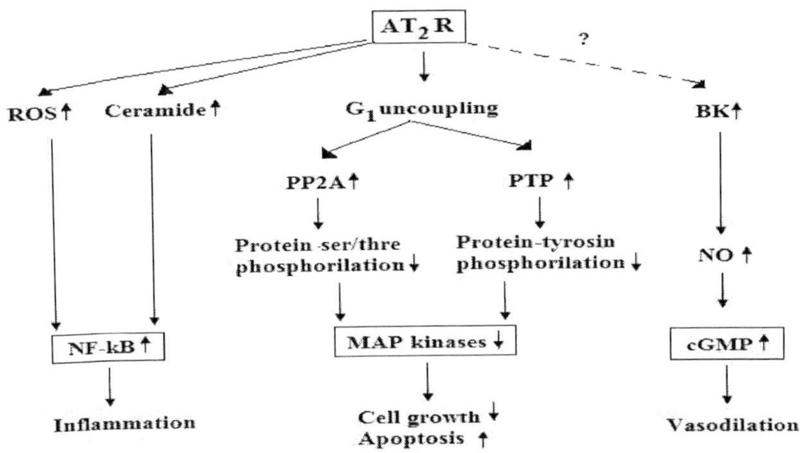

Figure 5. Schematic overview of AT2 receptor signal transduction [21]. AT2R: Angiotensin II type 2 receptor; BK: Bradykinin; cGMP: Cyclic GMP; MAP: Mitogen-activated protein; NF-kB: Nuclear factor kappa-B; NO: Nitric oxide; PP2A: Serin/threonin phosphatase 2A; PTP: Phosphotyrosine phosphatase; ROS: Reactive oxygen species.

Hypertension. The AT1 receptor is apparently related to essential hypertension. Although no causal relationship has yet been established, the relationship is suggested because AT1 receptor blockers effect essential hypertension. Moreover, several studies have shown that Ang II can induce different mechanisms involved in the complex physiology of essential hypertension. It leads to direct vasoconstriction via AT1 receptor stimulation in vascular smooth muscle cells. Superoxide is produced after AT1 receptor stimulation and inactivates nitric oxide (NO), decreasing an artery's vasodilative capacity. In endothelial cells, this stimulation also leads to production of reactive oxygen species (ROS), F2-isoprostanes and endothelin, substances which can potentiate the vasoconstrictive effects of Ang II. The activated RAAS leads to a higher media width to lumen diameter ratio (so-called vascular remodeling) in small arteries, independent of its effects on blood pressure. This effect is mediated via the AT1 receptor, which is blocked by the AT1 receptor blocker losartan. Finally, the RAAS effects blood pressure via the kidneys (water and salt control), the brain (thirst) and the sympathetic nervous system [24].

Atherosclerosis. ACE inhibitors and more recently AT1 receptor blockers have been shown effective in preventing events associated with atherosclerosis, or vascular dysfunction. The RAAS plays a role in different processes in the evolution of atherosclerosis. Both Ang II-forming enzymes (ACE, chymase) and Ang II itself occur at higher levels in atherosclerotic plaques. The various effects of Ang II in the atherosclerosis process are mediated by its AT1 receptor, suggesting angiotension II type 1 receptor blocker fulfill an important role in atherosclerosis. As mentioned above, both the AT1 and AT2 receptors can induce macrophage infiltration via the NFκB (transcription regulator) pathway. Infiltration of macrophages into the vessel wall is a necessary step in atherosclerosis onset and progression. Ang II also induces production of ROS, which decreases NO availability, leading to endothelial dysfunction, an early step in the atherosclerotic process. ROS also stimulate macrophage-mediated oxidation of low-density lipoprotein (LDL). Oxidized LDL may play a role in accelerated atherosclerosis because it promotes cellular cholesterol accumulation and foam cell formation. Ang II also increases oxidized LDL receptor density via the AT1 receptor. In humans, AT1 receptor blockade reduces oxidative stress markers in patients with essential hypertension as well as in those with coronary artery disease. AT1 stimulation leads to proliferation and migration of vascular smooth muscle cells, and consequently neointimal formation, another vital part of the atherosclerotic process. Plasminogen activator inhibitor-1 (PAI-1) is increased by Ang II, meaning that Ang II is able to inhibit fibrinolysis, producing a predisposition to coronary thrombosis. Stimulation by Ang II leads to up-regulation of intercellular adhesion molecule-1 (ICAM-1), vascular cellular adhesion molecule-1 (VCAM-1) and E-selectine. These molecules support monocyte adhesion to endothelial cells and may play a crucial role in the pathogenesis of atherosclerosis. Production of VCAM-1 can be suppressed by AT1 receptor blockade [25].

Restenosis. The AT1 receptor is involved in restenosis after vascular angioplasty in animal models. Balloon injury of the carotid artery in rats results in smooth muscle cell proliferation, which is AT1-dependent. Via its AT1 receptor, the RAAS is also involved in other processes constituting part of post-balloon angioplasty restenosis, which are the same as the atherosclerotic processes mentioned above. However, the RAAS has no effect on vessel recoil, an important restenosis mechanism after coronary balloon angioplasty. Restenosis in stented human coronary arteries differs histologically from restenosis after balloon angioplasty, because in-stent restenotic lesions contain mainly smooth muscle cells and exhibit more active proliferation of smooth muscle cells than post-balloon angioplasty restenotic lesions. As stated, AT1 receptor stimulation in animal models leads to proliferation and migration of vascular smooth muscle cells, and thus to neointimal formation in the stent. In specimens taken from human coronary arteries with an atherectomy catheter, smooth muscle cells from in-stent restenotic lesions contained abundant AT1 receptors. In humans, the AT1 receptor blocker valsartan appears to reduce the in-stent restenosis rate [26].

Left ventricular hypertrophy. In patients with hypertension, AT1 receptor stimulation is involved in development of left ventricular hypertrophy (LVH) because it plays a role in different processes associated with LVH, such as cardiac fibrosis, cardiac myocyte hypertrophy and apoptosis. Ang II leads to cardiac fibrosis by stimulating collagen synthesis and fibroblast growth. It can also cause down-regulation of matrix metalloproteinase-1 (MMP-1) in patients with essential hypertension. MMP-1 is a rate-limiting enzyme which participates in degradation of extracellular collagen. Indeed, the ACE inhibitor lisinopril was able to mediate myocardial fibrosis regression in patients with mild hypertension. In cardiomyopathic hamsters, an Ang II receptor blocker inhibited MMP-1 down-regulation. In animal models, Ang II has been demonstrated to induce cardiac myocyte hypertrophy, which was inhibited with AT1 receptor blockers. NF-κB, induced by Ang II, is critical in this hypertrophic growth. In patients with essential hypertension, the AT1 receptor blocker valsartan produced regression of left ventricular mass (as estimated with echocardiography). In another study, losartan (an AT1 receptor blocker) reduced electrocardiographic LVH parameters. Additional studies have suggested that other AT1 receptor blockers also have the ability to regress LVH. Finally, in rat studies, Ang II was shown to induce apoptosis via the AT1 receptor, an effect not observed in human hearts. Unlike in some animal studies, Ang II did not influence cardiac contractility in preparations of human ventricular myocytes [27].

Chronic heart failure. The RAAS system plays a role in chronic heart failure (CHF), since the processes mentioned above leading to LVH are also involved in deterioration to a clinical CHF diagnosis. Peripheral vasoconstriction, another important feature of CHF, is also caused by AT1 receptor stimulation. The Valsartan Heart Failure Trial (Val-HeFT) study recently demonstrated that AT1 receptor blockade may have a beneficial role in chronic heart failure. Finally, in a meta-analysis angiotensin receptor blockers were concluded to be a promising option in heart failure treatment [28].

Atrial fibrillation. ACE is up-regulated during atrial fibrillation (AF), leading to possible dependence of AF on AT1 receptors. In a dog model, AT1 receptor stimulation also led to shortening of the effective atrial refractory period, consequently increasing AF inducibility and stability. These findings suggest renin-angiotensin system involvement in atrial fibrillation via its AT1 receptor, which was confirmed in a recent study in which the AT1 receptor blocker irbesartan reduced recurrence of AF [29].

Angiotensin-Converting Enzyme Inhibitors

Before 1968, the only known ACE inhibitors were non-specific metal chelators such as EDTA. Ferreira [30] showed that a non-toxic ethanol extract of venom from the Brazilian arrowhead viper, *Bothrops jararaca*, potentiated smooth muscle contraction, produced hypotension and increased capillary permeability induced by bradykinin, a nonapeptide originally isolated after incubation of plasma with the same venom. Various properties of this bradykinin potentiating factor (BPF), including its inactivation by trypsin, indicated it to be a peptide or mixture of peptides. At least a portion of BPF's potentiating activity was apparently to due to its inhibition of bradykinin enzymatic degradation in the plasma. It took several years to determine that ACE was the bradykininase inhibited by BPF. Initial testing of the ACE inhibiting properties of BPF was done under a mistaken assumption about the relationship of this enzyme to the BPF-inhibited plasma bradykininase. In 1968, the best characterized plasma bradykinin-degrading enzyme was a carboxypeptidase referred to as kininase I, which cleaves the carboxyl-terminal arginine residue from bradykinin. This enzyme and ACE both cleaved bonds in their peptide substrates following the Pro-Phe sequence, leading to the suggestion that they could be identical. Although not quite correct, this logic led to testing of BPF as an ACE inhibitor, a nexus in development of ACE inhibitors. Structure-activity correlations between BPP analogs suggest that these snake venom peptide inhibitors compete with substrates for binding to the ACE active site by binding in the same manner as the substrates to the obligatory ACE binding site (subsites S1, S1′, and S2′). The snake venom peptide inhibitors' affinity surpassed that normally observed with peptide substrates, probably due to additional interactions with a region adjacent the ACE active site (subsites S_0, to S_9) which acts as an auxiliary binding site [31].

Current annual sales of ACE inhibitors exceed US$6 billion, making them a major protease inhibitor success story. ACE inhibitors have been on the market for over 20 years, with 13 currently approved for clinical use and several others in clinical trials (Table 1) [32]. They are widely used to treat cardiovascular conditions including hypertension, heart failure and heart attack [33].

Table 1. ACE inhibitor posology and pharmacokinetic

ACE inhibitor	Clinical use	Dose per day (mg)	Administration (times per day)	t_{max} (h)	Elimination half-life (h)	PPU (%)	Effect duration (h)	Excretion path
Benazapril	AHT	20-40	1/2	1-2	1-3	95-97	> 24	Renal/ hepatic
Captopril	AHT/CCI	50-100 25-150	2/3	0.9	2	30	4-6	Renal
Enalapril	AHT/CCI	2.5-5	1	3-4	11	< 50	12-24	Renal
Fosinopril	AHT	20-40	1	3	4	95	> 24	Renal/ hepatic
Lisinopril	AHT/CCI	20-40	1	6	12	< 10	> 24	Renal
Perindopril	AHT	4-8	1	4	30	20	20	Renal
Quinapril	AHT	20-80	1/2	2	2.5	95	> 24	Renal
Ramipril	AHT	5-10	1/2	2-3	2	60	> 24	Renal

tmax = Maximum time of inhibitor.
PPU = Plasmatic protein union.
AHT = Arterial hypertension.
CCI = Chronic cardiac insufficiency.

Development of the current generation of ACE inhibitors was a unique process since 30 years ago neither ACE's sequence nor their three-dimensional structures were understood. Instead, the structure of carboxypeptidase A, now known to be considerably different from that of ACE, was used for drug design. The ACE inhibitors share a number of common features: low molecular mass; a metal-chelating group (phosphinate, thiol ligand or carboxylate) that binds to the zinc moiety in the enzyme's active site; and they target only the S1, S1' and S2' ACE subsites, with high affinity (IC_{50} = 0.4-23 nM for the active metabolite). To achieve good oral bioavailability, most ACE inhibitors (except captopril, lisinopril and enalapril) are synthesized as ester prodrugs. With the exception of captopril, they require only a single daily dose, although they exhibit efficacy in a limited number of people and have side effects such as coughing and angioedema [34]. When ACE's crystal structure was finally solved, it revealed the enzyme to be composed of two highly homologous but not identical domains with somewhat different functions and specificities. This finding could explain some side effects of the early ACE inhibitors, which were relatively non-selective and inhibited both domains with similar affinities. However, the C-terminal and N-terminal domains apparently have different functions. The C-terminal domain seems to be primarily responsible for converting Ang I to Ang II, with a major effect on blood pressure regulation. The N-terminal domain is apparently involved in haemoregulation, a hypothesis recently confirmed in a preconstricted porcine coronary microartery model using a new generation of inhibitors specific to the C-terminal (RXPA380) and N-terminal (RXP407) domains. These new inhibitors were designed based on structural differences between the two domains, are much more selective (*K*i (C-term)/*K*i (N-term) = 25,000 for RXPA380) and should offer improved control of different physiological processes while improving the drug safety profile [35].Another approach to ACE inhibition is generation of inhibitors targeting ACE as well as neutral endopeptidase (NEP). Similar to ACE, NEP is a zinc metalloproteinase responsible for degrading various natriuretic peptides (atrial, brain-derived natriuretic peptide and C-type natriuretic peptide), and cleaving Ang I and BK. Simultaneous potentiation of atrial natriuretic peptide via NEP inhibition and Ang II attenuation via ACE inhibition produces complementary effects in hypertension and congestive heart failure management. Omapatrilat® (Bristol-Myers Squibb), a bicyclic thiazepinone peptidomimetic, is the most advanced of the dual ACE/NEP inhibitors in development. It was shown to surpass existing agents in reducing hypertension, but its registration was halted by the United States Food and Drug Administration (FDA) due to side effects (e.g. severe angioedema) in Phase III trials; additional testing has been requested [36].

Functional Foods in Angiotensin-Converting Enzyme Inhibition

Synthetic ACE inhibitors cause side effects such as dry cough, rash or itching, allergic reaction with generalized swelling (angioedema), and in rare cases swelling of the upper airway and excess potassium retention (hyperkalemia), especially in people with kidney failure. As a result, natural ACE inhibitors have attracted increasing attention from food and medical researchers as alternatives to synthetic drugs. Peptides from partial enzymatic hydrolysis of food proteins are being studied extensively by food scientists. A number of beneficial biological peptides have been identified and classified from food protein hydrolysates. Inactive within the parent protein sequence, enzymatic digestion or food processing can release these biologically-active peptides. Depending on their amino acid sequence, they can exert *in vivo* activities affecting nutrient utilization as well as the cardiovascular, endocrine, immune and nervous systems, among others [37].

Synthetic ACE inhibitors are commonly used in drug preparations aimed at treating hypertension, but lowering blood pressure to analogous levels using commonly consumed foods represents a significant advantage, especially for people unaware of their hypertensive condition. ACE-inhibitory peptides have been identified in food protein sources such as legumes seeds [38], egg [39], and milk proteins, all considered to be particularly good bioactive peptide sources. Enzymatic hydrolysis is now used widely in biotechnological processes to improve milk protein functional properties and/or to produce bioactive milk protein hydrolysates. Notable progress has been made to date, and products such as casein phosphopeptide and antihypertensive peptides are currently on the market. The physiological effect of biopeptides depends on their ability to reach the target site. Biofunctional peptides have potential applications in the formulation of health-enhancing nutraceutical compounds with well-defined pharmaceutical effects [40]. One possible indication of the health benefits of peptides from milk is that many studies link higher milk and milk product intake with lower blood pressure and reduced risk of hypertension. For example, a study of 5000 men found that those with normal blood pressure reported a higher intake of whole milk than did hypertensive men. Similarly, the Puerto Rico Heart Study found an inverse association between milk intake and both systolic and diastolic pressure in men [41].

Particular attention has been given Ameal S cultured milk (Calpis®), a sour milk drink fermented with *Lb. helveticus* and *S. cerevisiae*, and containing the ACE inhibitory peptides IPP and VPP. Ameal S is reported to exhibit hypotensive properties in both spontaneously hypertensive rats (SHR) and humans. Single oral doses of this sour milk product in SHR resulted in drops in systolic blood pressure (SBP) of up to 21 mm mercury (Hg) at 5 mg/kg body weight (BW) and 26 mmHg at 10 mg/kg BW. Also in SHR, oral ingestion of IPP (0.3 mg/kg BW) lowered SBP to 28 mmHg while VPP (0.6 mg/kg BW) lowered it to 32 mmHg [42]. Eight hours after intravenous administration of IPP and VPP, similar effects have been reported in SHR: IPP (1.8 mg/kg BW) lowered SBP to 29.5 mmHg; and VPP (3.6 mg/kg BW) lowered it to 25 mmHg. Use of Ameal S in SHR is also reported to lower SBP (-10 to -19 mmHg) in long-term studies (14-23 weeks duration). In human studies, Ameal S has produced inconclusive results as to its hypotensive effect. After daily ingestion of 95 mL Ameal S for 8 weeks, mildly hypertensive volunteers experienced a decrease in SBP of up to 14 mmHg compared to a control group ingesting acidified milk [43].

A full understanding of the potential role of bioactive peptides in the prevention and treatment of cardiopathies will require more complete knowledge of the biological mechanisms surrounding cardiovascular control and how these are modulated by peptides. More specifically, further study is needed on the mechanisms involved in the interaction between angiotensin-converting enzyme active sites, ACE-inhibiting peptides and/or the amino acids within these peptides. Development of products containing food-origin ACE-inhibiting peptides entails going beyond a food's basic nutritional benefits and understanding the mechanisms behind the beneficial effect. An area of particular interest in the future may be application of enrichment protocols such as membrane processing and chromatographic isolation for extraction of highly potent biologically-active peptide fractions from hydrolysates of different sources for subsequent use as functional food ingredients.

REFERENCES

[1] Hooper, N.M. and Turner, A.J. (2003). An ACE structure. *Nature Structural and Molecular Biology*, 10, 155-157.

[2] Tzakos, A.G., Galanis, A.S., Spyroulias, G.A., Cordopatis, P., Manessi-Zoupa, E., Gerothanassis, I.P. (2003). Structure-function discrimination of the N and C-catalytic domains of human angiotensin-converting enzyme: implications for Cl^- activation and peptide hydrolysis mechanisms. *Protein Engineering*, 16, 993-1003.

[3] Carey, R.M., Siragy, H.M. (2003). Newly recognized components of the renin-angiotensin system: potential roles in cardiovascular and renal regulation. *Endocrine Reviews*, 24, 261-271.

[4] Donoghue, M., Hsieh, F., Baronas, E., Godbout, K., Gosselin, M., Stagliano, N. (2000). A novel angiotensin-converting enzyme-related carboxypeptidase (ACE2) converts angiotensin I to angiotensin 1-9. *Circulation Research*, 87, E1-E9.

[5] Van Sande, M.E., Scharpé, S.L., Neels, H.M., Van Camp, K.O. (1985). Distribution of angiotensin-converting enzyme in human tissues. *Clinical Chemical Acta*, 147(3), 255-260.

[6] Krassnigg, F., Niederhauser, H., Fink, E., Frick, J., Schill, W.B. (1989). Angiotensin-converting enzyme in human seminal plasma is synthesized by the testis, epididymis and prostate. *International Journal of Andrology*, 12, 22-28.

[7] Metzger, R., Franke, F.E., Bohle, R.M., Alhenc-Gelas, F., Danilov, S.M. (2011). Heterogeneous distribution of angiotensin I-converting enzyme (CD143) in the human and rat vascular systems: vessel, organ and species specificity. *Microvascular Research*, 81(2), 206-215.

[8] Diet, F., Pratt, R.E., Berry, G.J., Momose, N., Gibbons, G.H., Dzau, V.J. (1996). Increased accumulation of tissue ACE in human atherosclerotic coronary artery disease. *Circulation*, 94(11), 2756-2767.

[9] Santeliz Contra, H., Romano Estrada, L., González Chávez, A., Hernández and Hernández, H. El sistema renina-angiotensina-aldosterona y su papel funcional más allá del control de la presión arterial. *Revista Mexicana de Cardiología*, 19(1), 21-28.

[10] Marcic, B., Deddish, P.A., Jackman, H.L., Erdös, E.G., and Tan, F. (2000). Effects of the N-Terminal Sequence of ACE on the Properties of Its C-Domain. *Hypertension*, 36, 116-121.

[11] Ehlers, M.R.W., Riordan, J.F. (1991). Angiotensin-converting enzyme: zinc- and inhibitor-binding stoichiometries of the somatic and testis isozymes. *Biochemistry*, 30, 7118-7126.

[12] Aziz, M., Rousseau, A., Ezan, E., Guyene, T.T., Michelet, S., Grognet, J.M., Lenfant, M., Corvol, P., Menard, J. (1996). Acute angiotensin-converting enzyme inhibition increases the plasma level of the natural stem cell regulator N-acetyl-seryl-aspartyl-lysyl-proline. *The Journal of Clinical Investigation*, 97, 839-844.

[13] Deddish, P.A., Marcic, B., Jackman, H.L., Wang, H.Z., Skidgel, R.A., Erdos, E.G. (1998). N-domain specific substrates and C-domain inhibitors of angiotensin-converting enzyme: angiotensin (1-7) and keto-ACE. *Hypertension*, 31, 912-917.

[14] Deddish, P.A., Wang, J., Michel, B., Morris, P.W., Davidson, N.O., Skidgel, R.A., Erdos, E.G. (1994). Naturally occurring active N-domain of human angiotensin I-converting enzyme. *Proceedings of the National Academy of Sciences of the U.S.A.*, 91, 7807-7811.

[15] Fuchs, S., Xiao, H.D., Cole, J.M., Adams, J.W., Frenzel, K., Michaud, A. (2002). Role of the N-terminal catalytic domain of angiotensin-converting enzyme investigated by targeted inactivation in mice. *Journal of Biological Chemistry*, 279, 15946-15953.

[16] Piepho, R.W., Beal, J. (2000). An overview of antihypertensive therapy in the 20th century. *Journal of Clinical Pharmacology*, 40, 967-977.

[17] Brown, M.J. (2006). Direct renin inhibition - a new way of targeting the renin system. *Journal of the Renin Angiotensin Aldosterone System*, 7(2), S7-S11.

[18] Morgan, L., Broughton, P.F., Kalsheker, N. (1996). Angiotensinogen: molecular biology, biochemistry and physiology. *International Journal of Biochemistry and Cell Biology*, 28, 1211-1222.

[19] Saavedra, J.M. and Nishimura, Y. (1999). Angiotensin and cerebral blood flow. *Cellular and Molecular Neurobiology*, 19(5), 553-573.

[20] Reudelhuber, T.L. (2005). The renin-angiotensin system: peptides and enzymes beyond angiotensin II. *Current Opinion of Nephrology and Hypertension*, 14,155-159.

[21] Wagenaar, L.J., Voors, A.A., Buikema, H., Van Glist, W.H. (2002). Angiotensin receptors in the cardiovascular system. *Canadian Journal of Cardiology*, 18(12), 1331-1339.

[22] Van Geel, P.P., Pinto, Y.M., Voors, A.A. (2000). Angiotensin II type 1 receptor A1166C gene polymorphism is associated with an increased response to angiotensin II in human arteries. *Hypertension*, 35, 717-721.

[23] Bullock, G.R., Steyaert, I., Bilbe, G., (2000). Distribution of type-1 and type-2 angiotensin receptors in the normal human lung and in lungs from patients with chronic obstructive pulmonary disease. *Histochemistry and Cell Biology*, 115, 117-124.

[24] Dahlöf, B., Devereux, R.B., Kjeldsen, S.E. (2002). Cardiovascular morbidity and mortality in the Losartan Intervention for endpoint reduction in hypertension study (LIFE): a randomized trial against atenolol. *Lancet*, 359, 995-1003.

[25] Prasad, A., Koh, K.K., Schenke, W.H. (2001). Role of angiotensin II type 1 receptor in the regulation of cellular adhesion molecules in atherosclerosis. *American Heart Journal*, 142, 248-253.

[26] Daemen, M.J., Lombardi, D.M., Bosman, F.T. (1991). Angiotensin II induces smooth muscle cell proliferation in the normal and injured rat arterial wall. *Circulation Research*, 68, 450-456.

[27] Dahlöf, B. (2001). Left ventricular hypertrophy and angiotensin II antagonists. *American Journal of Hypertension*, 14, 174-182.

[28] Jong, P., Demers, C., McKelvie, R.S. (2002). Angiotensin receptor blockers in heart failure: meta-analysis of randomized controlled trials. *Journal of the American College of Cardiology*, 39, 463-470.

[29] Hernández-Madrid, A., Rebollo, J.G., Rodríguez, A., (2002). A prospective and randomized study on the effect of an angiotensin II type 1 receptor blocker irbesartan in

maintaining sinus rhythm in patients with persistent atrial fibrillation. *Journal of the American College of Cardiology*, 39, 103A.

[30] Ferreira, S.H. (1965). A bradykinin-potentiating factor (BPF) present in the venom of *Bothrops jararaca. British Journal for Pharmacology,* 24, 163-169.

[51] Cushman, D.W., Cheung, H.S., Emily F., Sabo, E.F., Ondetti, M.A. (1981). Angiotensin-Converting Enzyme Inhibitors: Evolution of a New Class of Antihypertensive Drugs. In: Angiotensin-Converting Enzyme Inhibitor Mechanisms of Action and Clinical Implications, Horovitz, Z.P. (ed), Urban and Schwarzenberg, Baltimore-Munich, pp. 3-25.

[52] Fernández Oropesa, C.M., Gallego Fernández, C. (1995). Utilidad terapéutica de los inhibidores de la enzima convertidora de angiotensina. *Farmacia Hospitalaria*, 19(1), 3-9.

[53] Zaman, M.A., Oparil, S., Calhoun, D.A. (2002). Drugs targeting the renin angiotensin aldosterone system. *Nature Reviews Drug Discovery*, 1, 621-636.

[54] Abbenante, G., Fairlie, D.P. (2005). Protease inhibitors in the clinic. *Journal of Medicinal Chemistry*, 1, 71-104.

[55] Van Esch, J.H.M., Tom, B., Dive, V., Batenburg, W.W., Georgiadis, D., Yiotakis, A., Van Gool, J.M.G., De Bruijn, R.J.A., De Vries, R., Jan Danser, A.H. (2005). Selective angiotensin-converting enzyme C-domain inhibition is sufficient to prevent angiotensin I-induced vasoconstriction. *Hypertension*, 45, 120-125.

[56] Kostis, J.B., Packer, M., Black, H.R., Schmieder, R., Henry, D., Levy, E. (2004). Omapatrilat and enalapril in patients with hypertension: the Omapatrilat Cardiovascular Treatment vs. Enalapril (OCTAVE) trial. *American Journal of Hypertension*, 17, 103-111.

[57] Zhao, X.H., Li, Y.Y. (2009). An approach to improve ACE-inhibitory activity of casein hydrolysates with plastein reaction catalyzed by Alcalase. *European Food Research and Technology*, 229,795-805.

[58] Li, G.H., Shi, Y.H., Liu, H., Le, G.W. (2006). Antihypertensive effect of Alcalase-generated mung bean protein hydrolysates in spontaneously hypertensive rats. *European Food Research and Technology*, 222(6), 733-736.

[59] Miguel, M., Alonso, M.J., Salaices, M., Aleixandre, A., López-Fandiño, R. (2007). Antihypertensive, ACE-inhibitory and vasodilator properties of an egg white hydrolysate: effect of a simulated intestinal digestion. *Food Chemistry*, 104(1), 163-168.

[60] Iwaniak, A., Minkiewicz, P., (2007). Proteins as the source of physiologically and functionally active peptides. *Acta Scientiarum Polonorum Technolgia Alimentaria*, 6(3), 5-15.

[61] Groziak, S.M., Miller, G.D. (2000). Natural bioactive substances in milk and colostrum: effects on the arterial blood pressure system. *British Journal of Nutrition*, 84(1), S119-S125.

[62] Nakamura, Y., Yamamoto, N., Sakai, K., Okubo, A., Yamazaki, S., Takano, T. (1995). Purification and characterization of Angiotensin I-converting enzyme inhibitors from sour milk. *Journal of Dairy Science*, 78, 777-783.

[63] Fitzgerald, R.J., Murray, B.A. (2006). Bioactive peptides and lactic fermentations. *International Journal of Dairy Technology*, 59, 118-125.

In: Angiotensin: New Research
Editors: S. Harada, I. Moi, pp. 165-179

ISBN: 978-1-62100-773-9

Chapter 7

REDOX REGULATION OF ANGIOTENSIN RECEPTOR SIGNALING IN THE HEART

Motohiro Nishida*[*], *Caroline Sunggip*, *Naoyuki Kitajima and Hitoshi Kurose
Department of Pharmacology and Toxicology, Graduate School of Pharmaceutical Sciences, Kyushu University, 3-1-1 Maidashi, Higashi-ku, Fukuoka 812-8582, Japan.

ABSTRACT

Cardiovascular diseases are leading cause of morbidity and mortality in developed countries. Renin-angiotensin system (RAS) and its effector molecule, angiotensin (Ang) II, play an important role in the pathophysiology of cardiovascular and kidney diseases. Most of the known pathophysiological effects of Ang II are mediated by Ang type 1 receptors (AT_1Rs), and up-regulation of AT_1Rs is an important event involves in undesired cardiovascular-renal crosstalk. Many lines of evidences have shown that reactive oxygen species (ROS) and reactive nitrogen species (RNS) play significant roles in regulation of AT_1R signaling. In our study, we reveal that AT_1R-stimulated ROS production mediates activation of mitogen-activated protein kinases (MAPKs), leading to hypertrophic growth of cardiomyocytes and excessive cytokine production by cardiac fibroblasts. These findings indicate that ROS work as a crucial second messenger in Ang II-induced signaling. Endogenous ROS apparently increase AT_1R expression level, while RNS down-regulates the expression of AT_1R. The differences in the effects of ROS and RNS on AT_1R expression can be explained by the local covalent modification of cysteine thiols that are found at active or allosteric sites of effector proteins. This review introduces the recent findings on molecular mechanisms underlying reduction/oxidation (redox)-dependent post-translational regulation of AT_1R signaling in the cardiovascular system. These findings will provide a new understanding on the importance of cross talk between Ang II signaling and ROS/RNS in the development of heart failure.

---

* Corresponding author: Motohiro Nishida, Ph.D.
Department of Pharmacology and Toxicology,
Graduate School of Pharmaceutical Sciences, Kyushu University,
3-1-1 Maidashi, Higashi-ku, Fukuoka 812-8582, Japan.
E-mail: nishida@phar.kyushu-u.ac.jp
Tel&Fax: +81-92-642-6878

INTRODUCTION

The renin-angiotensin system (RAS) plays an important role in maintaining blood pressure and salt homeostasis in mammals [1, 2]. RAS initiates through well-regulated secretion of renin from the kidney. Tigerstedt and Bergman first identified renin as a pressor substance in 1898 [3]. They demonstrated that intravenous injection of rabbit kidney's extract (but not other tissue extracts) to animals cause a rise in arterial blood pressure. They named the extract substance 'renin'. Several decades later, renin was identified, not as a vasoconstricting substance, but rather as an enzyme that catalyzed the formation of a substance responsible for increasing blood pressure, namely Ang (however, Ang was referred to as angiotonin or hypertensin at that time) [4, 5]. In 1956, Skeggs *et al.* identified two distinct forms of Ang, Ang I and II. They discovered that by the action of Ang-converting enzyme (ACE), the inactive Ang I is converted to a potent vasoconstrictor, Ang II [6]. Since then, Ang II was recognized as the main effector substance of RAS. In 1980s, several Ang II receptor isoforms were identified and AT_1R was postulated to be an isoform which responsible for the undesirable effects of Ang. [7, 8].

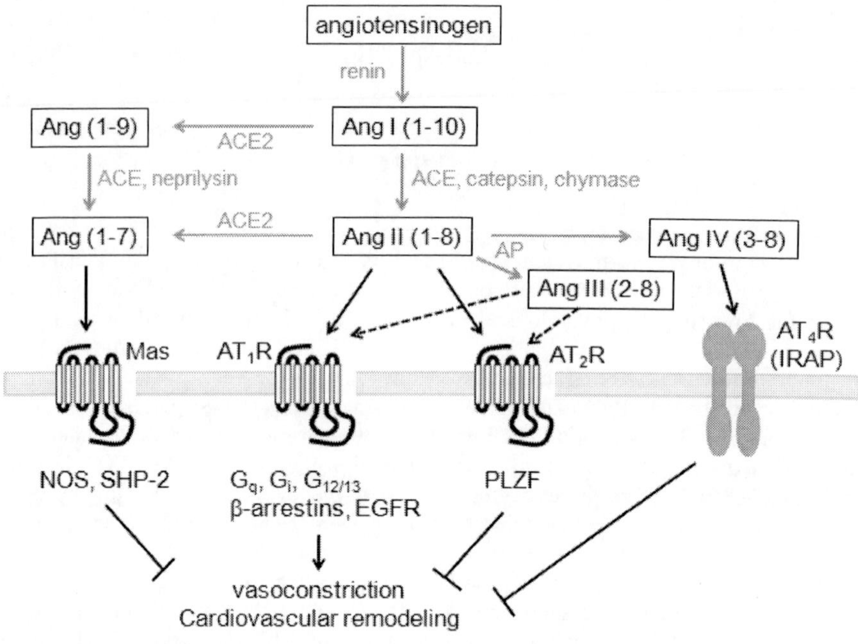

Figure 1. The major components of RAS and regulation of cardiovascular functions by the respective Ang receptors. ACE2; Ang converting enzyme 2, AP; aminopeptidase, EGFR; epidermal growth factor receptor, IRAP; insulin-regulated aminopeptidase, NOS; nitric oxide synthase, PLZF; promyelocytic leukaemia zinc finger protein, SHP-2; Src homology 2 domain-containing protein tyrosine phosphatase type 2.

In later years, the elementary understanding of RAS has continued to expand to a much-adopted theory nowadays (Figure 1). The RAS activation starts with the protease renin cleavage of circulating angiotensinogen from liver to yield a 10 amino-acid polypeptide, Ang

I (1-10). Angiotensin converting enzyme (ACE) in the lung or vascular endothelium then cleaves Ang I to produce an active octapeptide, Ang II (Ang (1-8)). Although there are other Ang II-generating enzymes (e.g cathepsins, chymase) [9, 10], ACE is believed to be the sole enzyme in the regulation of Ang II production in the RAS [1, 2]. Ang II is degraded to Ang (1-7), Ang III (2-8) or Ang IV (3-8) by the action of ACE2 [11] and aminopeptidase. These Ang-derived metabolites exert biological activities through binding to seven transmembrane-spanning receptors (AT_1R, AT_2R and Mas) or insulin-regulated aminopeptidase (IRAP; originally defined as AT_4R by an international nomenclature committee) [14-16]. Several reports outlined counter-regulatory role of Ang (1-7) by opposing many AT_1R-mediated actions [12, 13]. Among the Ang-derived metabolites, Ang II is the key regulator of cardiovascular functions, and most of its biological effects are mediated via AT_1R.

1. Phenotypes of RAS Component-Deficient Mice

Gene targeting experiments have provided several important insights into the pathophysiological roles of RAS. Deletion of genes encoding angiotensinogen and ACE results in hypotension, reduced survival, and abnormal renal development associated with plasma Ang II deficiency [17-20]. ACE-deficient male mice have impaired fertility [19, 20]. This was due to lost of a testis-specific ACE isozyme expressed in spermatids, which play important roles in sperm transport and binding to zona pellucid of oocytes. ACE2 gene knockout mice are generally viable, fertile and do not appear to have significant cardiac abnormality nor impaired Ang II plasma level [21]. However, adult knockout mice show modest glomerulosclerosis and albuminuria. As these effects can be reverse by AT_1R blockade, ACE2 deficiency may cause renal injury via impaired degradation of Ang II and its subsequent activation of AT_1Rs.

Mice lacking functional $AT_{1a}R$ exhibit no major impairment in the heart, vascular system, and kidney, although a reduction of resting blood pressure observed [22-24]. Tubuloglomerular feedback loop, which regulates Na^+ delivery to the distal tubule, was undetectable in $AT_{1a}R$ knockout mice, indicating that AT_1R plays an essential role in regulation of renal hemodynamic [25]. Deletion of $AT_{1b}R$, which is highly expressed in adrenal zona glomerusa and testis spermatic cells, showed no phenotypes abnormalities in mice [26]. Similarly, AT_2R-knockdown mice develop normally, but exhibit impaired drinking response to water deprivation as well as a reduction in spontaneous movements [27]. Deletion of AT_2R increases vasopressor response to Ang II injection, indicating AT_2R as a negative regulator for Ang II-induced vasopressor response. Furthermore, AT_2R signaling was found to attenuate aortic aneurysm in a mouse model of Marfan syndrome, an autosomal dominant connective tissue disorder. This achieved through inhibition of AT_1R-stimulated activation of extracellular signal-regulated kinase (ERK) [28], thus suggesting a protective nature of AT_2R signaling in vascular diseases (Figure 1). Interestingly, Inagami's group reported that AT_2R contributes to the development of cardiac hypertrophy in response to pressure overload or to chronic Ang II infusion [29, 30]. This group also showed that C-terminus of AT_2R binds to the transcription factor, promyelocytic zinc finger protein (PLZF), and AT_2R internalization induced by Ang II translocates PLZF into the nucleus, leading to expression of phosphatidylinositol-3 kinase (PI3K) p85α subunit, consequently led to cardiac hypertrophy

[31]. These findings suggest that AT_2R contributes to the cardiac adaptive hypertrophic response against hemodynamic stress.

The phenotype of Mas knockout mouse appears to be highly dependent on strain. Mas knockout on a C57BL/6 genetic background mice (but not mixed 129xC57BL/6) shows impaired cardiac and renal function that is partially due to fibrosis [32, 33]. As Mas receptor stimulation by Ang (1-7) opposes many of the AT_1R-mediated actions including vasoconstriction, hypertrophy and fibrosis, it may have a role in preventing the advancement of heart failure [32]. AT_4R is mainly expressed in the brain, especially in the CA1 and CA3 regions of Ammon's horn in the hippocampus [16]. Inhibitions of IRAP activities were found to have benefit on memory enhancement. However, genetic ablation of AT_4R genes causes age-related deterioration of spatial memory in mice [34]. In the cardiovascular system, ablation of AT_4R has been reported to attenuate hypofibrinolysis via PAI-1 down regulation and reduces occlusive arterial thrombosis [35], indicating that AT_4R protect against vascular injury.

2. G PROTEIN-DEPENDENT AT_1R SIGNALING PATHWAYS

Stimulation of AT_1R induces G protein-dependent and G protein-independent signaling pathways [36]. AT_1Rs couple with three G protein subfamilies; G_q, G_i, G_{12} [36, 37], and activation of $G\alpha_{q/11}$ and $G\alpha_{12/13}$-mediated signaling pathways contribute to development of cardiac hypertrophy and fibrosis [38, 39]. The G_q family protein induce activation of phospholipase C (PLC), which in turn induces increase in intracellular Ca^{2+} concentration ($[Ca^{2+}]_i$) through production of inositol-1,4,5-trisphosphate (IP_3) and diacylglycerol (DAG) from phosphatidylinositol 4,5-bisphosphate (PIP_2). Sustained increase in $[Ca^{2+}]_i$ in cardiomyocytes activates calmodulin (CaM)-dependent protein phosphatase 2B (calcineurin), and prompt increase expression of hypertrophic genes mainly through activation of nuclear factor of activated T cells (NFAT) [40]. We revealed that DAG-activated transient receptor potential canonical channels (TRPC3 and TRPC6) mediate Ang II-induced Ca^{2+} influx through voltage-dependent Ca^{2+} channel (VDCC), which consequently led to cardiac hypertrophy in *in vivo* and *in vitro* model [41, 42]. Activation of extracellular signal-regulated kinase (ERK) signaling pathway also participates in G_q-mediated cardiac hypertrophy. Lorenz *et al.* [43] has reported that $G\beta\gamma$ released from $G\alpha_q$ induces autophosphorylation of ERK1/2 at Thr^{188} residue and subsequent nuclear translocation of ERK1/2, resulting in expression of hypertrophic genes. On the other hand, we found that G_{12} family proteins mediate Ang II-induced ROS production/activation of c-Jun NH_2-terminal kinase (JNK) and p38 MAPK [44,45]. A study showed that activation of JNK and p38MAPK occur in response to activation of apoptosis signal-regulated kinase (ASK), which is interceded by ROS-mediated thioredoxin oxidation [46]. These indicate that ROS work as a critical mediator for $G_{12/13}$ signaling in cardiomyocytes. Furthermore, the inhibition of $G\alpha_{12/13}$ signaling in cardiomyocytes attenuates pressure overload-induced collagen deposition in the heart (fibrosis), which was shown in transgenic mice with cardiomyocytes-specific overexpression of $G\alpha_{12/13}$-specific inhibitory polypeptide [39]. Thus, $G\alpha_{q/11}$ and $G\alpha_{12/13}$ work through different signaling cascades in regulating heart morphological changes in response to pressure overload.

3. Mechanism of ROS Production by AT_1R Stimulation

Stimulation of AT_1R generates ROS through NADPH oxidase (Nox) activation [47,48]. Although seven mammalian Nox isoforms have been identified, only two isoforms (Nox2 and Nox4) are expressed in the heart [49, 50]. As the deletion of Nox2 or Nox4 improves heart failure after myocardial infarction or pressure overload, Nox-derived ROS may contribute to the progression of cardiovascular remodeling [47-50]. In addition, Ang II-induced ROS production through Nox activation attenuates basal endothelial nitric oxide (NO) synthase (eNOS) activity through proline-rich tyrosine kinase (Pyk2)-dependent phosphorylation of eNOS at Tyr657 [51], suggesting the mechanism of endothelial dysfunction observed in cardiovascular diseases is associated with increased activity of the RAS. Ang II may specifically generate ROS in the cardiovascular, but not NO (or RNS).

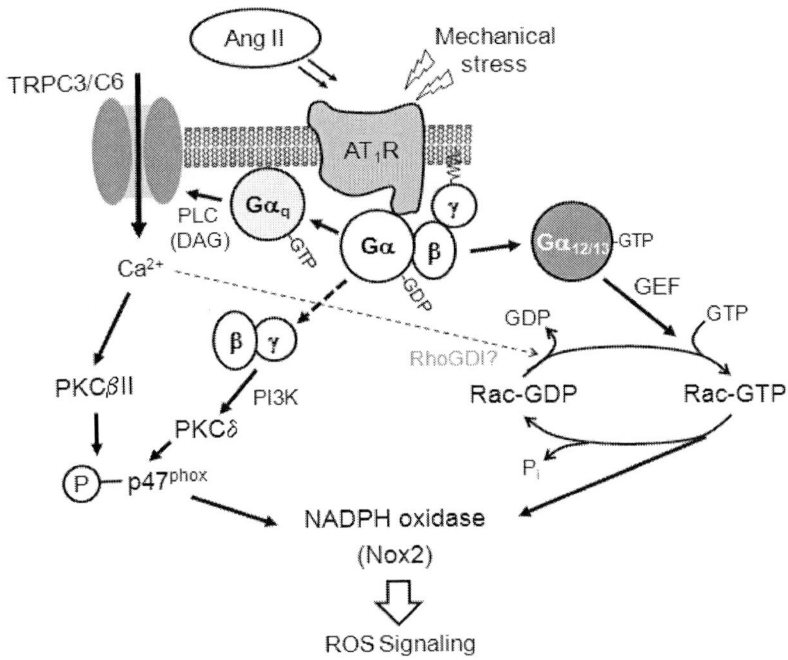

Figure 2. The putative mechanism of AT_1R-stimulated ROS production in the heart. Stimulation of AT_1R by Ang II or mechanical stress induces activation of G_q-, G_i- and $G_{12/13}$-dependent signaling pathways. The $G\alpha_q$-mediated phospholipase C (PLC) activation induces Ca^{2+} influx through diacylglycerol (DAG)-activated TRPC3/TRPC6 channels. This Ca^{2+} influx then activates conventional protein kinase C (PKCβII) and phosphorylates $p47^{phox}$, an essential NADPH oxidase subunit. The βγ subunit released from G_i family proteins activates PLCδ via PI3K, leading to Ca^{2+}-independent phosphorylation of $p47^{phox}$. The $G\alpha_{12/13}$ mediate promotion of GTP/GDP exchange of Rac GTPase, leading to activation of NADPH oxidase (Nox2) in the heart.

The Ang II-induced ROS production in the heart is regulated by G protein-dependent signaling pathways (Figure 2). The activation of Nox2 primarily depends on intracellular Ca^{2+} concentration, where an increase activates a small GTP-binding protein, Rac, and protein kinase C (PKC)-mediated phosphorylation of p47^{phox} [52, 53]. Our recent findings indicate that activation of G$\alpha_{12/13}$ upon AT_1R stimulation increases Rac activity in rat neonatal cardiomyocytes [44, 45], while inhibition of G$\beta\gamma$ suppresses Ang II- stimulated ROS production. As PIP_3-dependent PKCδ activation participates in Nox2 activation [53], there is a possibility that G$\beta\gamma$ mediates PI3K activation by Ang II stimulation. In addition, TRPC3 channel has been shown to contribute to Nox-mediated ROS production in rodent cardiomyocytes [54]. TRPC channels have two functions: to act as a sensor for various extracellular stresses, and to act as a protein scaffold at the plasma membrane to control the amplification and co-ordination of receptor signaling [55]. TRPC3 functionally interacts with protein kinase C (PKC) βII [56], and Ca^{2+}-dependent activation of PKCβII may induce Nox2 activation through phosphorylation of the p47^{phox} subunit [52]. Interestingly, inhibition of TRPC3-mediated Ca^{2+} influx also suppresses Rac1 activity in the cardiomyopathic mouse heart [54]. As Price et al. [57] had previously reported that PKC-mediated phosphorylation of Rho GDP dissociation inhibitor (GDI) α, induces Ca^{2+}-dependent Rac activation, it is possible that TRPC3-mediated Ca^{2+} influx dissociates RhoGDIα from Rac through PKCβII-dependent phosphorylation of RhoGDIα. The AT_1Rs are activated by mechanical stretch in a ligand-independent manner [58, 59]. Upon mechanical stretch, AT_1R undergoes an anticlockwise rotation and a shift of its transmembrane domain 7 (TMD7) into the ligand binding pocket, as shown by using substituted cysteine accessibility mapping (SCAM) method [60]. Thus, the AT1R-induced ROS-generating mechanism might participate in mechanical stress-induced ROS production.

4. Regulation of AT_1R Functions by Oxidative Modification

Numerous mutagenesis studies had revealed that an interaction between Asn111 in TMD3 and Tyr292 in TMD7 maintain AT_1R in inactive conformation. Disruption of this interaction by Ang II may promote an active conformation site. In addition, SCAM method provided evidences that constitutive activation of AT_1R causes TMD2 to pivot, bringing the top of TMD2 closer to the binding pocket and pushing the bottom of TMD2 away from the binding pocket [61]. The activation of AT_1R apparently causes counterclockwise rotation of TMD5 as viewed from the extracellular side [62]. The AT_1R activity is negatively regulated by oxidation or reduction of the AT_1Rs. Disulfide bridges between N-terminal region and third extracellular loop, and between the first and second extracellular loops are form to maintain the conformation of AT_1R protein [61-63]. AT_2R is resistant to inactivation by reducing agents due to the absence of disulfide bridges between the N-terminal region and third extracellular loop. Zhang *et al.* [64] has recently reported that nitro-oleic acid specifically binds to AT_1R, reduces G_q protein coupling, and inhibits inositol-1,4,5-trisphosphate production and Ca^{2+} mobilization, without inhibiting Ang II binding to the receptor.

ROS and RNS also regulate AT_1R transcriptional activity. We recently reported that endogenous ROS generated through *Pertusis* toxin (PTX) stimulation on Toll-like receptor 4 (TLR4) increase AT_1R density in rat cardiac fibroblasts [65]. PTX, a major virulence factor of Gram-negative bacillus *Bordetella* pertussis, which causes whooping cough, is a well-established pharmacological tool as specific inhibitor of receptor-$G_{i/o}$ protein coupling. PTX structurally composed of A-promoter and B-oligomer region. The A-promoter exerts ADP-ribosyltransferase activity on the α-subunit of heterotrimeric G_i proteins ($G\alpha_i$), consequently hinder receptor- G protein coupling. Meanwhile, the B-oligomer region recognizes and binds to carbohydrate-containing receptors that deliver A-protomer into the cytosol. In our study, 24 hr treatment with PTX B-oligomer or denatured PTX protein results in 2-fold increase in maximal ^{125}I-Ang II binding activity, indicating that PTX increases AT_1R density independently of ADP ribosylation. This response was similarly demonstrated with lipopolysaccharide (LPS) treatment.

TLR4 stimulation by PTX activates Rac through Syk tyrosine kinase, and subsequently induces NF-κB activation through ROS-dependent IκBα phosphorylation and degradation. Activation of NF-κB increases expression of IL-1β, which in turn activates Rac through IL-1β receptor stimulation. As IL-1β neutral antibody or IL-1β knockdown significantly suppress the increase in AT_1R density by PTX, IL-1β-dependent amplification of ROS-mediated NF-κB signaling is essential for the PTX-induced AT_1R up-regulation. We have yet to uncover the mechanism underlying ROS-mediated phosphorylation and degradation of IκBα, but other groups had reported that stress-induced Ca^{2+} mobilization induces nuclear accumulation of IκBα, resulting in IκBα degradation without N-terminal phosphorylation [66, 67]. In addition, a study on macrophages has found that TLR4-stimulated ROS production occur independent of MyD88 signaling pathways [68]. As AT_1R signaling contributes to various inflammatory responses including heart [13-15], ROS-mediated signaling may play a critical role in TLR4-induced inflammatory responses in mammalian cells.

It has been reported that NO and nitro-unsaturated fatty acids decrease Ang II signaling in the heart [31, 43]. We recently found that long-term treatment of adenosine 5'-triphosphate (ATP) in rat neonatal cardiac fibroblasts decreases AT_1R density. This so-called 'heterologous down-regulation' phenomenon is suggesting that over stimulation of one GPCR may reduce the expression levels of other GPCRs [51]. Cross talk between different GPCR signaling pathways may serve to fine-tune cell signaling [52], but the molecular mechanism(s) underlying heterologous down-regulation is still largely unknown. The ATP-induced AT_1R down-regulation was abolished by treatment with cyclosporine A or siRNAs for $P2Y_2R$, indicating that $P2Y_2R$-stimulated sustained increase in intracellular Ca^{2+} concentration and subsequent activation of calcineurin-NFAT signaling, participate in ATP-induced AT_1R down-regulation. Interestingly, the ATP-induced suppression of AT_1R signaling was completely diminished by 1400W, a selective inhibitor of inducible NO synthase (iNOS). iNOS promoter region contains NFAT-binding sequences and activation of calcineurin-NFAT signaling pathway has been reported to induce expression of iNOS proteins in cardiomyocytes and *in vivo* mouse hearts [53]. In fact, ATP increased expression of iNOS proteins in a concentration-dependent manner, and ATP-induced iNOS expression is completely suppressed by cyclosporine A. The expression of constitutively active mutant of NFAT also decreased AT_1R density, which canceled by 1400W. Thus, NFAT-dependent iNOS expression is required for ATP-induced suppression of AT_1R signaling.

We focused on the conserved cysteine (Cys) residue in the Rel homology domain of NF-κB [54, 55]. The Cys wedged between acidic and basic amino acids is nucleophilic, acidic and redoxly active, and numerous reactions may occur on this Cys thiol side chain [56]. As the reactive Cys located in the Rel homology domain involves in DNA binding or dimer formation of p65, the NO-mediated Cys modification (S-nitrosylation) of p65 may decrease transcriptional activity of NF-κB [54, 55]. Using biotin-switch assay method shown in Figure 3A, we found that treatment of rat cardiac fibroblasts with ATP for 24 hours actually induced S-nitrosylation of p65 subunit at Cys38. The promoter region of iNOS does not only contain NF-κB binding sequences but also NFAT binding sequences (Figure 4B). Treatment of cardiac fibroblasts with ATP induced iNOS expression, and the iNOS protein and p65 subunit were co-localized around the perinuclear regions (Figure 4C). Immunoprecipitation study confirmed that ATP-induced iNOS forms a complex with p65. In contrast, treatment with IL-1β strongly increases expression of iNOS protein but do not induce iNOS interaction with p65. This is due to translocation of p65 from cytosol to the nucleus by IL-1β itself. We found that flavin-binding domain of iNOS protein is a hot spot for the interaction with p65, and overexpression of iNOS fragment including flavin-binding domain completely suppressed the ATP-induced suppression of AT_1R signaling. Therefore, the formation of signaling complex between iNOS and p65 around the perinuclear region may be essential for the ATP-induced AT_1R down-regulation.

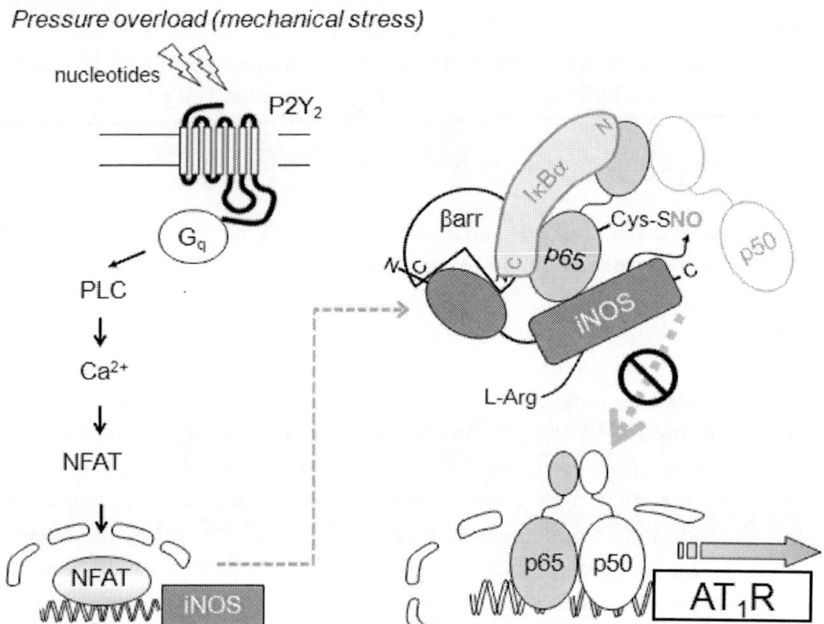

Figure 3. Heterologous crosstalk between AT_1R and $P2Y_2R$ via NO-mediated posttranslational modification (S-nitrosylation) of NF-κB. ATP stimulates purinergic G_q-coupled $P2Y_2R$ and activates calcineurin-NFAT signaling, which leads to induction of iNOS proteins. The NF-κB p65 subunit localizes both in the cytosol and nucleus, and cytosolic p65 interacts with iNOS proteins via flavin-binding domain of iNOS. The locally generated NO induces S-nitrosylation of p65 at Cys38, leading to decrease in DNA binding affinitiy, resulting in decrease in transcription rate of AT_1R gene. As the IκBα and β-arrestins are also known to interact with iNOS and p65, β-arrestins may anchor the formation of p65/IκBα/β-arrestins/iNOS quaternary complex.

5. Conclusion

There is no doubt that RAS plays essential roles in the pathogenesis of cardiovascular and kidney diseases. AT_1Rs in the kidney alone were sufficient to induce hypertension and cardiac hypertrophy in response to Ang II infusion in mice [78]. A couple of study however, reported that $AT_{1a}R$-mediated Ang II signaling is not crucial for the development of pressure-overload induced cardiac hypertrophy [58, 79]. Antagonizing $AT_{1a}R$ using candesartan suppresses pressure overload-induced cardiac hypertrophy in angiotensinogen-deficient mice model. These suggest that $AT_{1b}R$ participate in the development of cardiac hypertrophy in response to pressure overload. In addition, cardiomyocyte-specific overexpression of constitutively active mutant of human AT_1R causes blood pressure-independent cardiac hypertrophy and dysfunction [80]. Collectively, blockade of AT_1R signaling will be effective for preventing cardiovascular remodeling. Our findings strongly suggest that endogenous ROS/RNS produced by receptor stimulation, fine-tune AT_1R signaling pathways in the heart. Thus, unraveling the regulation of Ang II signaling by diverse Cys modification (thiol oxidation, S-glutathionation, S-nitrosylation, S-alkylation, S-sulfhydration etc.) may provide new therapeutic targets with great potential to ameliorate heart failure.

References

[1] Skeggs, L.T. Jr, Dorer, F.E., Levine, M., Lentz, K.E., & Kahn, J.R. (1980) The biochemistry of the renin-angiotensin system. *Adv Exp Med Biol* 130, 1-27.

[2] Turner, A.J., & Hooper, N.M. (2002) The angiotensin-converting enzyme gene family: genomics and pharmacology. *Tends Pharmacol Sci* 23, 177-183.

[3] Tigerstedt, R., & Bergman, P.G. (1898) Niere and Kreislauf. *Scand Arch Physiol* 8, 223-271.

[4] Braun Menéndez, E., Fasciolo, J.C., Leloir, L.F., & Muñoz, J.M. (1939) La substancia hipertensora de la sangre del riñón isquemiado. *Rev Soc Arg Biol* 15, 420-425.

[5] Page, I.H., & Helmer, O.M. (1939) A crystalline pressor substance, angiotonin. *Proc Center Soc Clin Invest* 12, 17.

[6] Skeggs, L.T. Jr, Lentz, K.E., Kahn, J.R., Shumway, N.P., & Woods, K.R. (1956) The amino acid sequence of hypertensin. II. *J Exp Med* 104, 193-197.

[7] Dinh, D.T., Frauman, A.G., Johnston, C.I., & Fabiani, M.E. (2001) Angiotensin receptors: Distribution, signaling and function. *Clin Sci* (London) 100, 481-492.

[8] Vinson, G.P., Ho, M.M., & Puddefoot, J.R. (1995) The distribution of angiotensin II type 1 receptors, and the tissue renin-angiotensin systems. *Mol Med Today* 1, 35-39.

[9] Belova, L.A. (2000) Angiotensin II-generating enzymes. *Biochemistry* (Mosc) 65, 1337-1345.

[10] Miyazaki, M., & Takai, S. (2006) Tissue Angiotensin II generating system by angiotensin-converting enzyme and chymase. *J Pharmacol Sci* 100, 391-397.

[11] Tipnis, S.R., Hooper, N.M., Hyde, R., Karran, E., Christie, G., & Turner, A.J. (2000) A human homolog of angiotensin-converting enzyme. Cloning and functional expression as a captopril-insensitive carboxypeptidase. *J Biol Chem* 275, 33238-33243.

[12] Santos, R.A., Frezard, F., & Ferreira, A.J. (2005) Angiotensin-(1-7): blood, heart, and blood vessels. *Curr Med Chem Cardiovas Hematol Agents* 3, 383-391.

[13] Ferrario, C.M. (2006) Angiotensin-converting enzyme 2 and angiotensin-(1-7): an evolving story in cardiovascular regulation. *Hypertension* 47, 515-521.

[14] de Gasparo, M., Catt, K.J., Inagami, T., Wright, J.W., & Unger, T.H. (2000) International union of pharmacology. XXIII. The angiotensin II receptors. *Pharmacol Rev* 52, 415-472.

[15] Oro, C., Qian, H., & Thomas, W.G. (2007) Type 1 angiotensin receptor pharmacology: signaling beyond G proteins. *Pharmacol Ther* 113, 210-226.

[16] Albiston, A.L., McDowall, S.G., Matsacos, D., Sim, P., Clune, E., Mustafa, T., Lee, J., Mendelsohn, F.A.O., Simpson, R.J., Connolly, L.M., & Chai, S.Y. (2001) Evidence that the angiotensin IV (AT4) receptor is the enzyme insulin-regulated aminopeptidase. *J Biol Chem* 276, 48623-48626.

[17] Tanimoto, K., Sugiyama, F., Goto, Y., Ishida, J., Takimoto, E., Yagami, K., Fukamizu, A., & Murakami, K. (1994) Angiotensinogen-deficient mice with hypotension. *J Biol Chem* 269, 31334-31337.

[18] Kim, H., Krege, J., Kluckman, K., Hagaman, J., Hodgin, J., Best, C., Jennette, J., Coffman, T., Maeda, N., & Smithies, O. (1995) Genetic control of blood pressure and the angiotensinogen locus. *Proc Natl Acad Sci USA* 92, 2735-2739.

[19] Krege, J., John, S., Langenbach, L., Hodgin, J., Hagaman, J., Bachman, E., Jennette, J., O'Brien, D., & Smithies, O. (1995) Male-female differencies in fertility and blood pressure in ACE-deficient mice. *Nature* (Lond) 375, 146-149.

[20] Escher, C.R., Marino, E.M., Howard, T.E., Machaud, A., Corvol, P., Capecchi, M.R., & Bernstein, K.E. (1997) The critical role of tissue angiotensin-converting enzyme as revealed by gene targeting in mice. *J Clin Invest* 15, 2375-2385.

[21] Oudit, G.Y., Herzenberg, A.M., Kassiri, Z., Wong, D., Reich, H., Khokha, R., Crackower, M.A., Backx, P.H., Penninger, J.M., & Scholey, J.W. (2006) Loss of angiotensin-converting enzyme-2 leads to the late development of angiotensin II-dependent glomerulosclerosis. *Am J Pathol* 168, 1808-1820.

[22] Ito, M., Oliverio, M.I., Mannon, P.J., Best, C.F., Maeda, N., Smithies, O., & Coffman, T.M. (1995) Regulation of blood pressure by the type 1A angiotensin II receptor gene. *Proc Natl Acad Sci USA* 92, 3521-3525.

[23] Sugaya, T., Nishimatsu, S., Tanimoto, K., Takimoto, E., Yamagishi, T., Imamura, K., Goto, S., Imaizumi, K., Hisada, Y., Otsuka, A., Uchida, H., Sugiura, M., Fukuta, K., Fukamizu, A., & Murakami, K. (1995) Angiotensin type 1a receptor-deficient mice with hypotension and hyperreninemia. *J Biol Chem* 270, 18719-18722.

[24] Oliverio, M.I., Best, C.F., Kim, H.S., Arendshorst, W.J., Smithies, O., & Coffman, T.M. (1997) Angiotensin II responses in AT1A receptor-deficient mice: A role for AT1B receptors in blood pressure regulation. *Am J Physiol* 272, F515-F520.

[25] Schnermann, J.B., Traynor, T., Yang, T., Huang, Y.G., Oliverio, M.I., Coffman, T., & Briggs, J.P. (1997) Absence of tubuloglomerular feedback responses in AT_{1A} receptor-deficient mice. *Am J Physiol* 273, F315-F320.

[26] Chen, X., Li, W., Yoshida, H., Tsuchida, S., Nishimura, H., Takemoto, F., Okubo, S., Fogo, A., Matsusaka, T., & Ichikawa, I. (1997) Targeting deletion of angiotensin type 1B receptor gene in themouse. *Am J Physiol* 272, F299-F304.

[27] Hein, L., Barsh, G.S., Pratt, R.E., Dzau, V.J., & Kobilka, B.K. (1995) Behavioural and cardiovascular effects of disrupting the angiotensin II type-2 receptor gene in mice. *Nature* 377, 744-747.

[28] Habashi, J.P., Doyle, J.J., Holm, T.M., Aziz, H., Schoenhoff, F., Bedja, D., Chen, Y., Modiri, A.N., Judge, D.P., & Dietz, H.C. (2011) Angiotensin II type 2 receptor signaling attenuates aortic aneurysm in mice through ERK antagonism. *Science* 332, 361-364.

[29] Senbonmatsu, T., Ichihara, S., Price, E.Jr., Gaffney, F.A., & Inagami, T. (2000) Evidence for angiotensin II type 2 receptor-mediated cardiac myocyte enlargement during in vivo pressure overload. *J Clin Invest* 106, R25-R29.

[30] Ichihara, S., Senbonmatsu, T., Price, E.Jr., Ichiki, T., Gaffney, F.A., & Inagami, T. (2001) Angiotensin II type 2 receptor is essential for left ventricular hypertrophy and cardiac fibrosis in chronic angiotensin II-induced hypertension. *Circulation* 104, 346-351.

[31] Senbonmatsu, T., Saito, T., Landon, E.J., Watanabe, O., Price, E.Jr., Roberts, R.L., Imboden, H., Fitzgerald, T.G., Gaffney, F.A., & Inagami, T. (2003) A novel angiotensin II type 2 receptor signaling pathway: possible role in cardiac hypertrophy. *EMBO J* 22, 6471-6482.

[32] Santos, R.A., Castro, C.H., Gava, E., Pinheiro, S.V., Almeida, A.P., Paula, R.D., Cruz, J.S., Ramos, A.S., Rosa, K.T., Irigoyen, M.C., Bader, M., Alenina, N., Kitten, G.T., & Ferreira, A.J. (2006) Impairment of in vitro and in vivo heart function in angiotensin-(1-7) receptor MAS knockout mice. *Hypertension* 47, 996-1002.

[33] Pinheiro, S.V., Ferreira, A.J., Kitten, G.T., da Silveira, K.D., da Silva, D.A., Santos, S.H., Gava, E., Castro, C.H., Magalhaes, J.A., da Mota, R.K., Botelho-Santos, G.A., Bader, M., Alenina, N., Santos, R.A., & Simoes e Silva, A.C. (2009) Genetic deletion of the angiotensin-(1-7) and the g protein-coupled receptor MAS are key players in renal inflammation. *Plos ONE* 4, e5406.

[34] Albiston, A.L., Fernando, R.N., Yeatman, H.R., Burns, P., Ng, L., Daswani, D., Diwakarla, S., Pham, V., & Chai, S.Y. (2010) Gene knockout of insulin-regulated aminopeptidase: Loss of the specific binding site for angiotensin IV and age-related deficit in spatial memory. *Neurobiol Learn Mem* 93, 19-30.

[35] Numaguchi, Y., Ishii, M., Kubota, R., Morita, Y., Yamamoto, K., Matsushita, T., Okumura, K., & Murohara, T. (2009) Ablation of angiotensin IV receptor attenuates hypofibrinolysis via PAI-1 downregulation and reduces occlusive arterial thrombosis. *Arterioscler Thromb Vasc Biol* 29, 2102-2108.

[36] Hunyady, L., & Catt, K.J. (2006) Pleiotropic AT1 receptor signaling pathways mediating physiological and pathogenic actions of Angiotensin II. *Mol Endocrinol* 20, 953-970.

[37] Sadoshima, J. & Izumo, S. (1997) The cellular and molecular response of cardiac myocytes to mechanical stress. *Annu Rev Physiol* 59, 551-571.

[38] D'Angelo, D.D., Sakata, Y., Lorenz, J.N., Boivin, G.P., Walsh, R.A., Liggett, S.B., & Dorn, G.W. 2nd. (1997) Transgenic $G\alpha_q$ overexpression induces cardiac contractile failure in mice. *Proc Natl Acad Sci USA*, 94, 8121-8126.

[39] Nishida, M., Sato, Y., Uemura, A., Narita, Y., Tozaki-Saitoh, H., Nakaya, M., Ide, T., Suzuki, K., Inoue, K., Nagao, T., & Kurose, H. (2008) $P2Y_6$ receptor-$G\alpha_{12/13}$ signalling

in cardiomyocytes triggers pressure overload-induced cardiac fibrosis. *EMBO J*, 27, 3104-3115.

[40] Heineke, J., & Molkentin, J.D. (2006) Regulation of cardiac hypertrophy by intracellular signaling pathways, *Nat Rev Mol Cell Biol* 7, 589-600.

[41] Onohara, N., Nishida, M., Inoue, R., Kobayashi, H., Sumimoto, H., Sato, Y., Mori, Y., Nagao, T., & Kurose, H. (2006) TRPC3 and TRPC6 are essential for angiotensin II-induced cardiac hypertrophy, *EMBO J* 25, 5305-5316.

[42] Kiyonaka, S., Kato, K., Nishida, M., Mio, K., Numaga, T., Sawaguchi, Y., Yoshida, T., Wakamori, M., Mori, E., Numata, T., Ishii, M., Takemoto, H., Ojida, A., Watanabe, K., Uemura, A., Kurose, H., Morii, T., Kobayashi, T., Sato, Y., Sato, C., Hamachi, I., & Mori, Y. (2009) Selective and direct inhibition of TRPC3 channels underlies biological activities of a pyrazole compound, *Proc Natl Acad Sci USA* 106, 5400-5405.

[43] Lorenz, K., Schmitt, J.P., Schmitteckert, E.M., Lohse, M.J. (2009) A new type of ERK1/2 autophosphorylation causes cardiac hypertrophy. *Nat Med* 15, 75-83.

[44] Nishida, M., Tanabe, S., Maruyama, Y., Mangmool, S., Urayama, K., Nagamatsu, Y., Takagahara, S., Turner, J.H., Kozasa, T., Kobayashi, H., Sato, Y., Kawanishi, T., Inoue, R., Nagao, T., & Kurose, H. (2005) $G\alpha_{12/13}$-and reactive oxygen species-dependent activation of c-Jun NH_2-terminal kinase and p38 MAPK by angiotensin receptor stimulation in rat neonatal cardiomyocytes. *J Biol Chem* 280, 18434-18441.

[45] Fujii, T., Onohara, N., Maruyama, Y., Tanabe, S., Kobayashi, H., Fukutomi, M., Nagamatsu, Y., Nishihara, N., Inoue, R., Sumimoto, H., Shibasaki, F., Nagao, T., Nishida, M., & Kurose, H. (2005) $G\alpha_{12/13}$-mediated production of reactive oxygen species is critical for angiotensin receptor-induced NFAT activation in cardiac fibroblasts. *J Biol Chem* 280, 23041-23047.

[46] Saitoh, M., Nishitoh, H., Fujii, M., Takeda, K., Tobiume, K., Sawada, Y., Kawabata, M., Miyazono, K., & Ichijo, H. (1998) Mammalian thioredoxin is a direct inhibitor of apoptosis signal-regulating kinase (ASK) 1. *EMBO J* 17, 2596-2606.

[47] Rajagopalan, S., Kurz, S., Munzel, T., Tarpey, M., Freeman, B.A., Griendling, K.K., & Harrison, D.G. (1996) Angiotensin II-mediated hypertension in the rat increases vascular superoxide production via membrane NADH/NADPH oxidase activation. Contribution to alterations of vasomotor tone. *J Clin Invest* 97, 1916-1923.

[48] Ushio-Fukai, M., Alexander, R.W., Akers, M., & Griendling, K.K. (1998) p38 Mitogen-activated protein kinase is a critical component of the redox-sensitive signaling pathways activated by angiotensin II. *J Biol Chem* 273, 15022-15029.

[49] Looi, Y.H., Grieve, D.J., Siva, A., Walker, S.J., Anilkumar, N., Cave, A.C., Marber, M., Monaghan, M.J., & Shah, A.M. (2008) Involvement of Nox2 NADPH oxidase in adverse cardiac remodeling after myocardial infarction. *Hypertension* 51, 319-325.

[50] Kuroda, J., Ago, T., Matsushima, S., Zhai, P., Schneider, M.D., & Sadoshima, J. (2010) NADPH oxidase 4 (Nox4) is a major source of oxidative stress in the failing heart. *Proc Natl Acad Sci USA* 107, 15565-15570.

[51] Loot, A.E., Schreiber, J.G., Fisslthaler, B., & Fleming, I. (2009) Angiotensin II impairs endothelial function via tyrosine phosphorylation of the endothelial nitric oxide synthase. *J Exp Med* 206, 2889-2896.

[52] Sumimoto, H. (2008) Structure, regulation and evolution of Nox-family NADPH oxidases that produce reactive oxygen species. *FEBS J* 275, 3249-3277.

[53] Brown, G.E., Stewart, M.Q., Liu, H., Ha, V-L., & Yaffe, M.B. (2003) A novel assay system implicates PtdIns(3,4)P_2, PtdIns(3)P, and PKCδ in intracellular production of reactive oxygen species by the NADPH oxidase. *Mol Cell* 11, 35-47.

[54] Kitajima, N., Watanabe, K., Morimoto, S., Sato, Y., Kiyonaka, S., Hoshijima, M., Ikeda, Y., Nakaya, M., Ide, T., Mori, Y., Kurose, H., & Nishida, M. (2011) TRPC3-mediated Ca^{2+} influx contributes to Rac1-mediated production of reactive oxygen species in MLP-deficient mouse hearts. *Biochem Biophys Res Commun* 409, 108-113.

[55] Nishida, M., Hara, Y., Yoshida, T., Inoue, R., & Mori, Y. (2006) TRP channels: Molecular diversity and physiological function. *Microcirculation* 13, 535-550.

[56] Numaga, T., Nishida, M., Kiyonaka, S., Kato, K., Katano, M., Mori, E., Kurosaki, T., Inoue, R., Hikida, M., Putney, J.W.Jr., & Mori, Y. (2010) Ca^{2+} influx and protein scaffolding via TRPC3 sustain PKCβ and ERK activation in B cells. *J Cell Sci* 123, 927-938.

[57] Price, L.S., Langeslag, M., ten Klooster, J.P., Hordijk, P.L., Jalink, K., & Collard, J.G. (2003) Calcium signaling regulates translocation and activation of Rac. *J Biol Chem* 278, 39413-39421.

[58] Zou, Y., Akazawa, H., Qin, Y., Sano, M., Takano, H., Minamino, T., Makita, N., Iwanaga, K., Zhu, W., Kudoh, S., Toko, H., Tamura, K., Kihara, M., Nagai, T., Fukamizu, A., Umemura, S., Iiri, T., Fujita, T., komuro, I. (2004) Mechanical stress activates angiotensin II type 1 receptor without the involvement of angiotensin II. *Nat Cell Biol* 6, 499-506.

[59] Mederos y Schnitzler, M., Storch, U., Meibers, S., Nurwakagari, P., Breit, A., Essin, K., Gollasch, M., & Gudermann, T. (2008) G_q-coupled receptors as mechanosensors mediating myogenic vasoconstriction. *EMBO J* 27, 3092-3103.

[60] Yasuda, N., Miura, S., Akazawa, H., Tanaka, T., Qin, Y., Kiya, Y., Imaizumi, S., Fujino, M., Ito, K., Zou, Y., Fukuhara, S., Kunimoto, S., Fukuzaki, K., Sato, T., Ge, J., Mochizuki, N., Nakaya, H., Saku, K., & Komuro, I. (2008) Conformational switch of angiotensin II type 1 receptor underlying mechanical stress-induced activation. *EMBO Rep*. 9, 179-186.

[61] Domazet, I., Holleran, B.J., Martin, S.S., Lavigne, P., Leduc, R., Escher, E., & Guillemette, G. (2009) The second transmembrane domain of the human type 1 angiotensin II receptor participates in the formation of the ligand binding pocket and undergoes integral pivoting movement during the process of receptor activation. *J Biol Chem* 284, 11922-11929.

[62] Domazet, I., Martin, S.S., Holleran, B.J., Morin, M-È., Lacasse, P., Lavigne, P., Escher, E., Leduc, R., & Guillemette, G. (2009) The fifth transmembrane domain of angiotensin II type 1 receptor participates in the formation of the ligand-binding pocket and undergoes a counterclockwise rotation upon receptor activation. *J Biol Chem* 284, 31953-31961.

[63] Ohyama, K., Yamano, Y., Sano, T., Nakagomi, Y., Hamakubo, T., Morishima, I., Inagami, T. (1995) Disulfide bridges in extracellular domains of Angiotensin II receptor type IA. *Regul Pept* 57, 141-147.

[64] Zhang, J., Villacorta, L., Chang, L., Fan, Z., Hamblin, M., Zhu, T., Chen, C.S., Cole, M.P, Schopfer, F.J., Deng, C.X., Garcia-Barrio, M.T., Feng, Y-H., Freeman, B.A.,

Chen, Y.E. (2010) Nitro-oleic acid inhibits angiotensin II-induced hypertension. *Circ Res* 107, 540-548.

[65] Nishida, M., Suda, R., Nagamatsu, Y., Tanabe, S., Onohara, N., Nakaya, M., Kanaho, Y., Shibata, T., Uchida, K., Sumimoto, H., Sato, Y., & Kurose, H. (2010) Pertussis toxin upregulates angiotensin type1 receptors through TLR4-mediated Rac activation. *J Biol Chem* 285, 15268-15277.

[66] Lao, Y., & Chang, D.C. (2008) Mobilization of Ca^{2+} from endoplasmic reticulum to mitochondria plays a positive role in the early stage of UV- or TNFalpha-induced apoptosis. *Biochem Biophys Res Commun* 373, 42-47.

[67] Tsuchiya, Y., Asano, T., Nakayama, K., Kato Jr.T., Karin, M., & Kamata, H. (2010) Nuclear IKKβ is an adaptor protein for IκBα ubiquitination and degradation in UV-induced NF-κB activation. *Mol Cell* 39, 570-582.

[68] Bae, Y.S., Lee, J.H., Choi, S.H., Kim, S., Almazan, F., Witztum, J.L., Miller, Y.I. (2009) Macrophages generate reactive oxygen species in response to minimally oxidized low-density lipoprotein: toll-like receptor 4- and spleen tyrosine kinase-dependent activation of NADPH oxidase 2. *Circ Res* 104, 210-218.

[69] Nishida, M., Ogushi, M., Suda, R., Toyotaka, M., Saiki, S., Kitajima, N., Nakaya, M., Kim, K-M., Ide, T., Sato, Y., Inoue, K., & Kurose, H. (2011) Heterologous down-regulation of angiotensin type 1 receptors by purinergic $P2Y_2$ receptor stimulation through S-nitrosylation of NF-κB. *Proc Natl Acad Sci USA* 108, 6662-6667.

[70] Kaiser, R.A., Oxhorn, B.C., Andrews, G., & Buxton, I.L.O. (2002) Functional compartmentation of endothelial P2Y receptor signaling. *Circ Res* 91, 292-299.

[71] Chuang, T.T., lacovelli, L., Sallese, M., & De Blasi, A. (1996) G protein-coupled receptors: heterologous regulation of homologous desensitization and its implications. *Trends Pharmacol Sci* 17, 416-421.

[72] Stamler, J.S., Toone, E.J., Lipton, S.A., & Sucher, N.J. (1997) (S)NO signals: translocation, regulation, and a consensus motif. *Neuron* 18, 691-696.

[73] Kelleher, Z.T., Matsumoto, A., Stamler, J.S., & Marshall, H.E. (2007) NOS2 regulation of NF-κB by S-nitrosylation of p65. *J Biol Chem* 282, 30667-30672.

[74] Marshall, H.E., & Stamler, J.S. (2001) Inhibition of NF-κB by S-nitrosylation. *Biochemistry* 40, 1688-1693.

[75] Gao, H., Sun, Y., Wu, Y., Luan, B., Wang, Y., Qu, B., & Pei, G. (2004) Identification of β-arrestin2 as a G protein-coupled receptor-stimulated regulator of NF-κB pathways. *Mol Cell* 14, 303-317.

[76] Witherow, D.S., Garrison, T.R., Miller, W.E., & Lefkowitz, R.J. (2004) β-arrestin inhibits NF-κB activity by means of its interaction with the NF-κB inhibitor IκBα. *Proc Natl Acad Sci USA* 101, 8603-8607.

[77] Kuhr, F.K., Zhang, Y., Brovkovych, V., & Skidgel, R.A. (2010) β-arrestin2 is required for B1 receptor-dependent post-translational activation of inducible nitric oxide synthase. *FASEB J* 24, 2475-2483.

[78] Crowley, S.D., Gurley, S.B., Herrera, M.J., Ruiz, P., Griffiths, R., Kumar, A.P., Kim, H-S., Smithies, O., Le, T.H., & Coffman, T.M. (2006) Angiotensin II causes hypertension and cardiac hypertrophy through its receptors in the kidney. *Proc Natl Acad Sci USA* 103, 17985-17990.

[79] Harada, K., Komuro, I., Shiojima, I., Hayashi, D., Kudoh, S., Mizuno, T., Kijima, K., Matsubara, H., Sugaya, T., Murakami, K., & Yazaki, Y. (1998) Pressure overload induced cardiac hypertrophy in angiotensin II type 1A receptor knockout mice. *Circulation* 97, 1952-1959.

[80] Ainscough, J.F.X., Drinkhill, M.J., Sedo, A., Turner, N.A., Brooke, D.A., Balmforth, A.J., & Ball, S.G. (2009) Angiotensin II type-1 receptor activation in the adult heart causes blood pressure-independent hypertrophy and cardiac dysfunction. *Cardiovas Res* 81, 592-600.

In: Angiotensin: New Research
Editors: S. Harada, I. Moi, pp. 181-193
ISBN: 978-1-62100-773-9

Chapter 8

CROSS TALK BETWEEN ANGIOTENSIN II AND PPAR-γ DURING CARDIAC REMODELING

***Laxmansa C. Katwa**[*,1] **and Cooduvalli S. Shashikant**[2]*

[1] Department of Physiology, Brody School of Medicine at East Carolina University, Greenville, North Carolina 27858, U.S.A.

[2] Department of Dairy and Animal Science, College of Agricultural Sciences, The Pennsylvania State University, University Park, PA 16802, U.S.A.

ABSTRACT

Cardiac remodeling is characterized by excessive production of extracellular matrix (ECM) proteins by specialized cells referred to as cardiac myofibroblasts. Cardiac myofibroblasts function both as autocrine and paracrine cell types secreting pro-fibrotic factors, which accelerates production of ECM proteins. Among these pro-fibrotic factors, Angiotensin II (Ang II) plays a predominant role by influencing multiple pathways that promote ECM production and adverse remodeling. Agents that block Ang II and its receptors reduce ECM synthesis and improve cardiac function.

These effects are similar to those obtained by peroxisome proliferators activated receptor–γ (PPAR-γ) agonists. Both Ang II receptor inhibitors and PPAR-γ agonists appear to have similar beneficial effects on cardiovascular diseases, diabetes and metabolic syndromes.

These similar effects suggest cross-regulatory interactions between Ang II and PPAR-γ pathways. The significance of these interactions regulating cardiac remodeling is discussed in this chapter.

[*] Address for correspondence: Dr. Laxmansa C. Katwa, PhD, Associate Professor, Department of Physiology, Mail Stop 634, The Brody School of Medicine, East Carolina University, 600 Moye Blvd., Greenville, NC 27834. Tel: 252-744-1906, Email : KatwaL@ecu.edu

INTRODUCTION

Cardiac remodeling generally refers to alterations in the structure and architecture of left ventricular heart under pathological conditions [1]. The process is maladaptive as in the case of hypertension, myocardial infarction (MI) and heart failure, which subsequently leads to death. At cellular level, cardiac remodeling is characterized by hypertrophy of cardiac myocytes, and excessive production of extracellular matrix proteins (ECM) by cardiac fibroblasts and myofibroblasts. Historically, the role of cardiac myocytes, the muscular compartment of the heart, has been extensively studied both *in vitro* and in animal models. In contrast, the role of cardiac fibroblasts, major non-muscular compartment of the heart, has been appreciated only in recent years [2-5]. Cardiac fibroblasts account for two thirds of the cells in the heart. Until recently, they were considered quiescent, monotonous and uniform cells, but considerable heterogeneity in fibroblast population is now being recognized. Cardiac fibroblasts secrete cytokines, growth factors and ECM proteins. They are mainly responsible for ECM homeostasis, maintenance of structural integrity and physiological environment in which cardiac myocytes function. They provide a mechanical scaffold for cardiomyocytes and coordinate the pump function of the heart. In pathological conditions, cardiac fibroblasts play an important role in regulating cardiac function. In response to injury, cardiac fibroblasts differentiate into a myofibroblast phenotype. Cardiac myofibroblasts acquire smooth muscle cell markers such as smooth muscle actin-α and become contractile [6-8]. They act as both paracrine and autocrine cells, producing growth factors, cytokines, pro-inflammatory and pro-remodeling factors. Cardiac myofibroblasts are proliferative, invasive and possess contractile and motile properties, allowing them to migrate to the site of injury and repair tissue damage. Under normal circumstances, cardiac myofibroblasts undergo apoptosis and disappear from the normal functioning heart. However, under pathological conditions due to continued stress on the heart, they fail to undergo apoptosis, producing excessive collagens and other ECM proteins [3, 5]. Thus, remodeling becomes excessive, maladaptive and causes considerable alterations in the structure and physiology of heart. These changes profoundly influence the function of cardiac myocytes, leading to heart failure and death. Consistent with the central role cardiac fibroblasts play in cardiac remodeling, several classes of drugs, which exert profound effects on cardiac fibroblasts are currently prescribed for treatment of cardiovascular diseases [3]. These include drugs that target Angiotensin II (Ang II) and peroxisome proliferator-activated receptor-γ (PPAR-γ), among others. Our understanding of various biochemical pathways affected by these drug targets largely comes from studies carried out with *in vitro* cultured cardiac fibroblasts and myofibroblasts. In this chapter, we will summarize recent findings on cross-regulatory interactions between Ang II and PPAR-γ pathways in cardiac fibroblasts and myofibroblasts.

ANGIOTENSIN-II (ANG II)

Ang II is the main mediator of the renin-angiotensin-aldosterone system (RAAS) [9, 10]. Ang II is first produced as biologically inactive Angiotensinogen (Ao), which is converted to Ang I by the action of aspertyl or serine proteases. Angiotensin converting enzyme (ACE), a membrane bound ectoenzyme, cleaves Ang I to biologically active Ang II peptide ([11-13]. A second enzyme, ACE2, further cleaves Ang II to a heptapeptide referred to as Ang-(1-7). Ang-(1-7) may antagonize effects of Ang II on cardiac remodeling and thus play a regulatory role. The effect of Ang II and Ang-(1-7) peptides are mediated through specific G-protein coupled receptors (GPCR). Ang II acts through Angiotensin II type 1 (AT1) and type 2 (AT2) receptors; whereas, Ang-(1-7) acts through another GPCR receptor, referred to as Mas, but its biological effects are unclear [14, 15]. Although Ang II, Ang-(1-7) and their receptors have been detected in fibroblasts at the site of fibrosis, most of the effects of RAAS system are mediated by Ang II through the AT1 receptor mediated signaling pathways.

Local RAAS systems are integral to the orderly and sequential nature of the repair process occurring in response to tissue injury [16]. Several lines of evidence suggest a central role for Ang II in the initiation and progression of cardiac remodeling [10, 17]. *De novo* production of Ang II significantly influences the post-infarction remodeling of the heart [9]. Drugs that inhibit RAAS activation have beneficial effects on the remodeling heart [18-19]. Clinical studies have shown that ACE inhibitors and angiotensin II type 1 receptor blockers (ARB's) reduce mortality and morbidity in patients with post-MI dysfunction and heart failure [6-8, 18, 20]. Ang II appears to have multiple, direct cytotoxic effects on myocytes including apoptosis, promoting cell hypertrophy and stimulating myocardial fibrosis [21].

Many of the effects of Ang II on cardiac remodeling are mediated through cardiac fibroblasts and myofibroblasts. Although activated macrophages and endothelial cells also produce Ang II and contribute to the initial process of remodeling, cardiac fibroblasts remain a major target cell type for Ang II mediated biological actions associated with cardiac remodeling [10, 17]. Consistent with this view, the distribution of AT1 receptors is predominant among cardiac fibroblasts compared to other cell types, including cardiomyocytes. The levels of cardiac fibroblast Ang II and AT1 receptors are elevated in post-MI hearts. Myofibroblasts remain the major cells expressing ACE and AT1 receptors in the fibrogenic stage of cardiac repair following MI [22, 23]. Both Ang II and AT1 receptor are expressed in cardiac myofibroblasts isolated from the site of MI [24, 25]. Myofibroblasts associated with the healing of infarct scars show increased production of Ang II and AT1 receptor [24, 26-29]. The levels of ACE are also elevated at the site of MI, co-localized with the myofibroblast population [11, 23, 30, 31].

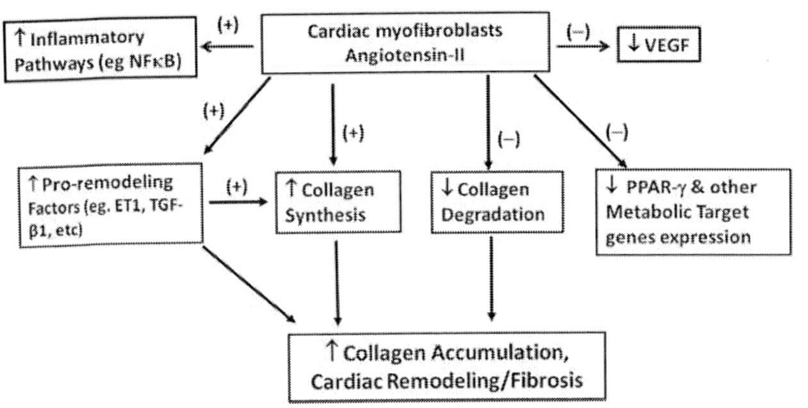

Figure 1. Effect of Ang II on various pathways operative in cardiac myofibroblasts.

Ang II influences multiple biochemical pathways in cardiac fibroblasts and myofibroblasts during remodeling (Figure 1). Ang II induces proliferation of myofibroblasts, which in turn participate in collagen synthesis [25, 32-35]. In a rat model of MI, Ang II induced hypertrophy of myofibroblasts at the infarct site. In sham operated control and non-infarct myofibroblasts, mitogenic activity of Ang II treatment was also detected [36]. There are several discrepancies in regards to the proliferative effects of Ang II, but a general consensus is that perhaps some of these effects are secondary due to the induced secretion of other growth factors, including TGF-β1, FGF2 and platelet derived growth factor-AA [10, 37-38].

Ang II induces differentiation of both neonatal and adult cardiac fibroblasts into myofibroblasts by activating TGF-β1 [28, 39-41]. Treatment of cardiac myofibroblasts *in vitro* with Ang II results in rapid accumulation of TGF-β1 mRNA and protein [28, 42-45]. Chronic administration of Ang II induces cardiac expression of TGF-β1 *in vivo* [46-48]. In contrast, blockade of AT1 receptor by antagonists reverses cardiac TGF-β1 expression, cardiac hypertrophy and fibrosis [48-51]. Ang II fails to induce cardiac hypertrophy and fibrosis in mice lacking in functional TGF-β1 [52]. Most of the effects of Ang II on cardiac function are likely mediated through TGF-β1 signaling [41]. Treatment of cardiac fibroblasts with anti-TGF-β1 antibodies reduces Ang II induced collagen I levels [52]. The mechanism by which Ang II induces TGF-β1 expression in cardiac myofibroblasts is not completely understood. However, studies in cardiomyocytes of hypetrtophied left ventricle indicate that Ang II regulates TGF-β1 expression at the level of transcription through nuclear activating protein 1(AP1) binding activity [48]. Ang II mediates its effect through AT1 receptor, which in turn activates NAD(P)H oxidase, protein kinase C (PKC), p38 MAP kinase and finally AP1 protein [41, 53]. Besides inducing TGF-β1, Ang II also induces secretion of other bioactive molecules such as endothelin-1, ET-1 [15, 40, 54, 55], leukemia inhibitory factor, LIF [15], osteopontin [56] vascular endothelial growth factor, VEGF [57], natriuretic peptides [53, 57, 58], and interleukin-6 [60].

Ang II promotes differentiation and proliferation of cardiac fibroblasts. It accelerates pro-fibrotic responses as indicated by increased production of ECM proteins. Ang II treatment increases synthesis of collagens I and II, fibronectin and integrin [15, 36, 42, 61-66]. Ang II is known to increase the synthesis of tissue inhibitor of metalloproteinase (TIMP) and reduce metalloproteinase (MMP) synthesis thereby inhibiting degradation of ECM proteins (65, 66, 67-69]. Many of these effects are probably indirect and mediated by induction of other pro-remodeling factors, such as ET1 and TGF-β1.

Ang II, also a potent pro-inflammatory agent, influences all stages of the inflammatory response. Through interaction with its AT1 receptor, Ang II activates NADPH oxidase and production of reactive oxygen species. This leads to activation of Ets-1, early growth response 1 and nuclear factor-κB(NF-κB). Some of the inflammatory responses by Ang II are mediated by the caspase-recruitment domain-9 (CARD-9) protein [70]. Ang II induces known mediators of inflammatory responses such as interferon-γ, INF-γ, and tumor necrosis factor-α, TNF-α [71].

In summary, cardiac myofibroblasts elaborate Ang II mediated multiple signaling pathways at the site of MI. These Ang II induced pathways result in pro-inflammatory and pro-fibrotic effects leading to increased synthesis and accumulation of collagen, a hallmark of fibrosis in MI and resulting heart failure.

PPAR-γ

In recent years, emerging evidence from different experimental systems suggest interactions between a xenobiotic activated transcription factor, peroxisome proliferators-activated receptor, PPAR-γ and various molecules that contribute to the remodeling process. Developing tools and reagents to manipulate PPAR-γ activity may represent a new paradigm in our understanding of cardiac remodeling. PPARs are implicated in the regulation of pathways that interface between intermediate metabolism and inflammation [72]. PPAR-γ plays a critical role in adipocyte differentiation, cellular energy homeostasis, insulin signaling, obesity and inflammation [72-75]. PPAR-γ agonists, such as thiazolidinediones (TZDs) that sensitize cells to insulin are used for their antidiabetic effects in liver, adipose tissue and skeletal muscle [73].

Diabetic patients treated with PPAR-γ agonists also show lower risks for CVD, demonstrating a potential beneficial role for PPAR-γ in modulating cardiac function. Consistent with this hypothesis, treatment with PPAR-γ agonists results in reduced infarct size [76-77], decreased inflammation [74,75], improved vasodialation [76] and decreased left ventricular hypertrophy [78,79]. Thus, PPAR-γ agonists are likely to promote several cellular responses relevant to tissue repair and remodeling.

PPAR-γ agonists could modulate several aspects of cardiac remodeling by affecting the activities of key players, especially in cardiac myofibroblasts (Figure 2). PPAR-γ agonist's show marked influences on collagen synthesis at several levels. When cultured myofibroblasts are treated with rosiglitazone, a decrease in collagen expression is observed [80]. The molecular mechanism, by which collagen synthesis in cardiac myofibroblasts is reduced, is yet to be elucidated.

The effect of PPAR-γ□ on collagen synthesis could be mediated by decreasing the activities of pro-fibrotic factors including Ang II, ET1, and TGF-β1. When cultured cardiac fibroblasts and myofibroblasts are treated with PPAR-γ agonists such as rosiglitazone or pioglitazone, there is a decrease in both AT1 receptor and the type I collagen expression [80, 81-83]. Rosiglitazone has been shown to significantly attenuate Ang II induced proliferation of cardiac fibroblasts [83]. Ang II and AT1 receptor induce oxidative stress in mouse cardiac fibroblasts. The inhibitory effect of pioglitazone on collagen synthesis is perhaps due to its anti-oxidant effect [82]. In vascular smooth muscle cells, PPAR-γ has been shown to suppress AT1 receptor gene transcription by the inhibition of the Sp1 binding to GC-box related element in the AT1 receptor cis-regulatory/promoter region [84]. Whether a similar mechanism is operative in cardiac myofibroblasts remains to be determined.

Rosiglitazone reduces ET1 expression and collagen synthesis in cultured cardiac myofibroblasts derived from the site of MI (Katwa unpublished observations). The mechanism by which PPAR-γ inhibits ET1 activity in cardiac myofibroblasts remains to be studied. However, in cardiac myocytes, both PPAR-γ overexpression and treatment with rosiglitazone have been shown to inhibit ET1 induced cardiac hypertrophy [85].

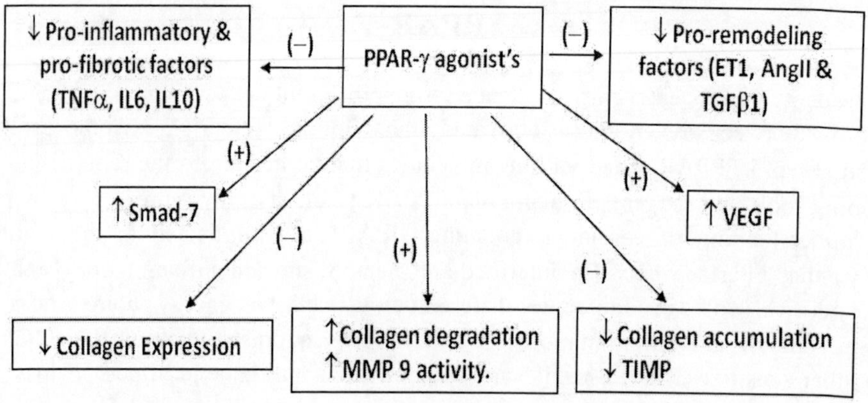

Figure 2. Effect of PPAR-γ agonists on cardiac collagen turn over, pro-angiogenic and pro-fibrotic factors.

Interaction between PPAR-γ and calcineurin/ nuclear factor of activated T cells (NFAT) has been implicated in the inhibition of ET1 activity. PPAR-γ has also been suggested to mediate conjugated linoleic acid mediated inhibition of ET1 activity in reducing cardiac hypertrophy [86]. Treatment of cardiac myofibroblasts with rosiglitazone also results in a decrease in TGF-β1 levels (Katwa, unpublished observations). The effect of rosiglitazone on TGF-β1, however, may not be direct but mediated through its effect on Ang II [6, 80, 83]. The effect of TGF-□β1 on collagen synthesis is mediated through the canonical Smad pathway [87]. Smads interact with transcriptional coactivator and histone acetyltransferase, p300, in the regulation of transcriptional activity of collagen promoter [88, 89]. PAPR-γ abrogates Smad-dependent pathways linked to stimulation of collagen synthesis by preventing p300 recruitment and histone H4 hyperacetylation in dermal fibroblasts [88]. In hepatic stellate cells, PPAR-γ inhibits p300 facilitated NF-1 binding to response elements present in the collagen promoter [90]. Although p300 is known to play a role in inflammation as well as cardiac hypertrophy, its role in the regulation of collagen synthesis in cardiac myofibroblasts is yet to be described. PPAR-γ is known to antagonize TGF-□β1 stimulated type 1 collagen synthesis in other fibroblast systems by antagonizing the effects of interferon-γ (IFN-γ, 91). PPAR-γ could also increase activities of matrix metalloproteinases, which promote collagen degradation. PPAR-γ agonists appear to cause a decrease in the levels of MMPs in various experimental systems [81, 92, 93].A similar decrease in the levels of MMPs and TIMPs was observed in cardiac myofibroblasts isolated from site of MI treated with rosiglitazone (Katwa, unpublished observation).

Interactions or Crosstalk between Ang II and PPAR Systems

Both Ang II and PPAR systems are implicated in metabolic syndrome and heart diseases, where they seem to have opposing effects. Increased frequency of left ventricular dysfunction and structural abnormalities are often observed in patients with metabolic syndrome [94-96]. In contrast, animal models of metabolic syndrome often show cardiac fibrosis [94, 97, 98].

Clinical strategies for treating both metabolic syndromes and cardiac failures often employ ACE inhibitors, ARB and PPAR agonists. Although molecular mechanisms that link fibrosis and metabolic syndrome are yet to be elucidated, several studies suggest a link between Ang II and PPAR systems [70, 80, 94, 99, 100]. Ang II and PPAR-γ mediated pathways intersect and modulate each other's activities in regulating cardiac collagen expression (Figure 3).

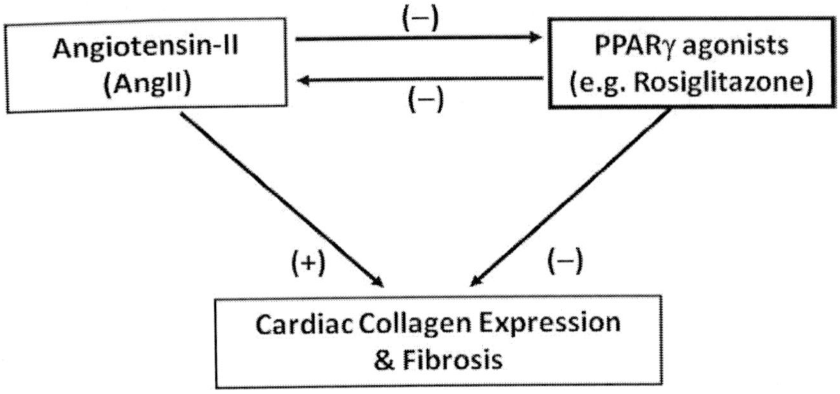

Figure 3. Cross talk between Ang II and PPAR-γ in post-MI remodeling and cardiac collagen expression.

In cardiac myofibroblasts, treatment with Ang II leads to decrease in PPAR- γ expression and activity, whereas treatment with ARB (losartan) leads to increase in PPAR- γ expression and activity (Figure 4).

In contrast, treatment with PPAR-γ agonist's leads to a decrease in AT1 receptor expression and activities in cardiac myofibroblasts isolated from the site of MI [80]. By mechanisms yet to be elucidated, these interactions affect collagen expression in cardiac myofibroblasts either directly or indirectly. Pro-inflammatory and pro-fibrotic factors could mediate some of the effects of Ang II and PPAR systems. Ang II decreases PPAR-γ expression with a concomitant increase in the expression of pro-inflammatory and pro-fibrotic agents in diabetics with MI and cardiac myofibroblasts [5, 6, 101, 102].

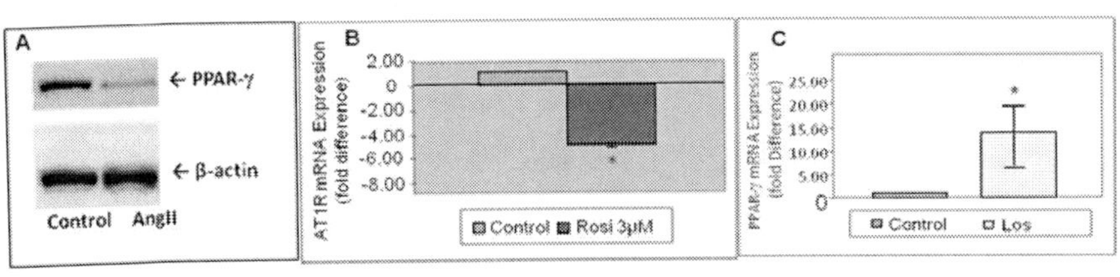

Figure 4. Cross talk between Ang II and PPAR-γ in cardiac myofibroblasts. Myofibroblasts (passage 4, 90% confluent) were treated in serum free DMEM medium with; (A) Ang II (10^{-7}M) for 24 hours and isolated protein (30μg/well) was analyzed by western blot resulted in the down regulation of PPAR-γ expression. Panel B &C are real-time PCR data of myofibroblasts treated with PPAR-γ agonist Rosiglitazone (3 μM). (B) demonstrates down regulation of AT1 receptor expression by PPAR-γ agonists and (C) results show effects of ARB (Los=Losartan) on myofibroblasts PPAR-γ expression (*p> 0.05).

In contrast, PPAR-γ agonists appear to decrease expression of pro-inflammatory and pro-fibrotic agents, including Ang II in cardiac myofibroblasts, and in diabetic heart tissue with MI [80,103, Katwa et al., unpublished data].

Combination of drugs such as PPAR-γ agonists and ARBs have shown beneficial effects in diabetes and cardiovascular diseases by decreasing infarct size and increasing metabolic activities of the cardiac tissue [104, 101,102]. Cardiac myofibroblasts treated with both PPAR-γ agonists and ARBs demonstrated significant decrease in not only collagen expression but also decreased levels of pro-inflammatory and pro-fibrotic agents. Our recent experimental findings on the effects of combination treatment with ARB (e.g. Lasortan) and PPAR-γ agonists (e.g. Rosiglitazone or Pioglitazone) demonstrated an increased PPAR-γ expression and decreased AT1 receptor expression and activity, as well as a significant reduction in collagen expression in cultured rat cardiac myofibroblasts isolated from the site of MI [80].

PPAR-γ agonists have recently been used to treat patients with diabetes and MI. These studies have revealed increased cardiovascular risks and mortality [95, 97, 98, 105]. The clinical relevance of combination therapy of ARBs and PPAR-γ agonists has yet to be determined. Since last decade, the experimental evidence from animal and clinical studies suggest that some of the drugs that interrupt the Ang II system may improve glucose and lipid metabolism and decrease the risk for type 2 diabetes [101,102, 104, 106, 107]. Some of the anti-diabetic properties of ARBs may be mediated by their ability to block adverse effects of Ang II on carbohydrate and lipid metabolism. The beneficial metabolic effects of certain ARBs may go well beyond just simple interruption of the Ang II action, as ARBs have been found to effectively activate PPAR-γ, a well-known target for insulin-sensitizing, antidiabetic drugs [102, 104]. Thus, the identification of ARBs selective PPAR-γ modulating ability suggests new opportunities for developing third-generation ARBs and PPAR-γ activators with enhanced potential for treating hypertension, diabetes and the metabolic syndrome.

ACKNOWLEDGMENTS

The authors wish to thank Paul Ferrell and Pranita Katwa for reading the manuscript. This work was supported in part by the National Institutes of Health grant (HL-60047) and East Carolina University Faculty Research Development grant awarded to LCK. CSS is supported by The Pennsylvania State University Experiment Station grant AES 4377.

REFERENCES

[1] Swynghedauw B., 1999, *Physiol. Rev.* 79, 215-262.
[2] Brown, R.D., Ambler, S.K., Mitchell, M.D., and Long, C.S. 2005, *Annu. Rev. Pharmacol. Toxicol.,* 45, 657-687.
[3] Porter, K.E., and Turner, N.A., 2009, *Pharmacol. Ther.,* 123, 255-278.
[4] Baum, J., and Duffy, H.S., 2011. *J. Cardiovasc. Pharmacol.* 57, 376-379.

[5] Katwa, L.C., and Shashikant, C.S. 2011, Cardiac remodeling and fibrosis: Role of myofibroblasts. In: N.A. Turner (ed), *The Cardiac Fibroblasts,* 29-52, Research Signpost. ISBN: 978-81-308-0435-4.
[6] Campbell, S.E., and Katwa L.C. 1997, *J. Mol. Cell. Cardiol.,* 29, 1947-1958.
[7] Chintalgattu, V., Harris, G.S., Akula, S.M., and Katwa, L.C. 2007, *Cardiovasc. Res.,* 74, 140-150.
[8] Petrov, V.V., Fagard, R.H., and Lijnen, P.J. 2002, *Hypertension,* 39, 258-263.
[9] Weber, K.T., Sun, Y., and Katwa, L.C. 1997, *Int. J. Biochem. Cell Biol.,* 29, 31-42.
[10] Cowling, R.T. and Greenberg, B. 2011. Angiotensin receptors and response to angiotensin peptides in cardiac fibroblasts. In: N.A. Turner (ed), The Cardiac Fibroblasts,173-195, *Research Signpost. ISBN:* 978-81-308-0435-4.
[11] Katwa, L.C., Ratajska, A., Cleutjens, J.P., Sun, Y., Zhou, G., Lee, S.J., Weber, K.T. 1995, *Cardiovasc. Res.,* 29, 57-64.
[12] Katwa, L.C., Tyagi, S.C., Campbell, S.E., Lee, S.J., Cicila, G.T., Weber, K.T. 1996, *Int. J. Biochem. Cell Biol.,* 28, 807-821.
[13] Katwa, L.C., Sun, Y., Campbell, S.E., Tyagi, S.C., Dhalla, A.K., Kandala, J.C., Weber, K.T. 1998, *J. Mol. Cell. Cardiol.,* 30, 1401-1413.
[14] Santos, R.A.S., Silva, A.C.S.E., Maric, C., Silva, D.M.R., Machado, R.P., de Buhr, I., Heringer-Walther, S., Pinheiro, S.V.B., Lopes, M.T., Bader, M., Randy T. Cowling and Barry Greenberg Mendes, E.P., Lemos, V.S., Campagnole-Santos, M.J., Schultheiss, H.P., Speth, R., and Walther, T. 2003, *Proc. Natl. Acad. Sci. U S A,* 100, 8258-8263.
[15] Iwata, M., Cowling, R.T., Gurantz, D., Moore, C., Zhang, S., Yuan, J.X., and Greenberg, B.H. 2005, *Am. J. Physiol Heart Circ. Physiol,* 289, H2356-H2363.
[16] Lijnen, P.J., Petrov, V.V. 2003, *Methods Find Exp. Clin. Pharmacol.,* 25, 541–64.
[17] Sun, Y., 2010. *J. Mol. Cell Cardiol.* 2010, 48, 483–489.
[18] Pfeffer, M.A., Lamas, G.A., Vaughan, D.E., Parisi, A.F., and Braunwald, E. 1988, *N. Engl. J. Med.,* 319, 80-86.
[19] Greenberg, B., Quinones, M.A., Koilpillai, C., Limacher, M., Shindler, D., Benedict, C., and Shelton, B. 1995, *Circulation,* 91, 2573-2581.
[20] Gabbiani, G., Hirschel, B.J., Ryan, G.B., Statkov, P.R., and Majno, G. 1972, *J. Exp. Med.* 135, 719-734.
[21] Gajarsa, J.J., Kloner, R.A. 2011, *Heart Fail Rev.,* 16, 13-21.
[22] Sun, Y., and Weber, K.T. 1996, *J. Mol. Cell. Cardiol.,* 28, 851-858.
[23] Sun, Y., Weber, K.T. 1996, *Cardiovasc Res,* 31, 518–525.
[24] Katwa, L.C., Campbell, S.E., Tyagi, S.C., Lee, S.J., Cicila, G.T., Weber, K.T. 1997, J. Mol. Cell. Cardiol., 29, 1375-1386.
[25] Chintalgattu, V., and Katwa, L.C. 2009, *Biochem. Biophys. Res. Commun.,* 386, 612-616.
[26] Sun Y, and Weber K.T. 1994, *Cardiovasc. Res.,* 28, 1623-1628.
[27] Weber, K.T., Sun, Y., Katwa, L.C., Cleutjens, J.P. 1995, *J. Mol. Cell. Cardiol.,* 27,107-120.
[28] Campbell, S.E., and Katwa L.C. 1997, *J. Mol. Cell. Cardiol.,* 29, 1947-1958.
[29] Sun, Y., and Weber K.T. 2000, *Cardiovasc. Res.,* 46, 250-256.
[30] Fabris, B., Jackson, B., Kohzuki, M., Perich, R., and Johnston, C.I. 1990, *Clin. Exp. Pharmacol. Physiol.,* 17, 309-314.

[31] Sun Y, Cleutjens J.P., Diaz-Arias, A.A., and Weber, K.T. 1994, *Cardiovasc. Res.,* 28, 1423-1432.

[32] Schorb, W., Booz, G.W., Dostal, D.E., Conrad, K.M., Chang, K.C., and Baker, K.M. 1993, *Circ. Res.,* 72, 1245-1254.

[33] Weber, K.T., Brilla, C.G., Campbell, S.E., Guarda, E., Zhou, G., and Sriram, K. 1993, *Basic Res. Cardiol.,* 88 Suppl 1:107-124.

[34] Kim, S., Ohta, K., Hamaguchi, A., Yukimura, T., Miura, K., Iwao, H., 1995, *Hypertension,* 25, 1252-1259.

[35] Bouzegrhane, F., and Thibault, G. 2002, Cardiovasc. Res., 53, 304-312.

[36] Staufenberger. S., Jacobs, M., Brandstätter, K., Hafner, M., Regitz-Zagrosek, V., Ertl, G., and Schorb, W. 2001, *J. Cell. Physiol.,* 187, 326-335.

[37] Simm, A. and Diez, C. 1999, *Basic Res. Cardiol.,* 94, 464-471.

[38] Santiago, J.J., Ma, X., McNaughton, L.J., Nickel, B.E., Bestvater, B.P., Yu, L., Fandrich, R.R., Netticadan, T., Kardami, E. 2011, Cardiovasc Res., 89, 139-147.

[39] Lee, A.A., Dillmann, W.H., McCulloch, A.D., and Villarreal, F.J. 1995, *J. Mol.Cell Cardiol.,* 27, 2347-2357.

[40] Gray, M.O., Long, C.S., Kalinyak, J.E., Li, H.T., and Karliner, J.S. 1998, *Cardiovasc. Res.,* 40, 352-363.

[41] Rosenkranz, S. 2004, *Cardiovasc. Res.,* 63, 423-432.

[42] Thibault, G., Lacombe, M.J., Schnapp, L.M., Lacasse, A., Bouzeghrane, F., and Lapalme, G. 2001, *Am. J. Physiol. Cell Physiol.,* 281, C1457-C1467.

[43] Klett, C.P., Palmer, A., Dirig, D.M., Gallagher, A.M., Riosecco-Camacho, N., and Printz, M.P. 1995, *J. Hypertens.,* 13, 1421-1431.

[44] Samuel, C.S., Unemori, E.N., Mookerjee, I., Bathgate, R.A., Layfield, S.L., Mak, J., Tregear, G.W., and Du, X.J. 2004, *Endocrinology,* 145, 4125-4133.

[45] Olson, E.R., Naugle, J.E., Zhang, X., Bomser, J.A., and Meszaros, J.G. 2005, *Am. J. Physiol. Heart Circ. Physiol.,* 288, H1131-H1138.

[46] Crawford, D., Chobanian, A., and Brecher, P. 1994, *Circ. Res.,* 74, 727-739.

[47] Kim, S., Ohta, K., Hamaguchi, A., Omura, T., Yukimura, T., Miura, K., Inada, Y., Ishimura, Y., Chatani, F., and Iwao, H. 1995, *J. Pharmacol. Exp. Ther.,* 273, 509-515.

[48] Wenzel, S., Taimor, G., Piper, H.M., and Schlu,¨ter, K.D. 2001, *FASEB. J.,* 15, 2291-2293.

[49] Tomita, H., Egashira, K., Ohara, Y., Takemoto, M., Koyanagi, M., Katoh, M., Yamamoto, H., Tamaki, K., Shimokawa, H., and Takeshita, A. 1998, *Hypertension,* 32, 273-279.

[50] Tokuda, K., Kai, H., Kuwahara, F., Yasukawa, H., Tahara, N., Kudo, H., Takemiya, K., Koga, M., Yamamoto, T., and Imaizumi T. 2004, *Hypertension,* 43, 499-503.

[51] Tsutsui, H., Matsushima, S., Kinugawa, S., Ide, T., Inoue, N., Ohta, Y., Yokota, T., Hamaguchi, S., and Sunagawa, K., 2007, *Hyperten. Res.* 30, 439-449.

[52] Schultz, J.J., Witt, S.A., Glascock, B.J., Nieman, M.L., Reiser, P.J., Nix, S.L., Kimball, T.R., and Doetschman, T. 2002, *J. Clin. Invest.,* 109, 787-796.

[53] Wang, S., Wang, X., Yan, J., Xie, X., Fan, F., Zhou, X., Han, L., and Chen, J. 2007, *Eur. J. Pharmacol.,* 567, 26-35.

[54] Fujisaki, H., Ito, H., Hirata, Y., Tanaka, M., Hata, M., Lin, M., Adachi, S., Akimoto, H., Marumo, F., and Hiroe, M. 1995, *J. Clin. Invest.,* 96, 1059-1065.

[55] Chao, H.H., Chen, J.J., Chen, C.H., Lin, H., Cheng, C.F., Lian, W.S., Chen, Y.L., Juan, S.H., Liu, J.C., Liou, J.Y., Chan, P., and Cheng, T.H. 2005, *Heart,* 91, 664-669.

[56] Ashizawa, N., Graf, K., Do, Y.S., Nunohiro, T., Giachelli, C.M., Meehan, W.P., Tuan, T.L., and Hsueh, W.A. 1996, *J. Clin. Invest.,* 98, 2218-2227.

[57] Chintalgattu, V., Katwa, L.C. 2003. *J. Mol. Cell. Cardiol.,* 35, 277-286.

[58] Calderone, A., Bel-Hadj, S., Drapeau, J., El-Helou, V., Gosselin, H., Clement, R., and Villeneuve, L. 2006, J. Cell. Physiol., 207, 165-173.

[59] Makino, N., Sugano, M., Satoh, S., Oyama, J., and Maeda, T. 2006, *Cell Biochem. Biophys.,* 44, 65-71.

[60] Sano, M., Fukuda, K., Sato, T., Kawaguchi, H., Suematsu, M., Matsuda, S., Koyasu, S., Matsui, H., Yamauchi-Takihara, K., Harada, M., Saito, Y., and Ogawa, S. 2001, *Circ. Res.,* 89, 661-669.

[61] Villarreal, F.J., Kim, N.N., Ungab, G.D., Printz, M.P., and Dillmann, W.H. 1993, *Circulation,* 88, 2849-2861.

[62] Crabos, M., Roth, M., Hahn, A.W., and Erne, P. 1994, *J. Clin. Invest.,* 93, 2372-2378.

[63] Zhou, G., Kandala, J.C., Tyagi, S.C., Katwa, L.C., and Weber, K.T. 1996, *Mol. Cell Biochem.,* 154, 171-178.

[64] Hafizi, S., Wharton, J., Morgan, K., Allen, S.P., Chester, A.H., Catravas, J.D., Polak, J.M., and Yacoub, M.H. 1998, *Circulation,* 98, 2553-2559.

[65] Lijnen, P.J., Petrov, V.V., and Fagard, R.H. 2001, *J. Renin. Angiotensin. Aldosterone. Syst.,* 2, 117-122.

[66] Peng, J., Gurantz, D., Tran, V., Cowling, R.T., and Greenberg, B.H. 2002, *Circ. Res.,* 91, 1119-1126.

[67] Stewart, J.A., Jr., Cashatt, D.O., Borck, A.C., Brown, J.E., and Carver, W.E. 2006, *J. Mol. Cell. Cardiol.,* 41, 97-107.

[68] Stacy, L.B., Yu, Q., Horak, K., and Larson, D.F. 2007, Perfusion, 22, 51-55.

[69] Pan, C.H., Wen, C.H., and Lin, C.S. 2008, *Exp. Physiol.,* 93, 599-612.

[70] Ren, J., Yang, M., Qi. G., Zheng, J., Jia, L., Cheng, J., Tian, C., Li, H., Lin, X., Du, J. 2011, Am. J. Hypertens., 24, 701-707.

[71] Sukumaran, V., Watanabe, K., Veeraveedu, P.T., Gurusamy, N., Ma, M., Thandavarayan, R.A., Lakshmanan, A.P., Yamaguchi, K., Suzuki, K., Kodama, M. 2011, *Int. J. Biol. Sci.,* 7, 154-167.

[72] Bensinger, S.J., Tontonoz, P. 2008, Nature, 454(7203), 470-477.

[73] Lehmann, J.M., Moore, L.B., Smith-Oliver, T.A., Wilkison, W.O., Willson, T.M., Kliewer, S.A. 1995, *J. Biol. Chem.,* 270,12953-12956.

[74] Wayman, N.S., Ellis, B.L., and Theimermann, C., 2002, *Med. Sci. Monit.,* 8, BR243-BR247.

[75] Diep, Q.N., Amiri, F., Benkirane, K., Paradis, P., Schiffrin, E.L. 2004, Can. J. Physiol. Pharmacol., 82, 976-985.

[76] Tabernero, A., Schoonjans, K., Jesel, L., Carpusca, I., Auwerx, J., Andriantsitohaina, R. 2002, BMC Pharmacol., 2:10, 1-10.

[77] Abdelrahman, M., Sivarajah, A., Thiemermann, C. 2005, Cardiovasc. Res., 65, 772-781.

[78] Asakawa, M., Takano, H., Nagai, T., Uozumi, H., Hasegawa, H., Kubota, N., Saito, T., Masuda, Y., Kadowaki, T., Komuro, I. 2002, Circulation, 105, 1240-1246.

[79] Sakai, S., Miyauchi, T., Irukayama-Tomobe, Y., Ogata, T., Goto, K., Yamaguchi, I. 2002, Clin. Sci (Lond)., 103 Suppl 48, 16S-20S.

[80] Katwa, L.C., and Gould, A.N., 2009, *FASEB J.,* 23, 776.9 (abstract).

[81] Chen, K., Li, D., Zhang, X., Hermonat, P.L., Mehta, J.L. 2004, J. Cardiovasc. Pharmacol., 44, 682-687.

[82] Chen, J., and Mehta, J.L. 2006, *Am. J. Physiol. Heart Circ. Physiol.,* 291, H1738-H1745.

[83] Hao, G.H., Niu, X.L., Gao, D.F., Wei, J., Wang, N.P. 2008, Br. J. Pharmacol., 153, 1409-1419.

[84] Sugawara, A., Takeuchi, K., Uruno, A., Ikeda, Y., Arima, S., Sato, K., Kudo, M., Taniyama, Y., Ito, S. 2001, Hypertens. Res., 24, 229-233.

[85] Bao, Y., Li, R., Jiang, J., Cai, B., Gao, J., Le, K., Zhang, F., Chen, S., Liu, P. 2008, Mol. Cell Biochem., 317, 189-196.

[86] Alibin, C.P., Kopilas, M.A., Anderson, H.D. 2008, *J. Biol. Chem.,* 283, 10707-10715.

[87] Massagué, J., Seoane, J., Wotton, D. 2005, Genes Dev., 19, 2783-2810.

[88] Ghosh, A.K., Bhattacharyya, S., Wei, J., Kim, S., Barak, Y., Mori, Y., Varga, J. 2009, FASEB J., 23, 2968-2977.

[89] Ghosh, A.K., Wei, J., Wu, M., Varga, J. 2008, Biochem. Biophys. Res. Commun., 374, 231-236.

[90] Yavrom, S., Chen, L., Xiong, S., Wang, J., Rippe, R.A., Tsukamoto, H. 2005, *J. Biol. Chem.,* 280, 40650-40659.

[91] Xu, Y., Farmer, S.R., Smith, B.D. 2007, J. Biol. Chem., 282, 26046-26056.

[92] Henderson, B.C., Sen, U., Reynolds, C., Moshal, K.S., Ovechkin, A., Tyagi, N., Kartha, G.K., Rodriguez, W.E., Tyagi, S.C. 2007, Int. J. Biol. Sci., 3, 385-392.

[93] Cao, Z., Ye, P., Long, C., Chen, K., Li, X., Wang, H. 2007, Pharmacology, 79, 184-192.

[94] Fujita, K., Maeda, N., Sonoda, M., Ohashi, K., Hibuse, T., Nishizawa, H., Nishida, M., Hiuge, A., Kurata, A., Kihara, S., Shimomura, I., Funahashi, T. 2008, Arterioscler Thromb Vasc Biol., 28, 863-870.

[95] Jain, R., Mullins, C.D., Lee, H., Wong, W. 2011, Res Social Adm Pharm., Jul 5. [Epub ahead of print] PMID: 21733760. doi:10.1016/j.sapharm.2010.12.003 .

[96] Nishio, K., Hosaka, M., Shigemitsu, M., Kobayashi, Y. 2011, *Cardiovasc. Revasc. Med.* Apr 11. [Epub ahead of print] PubMed PMID: 21489889.

[97] Sarafidis, P.A., Georgianos, P.I., Lasaridis, A.N. 2010, *Cardiovasc. Ther.,* Sep 15. doi:10.1111/j.1755-5922.2010.00222.x. [Epub ahead of print] PubMed PMID: 20840193.

[98] Berthet, S., Olivier, P., Montastruc, J.L., Lapeyre-Mestre, M.2011, *BMC Clin. Pharmacol.,* 11, 5. PubMed PMID: 21609444.

[99] Zhang, H., Pi, R., Li, R., Wang, P., Tang, F., Zhou, S., Gao, J., Jiang, J., Chen, S., Liu, P. 2007, Arch. Biochem. Biophys., 460, 25-32.

[100] Maejima, Y., Okada, H., Haraguchi, G., Onai, Y., Kosuge, H., Suzuki, J., Isobe, M. 2011, Lab. Invest., 91, 932-944.

[101] Goyal, S., Arora, S., Bhatt, T.K., Das, P., Sharma, A., Kumari, S., Arya, D.S. 2010, *Chem. Biol. Interact.,* 185, 271-280.

[102] Goyal, S.N., Bharti, S., Bhatia, J., Nag, T.C., Ray, R., Arya, D.S. 2011, *Diabetes Obes. Metab.,* 13, 533-541.

[103] Geng, D.F., Wu, W., Jin, D.M., Wang, J.F., Wu, Y.M. 2006, *Int. J. Cardiol.,* 113, 86-91.
[104] Kunz, T.W., and Pravenec, M. 2004, *Journal of Hypertension.* 22, 2253-2261.
[105] Graham, D.J., Ouellet-Hellstrom, R., MaCurdy, T.E., Ali, F., Sholley, C., Worrall, C., Kelman, J.A. 2010, *JAMA.*, 304, 411-418.
[106] Fliegner, D., Westermann, D., Riad, A., Schubert, C., Becher, E., Fielitz, J., Tschöpe, C., Regitz Zagrosek, V. 2007, *Eur. J. Heart Fail.,* 10, 30-38.
[107] Yamagishi, S., Ueda, S., Matsui, T., Nakamura, K., Okuda, S. 2008, *Curr. Pharm. Des.,* 14, 962-968.

In: Angiotensin: New Research
Editors: S. Harada, I. Moi, pp. 195-204

ISBN: 978-1-62100-773-9

Chapter 9

CELL SWELLING ACTIVATES IONIC CHANNELS AND DECREASES THE GAP JUNCTION PERMEABILITY: IMPLICATIONS FOR METABOLIC COOPERATION BETWEEN CELLS AND FOR CARDIAC ARRHYTHMIAS

Walmor C. De Mello*
School of Medicine, Medical Sciences Campus, UPR
San Juan, PR 00936-5067, U.S.A.

ABSTRACT

The regulation of cell volume is fundamental to cell survival. Here I discuss the factors involved in the regulation of cell volume in cardiac cells of the failing heart and the influence of cell swelling on the activation of ionic channels, particularly of the swelling-activated chloride channels. Emphasis is given to the novel finding that angiotensin II causes cell swelling in cardiac cells .Finally, the role of cell swelling on gap junction permeability and its consequence for impulse propagation and generation of cardiac arrhythmias is discussed.

1. ON THE PROCESS OF CELL VOLUME REGULATION

It is well known that preservation of cell volume is fundamental to cell survival. Because anionic macromolecules are within the cell, there is a constant danger of colloid osmotic cell swelling due to entrance of water and diffusible ions. The "pump and leak " concept implies that cell swelling is avoided because of two major factors: a) a low sodium permeability; b) an active extrusion of sodium ions made possible by the activation of Na+-K+ ATPase [1,2,3].

* Corresponding author: Walmor C De Mello. School of Medicine, Medical Sciences Campus,UPR, San Juan, PR 00936-5067,USA. Telephone 787-766-4441. Fax 787-766-4441. E-mail : walmor.de-mello@upr.edu.

Immediately after cell swelling, the cells release release KCl ,water and other osmolites with consequent reduction of cell volume to its initial value- a phenomenon called regulatory volume decrease (RVD) (see 4).Specific conditions or stimuli modulate the cell volume whose variations triggers several responses including cell migration, cell proliferation and release of hormones and transmitters [4].

Cell swelling occurs during hypoxia/ischemia, hyponatremia, hypothermia, which inhibits the Na^+-K^+-ATPase, increase in the extracellular K^+ concentration ($[K^+]_o$ as well as intracellular acidosis/diabetic ketoacidosis. According to these model analyses, the $[K^+]$ gradient, created by the Na^+/K^+ pump across the membrane, is the main determinant of a negative *membrane potential* and this negative V_m expels Cl^- out of the cell through Cl^- channels, compensating for the continuous Cl^- influx via Cl^--coupled transporters, such as NKCC1. Thereby, the pump maintains cellular osmolarity at the physiological level to keep the cell volume intact [6].The time course of cell swelling caused by blocking the Na^+/K^+ pump largely depends on redistribution of Cl^- across the membrane and on the membrane Cl^- permeability[6].

Conversely, cell shrinkage occurs during hypernatremia, following excessive Na^+ intake or water loss, reduced $[K^+]_o$ as well as hyperglycemia and alkalosis (see 5).The hypotonic stress induced by myocardial ischemia, for instance, leads to accumulation of metabolites intracellularly with consequent cell swelling due to water entering the cells [7]. Cell swelling is counteracted by decreasing intracellular osmolarity usually achieved by releasing inorganic or organic osmolytes [5]. Previous studies indicated that to accomodate the expanding volume the animal cells change their shape and increases surface area by drawing extra membrane from surface[8].

Cell swelling activates ionic channels including the swelling-dependent outward current ($I_{Clswell}$). The ClC family comprises 9 proteins-some are transporters and others are channels.

Four different types of Cl– channels have been decribed in cardiac cells [9]: a channel activated by PKA-dependent phosphorylation, which is probably identical to the channel activated by PKC, a $[Ca^{2+}]_i$-activated channel, a $[ATP]_o$-activated channel, and a stretch- or swelling-induced channel. All channels, except the PKA-induced Cl – channel, are blocked by disulfonic stilbene compounds (DIDS and SITS); the PKA-activated channel is blocked by 4,4'-dinitrostilbene-2,2'-disulfonic acid (DNDS). Two channels have been cloned and expressed: the CFTR channel, which is responsible for the PKA-stimulated channel [10] and ClC-3, which accounts for the swelling-induced current [11].

Because the E_{Cl} is positive to the resting potential, activation of Cl current causes depolarization of the resting potential and accelerates repolarization early during the action potential [12]. The physiological role of Cl currents, however, cannot be clearly determined and currents like I_{ClCa} that is activated by a physiological processes, i.e., the release of Ca^{2+} from the SR, does not seem to be expressed in all cells [13]. The density and expression of the currents is very variable; in general, I_{ClPKA} is better represented in ventricular cells and $I_{Clswell}$ in atrial cells. PKA- and PKC- dependent Cl – channel. The PKA-activated Cl – current [14] is typically present in the ventricle, less in the atrium, it is not present in the rabbit SAN or atrium, the dog atrium and ventricle, or the mouse and rat ventricle [15].

2. On the Process of Cell Communication and Metabolic Cooperation

Heart cells are communicated by gap junctions which permit the electrical synchronization and the exchange of metabolites and other signal molecules from cell to cell. Each cell of the pair contributes six connexins to form an oligomerized hemichannel (connexon) and the fusion of the two adjacent hemichannels forms the gap junction. The connexon is a hexameric arrangement of proteins (connexins) surrounding a central aqueous pore. Confocal microscopy with immunolocalization has shown that there are substantial changes in connexin43(Cx43) distribution in healed infarcts [16].Cx43 is absence from the infarct zone and is overexpressed forming a disorganized pathway along the border zone [17].Changes in distribution of Cx43 correlate with alteration in impulse conduction pathways [16].

The gap junction channel conductance or permeability is modulated by different factors including the intracellular calcium [18] , cAMP and activation of PKA with consequent phosphorylation of junctional proteins [19,20] or intracellular pH [21,22]. Recently, it was found that angiotensin II plays an important on the regulation of gap junction conductance in the failing heart [23,24] -a finding of particular interest because the renin angiotensin system is activated during this pathological condition.

It was proposed that metabolic cooperation among cells occurs through gap junctions and that there is a strict correlation between electrical coupling, dye transfer and metabolic cooperation [25]. The role of gap junctions in metabolic cooperation is supported by the finding that the effects on immunoglobulin synthesis by B lymphocytes are likely to be a consequence of the requirement for direct and protracted cross-talk with T lymphocytes involving, among other mechanisms, the formation of gap junction channels [26]. Moreover, when a mutant cell line deficient in an enzyme and a wild-type cells are grown together in presence of a labeled base, the autoradiographic grains are found in all cells [27].It is then possible that coordination of tissue function can be achieved through the exchange of regulatory intercellular signal molecules including cyclic nucleotides, small peptides, or high energy phosphates. The finding that cell swelling reduces the gap junction permeability [31] might indicate that variations in cell volume can alter the metabolic cooperation between cells. Unfortunately, our knowledge of the physiopathological role of metabolic cooperation in cardiac muscle is scanty.

3. Renin Angiotensin System as a Regulator of Cell Volume and Communication

Recently, it was found that the renin angiotensin system is involved in the regulation of heart cell volume [28].Angiotensin II or renin, for instance, cause cell swelling - an effect related to the inhibition of the sodium pump and activation of the Na-K-2Cl cotransporter [29].Cell swelling which causes the activation of ionic channels like the swelling-activate chloride current ($I_{Cl,swell}$), have electrophysiologic effects including membrane depolarization and reduction of action potential duration [29,13,30] what facilitates the generation of cardiac arrhythmias. Indeed, the activation of this current seems to be involved in generation of early afterdepolarizations in the failing ventricle exposed to hypotonic solution [30]. Ang (1-7) which counteracts many effects of Ang II in the cardiovascular system [31], reduces the cell volume and the swelling-activate chloride current ($I_{Cl,swell}$) [30].Because Ang (1-7) formed from Ang II through ACE2 [32], decreases the incidence of cardiac arrhythmias during ischemia/reperfusion [33,34] it is reasonable to think that the decrease in the $I_{Cl,swell}$ might explain, in part, the antiarrhythmic effect of the heptapeptide.

The K(v) 4.2/4.3 channels, which are the primary subunits of I(to, fast), are regulated by cell volume through phosphorylation/dephosphorylation of serine/threonine phosphatases [47] and their activation by cell swelling facilitates the generation of cardiac arrhythmias.

These observations indicate that cell swelling induced by myocardial ischemia, heart failure or drugs like ouabain, represents an important arrhythmogenic mechanism which are potentiated by Ang II which increases the heart cell volume [28]. On the other hand, recent findings indicate that cyclical mechanical stretch increases angiotensin II production and Cx43 gene expression in cultured cardiomyocytes, partially through mediation of the AT1 receptors, establishing a link between the local renin-angiotensin system activation and Cx43 expression in response to stretch [47].

4. Cell Swelling Causes a Drastic Decline in Gap Junction Permeability

Next to genome the cell surface is involved in the control of differentiation, growth and in all aspects of cell communication and cell recognition. Recently, evidence has been provided that cell swelling causes a severe impairment of dye coupling in cardiomyocytes from adult rat ventricle [35]. Indeed, when Lucifer Yellow CH was dialyzed into a swollen cardiomyocyte cell pair of adult rat ventricle, the intercellular diffusion of the dye was severely impaired. Since the dye does not cross the surface cell membrane but flows easily through gap junctions [36] the conclusion was that the gap junction permeability was drastically reduced. Moreover, the intracellular diffusion of the dye was not altered by cell swelling. Connexin43 which the most important connexin in mammalian ventricle, is permeable to Lucifer Yellow CH- a known fluorescent tracer with properties suitable for the determination of junctional permeability (Mw 443,valence =2 and about 10 μm in diameter).

Estimation of gap junction permeability (Pj) indicated that cell swelling reduced Pj to Lucifer Yellow CH significantly Pj calculated taking V_{cell} as 12% of total cell volume, was appreciably reduced from $0.16 \pm 0.04 \times 10^{-4}$ cm/s (n=35) in the control, to $0.89 \pm 1.1 \times 10^{-5}$ cm/s (n=40) after 35 minutes of exposure to hypotonic solution (see Table 1). Similar results were found assuming V_{cell} as 20% and 30 % of total cell volume, respectively [35] (see Table 1).

The mechanism by which cell swelling causes dye uncoupling is not known but it is probably multifactorial. The hydrated pore radio for Cx43 was observed to increase nonlinearly when increasing the KCl concentration from 115 mM to 140 mM and is consistent with the hypothesis that the intracellular K+ concentration in mammalian cells is responsible for the electrical coupling (see 37). Assuming that the junctional permeability is also dependent on the intracellular K concentration, it is possible that the dilution of the intracellular medium generated by cell swelling might be involved in the decline of junctional permeability.

Table 1. Influence of hypotonic solution on cell volume and gap junction permeability (P_J) cm/s

	Control		Hypotonic solution
Total cell volume	36000 ± 1100 (μm^3) (n=30) (5 animals)	P<0.05	57600 ± 980 (μm^3) (n=34) (5 animals)
	Pj		Pj
V_{cell} 12%	0.16 ± 0.04 x 10^{-4} (n=35) (6 animals)	P<0.05	0.89 ± 1.1 x 10^{-5} (n=40) (6 animals)
V_{cell} 20%	0.27 ± 0.05 x 10^{-4}	P<0.05	1.4 ± 1.3 x 10^{-5}
V_{cell} 30%	0.37 ± 0.04 x 10^{-4}	P<0.05	2.2 ± 1.6 x 10^{-5}

V_{cell} is the fraction of total cell volume occupied by Lucifer Yellow CH inside the cell and taken as 12%,20% and 30 % respectively of the total cell volume (13). Aj was taken as 17% of the cross sectional area of the rat cardiomyocyte (177 μm^2)[15] .

Cell swelling, on the other hand, stimulates protein kinase C [38 57] and enhances tyrosine phosphorylation of several proteins, a finding particularly relevant because it is known that Ang II changes the gap junction conductance as well as the inward calcium current in the heart through the activation of PKC and tyrosine kinases [39].It is well known that ion channel proteins may be phosphorylated and that this phosphorylation can change the functional properties of ion channels [40].Connexin43 which is the most important connexin in mammalian heart ventricle, is a phosphoprotein [41]. Previous studies, indicated that cAMP and consequent PKA activation increases the gap junction conductance and permeability in the heart [19,20]. It is known on the other hand, that an increase in the intracellular free calcium reduces the junctional conductance in cardiac muscle [18] and that cell swelling increments the intracellular calcium [42]. The role of the increase in free Ca^{2+}_i in the decline in dye coupling elicited by cell swelling, however, seems unlikely due to the use of EGTA (10 mM) in the pipette solution [35].An additional possibility is that cell swelling alters the structure of the gap junctions. Further studies will be needed to clarify the mechanisms involved in the decline of junctional permeability in cardiac muscle induced by cell swelling.

5. On the Arrhythmogenic Action of Cell Swelling

Evidence is available that a decline in cell coupling causes slow conduction and facilitates the generation of reentrant rhythms [43]. On the other hand, electrophysiological studies performed on cells and tissues isolated from the failing heart show an increase in duration of the action potential and a decrease of conduction velocity [43, 44]. Downregulation of K currents as well as abnormalities of calcium and sodium currents, for instance, have been found in animal models as well on the human failing heart [44]. Significant decrease of gap junctional conductance [45] and abnormalities of connexin43 distribution [45] are in part responsible for the impairment of impulse propagation and the generation of reentrant rhythms.

Evidence is available that atrial fibrillation, which is most common arrhythmia, generates structural and electrophysiological remodeling of the atria. Cellular electrophysiological studies have shown marked reductions in the densities of the L-type voltage-gated Ca^{2+}current and in K currents including I_{TO}, and IKur, in atrial cardiomyocytes isolated from patients with chronic atrial fibrillation. In animal models as well as in patients with atrial fibrillation, the decline in $I_{Ca,L}$ seems to explain the decreases in action potential duration as well as the refractory period that are related to atrial remodeling [51]. It is also known that angiotensin II enhances the incidence of arrhythmias [52,53] particularly during ischemia/reperfusion [48] and that the blockade of AT1 receptor (AT1R) reduces the incidence of arrhythmias as well as the mortality after myocardial infarction. Since the AT1R is upregulated after myocardial ischemia, it is reasonable to think that the level of AT1R expression would mediate the response to AT1R blockade.

The K(v) 4.2/4.3 channels, which are the primary subunits of I(to, fast), are regulated by cell volume through phosphorylation/dephosphorylation of serine/threonine phosphatases [46] and their activation by cell swelling facilitates the generation of cardiac arrhythmias. The activation of $I_{Clswell}$ is also arrhythmogenic [30]. Taken together, the activation of ionic channels and the decline of intercellular communication elicited by cell swelling establishes the conditions for the generation of cardiac arrhythmias (see Fig 1).

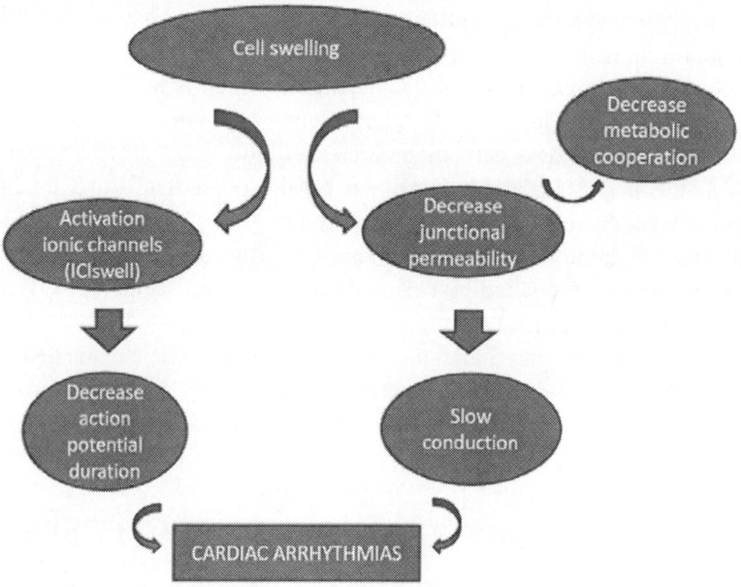

Figure 1. Diagram showing the influence of cell swelling on activation of ionic channels and gap junction permeability in cardiac muscle and its consequences including changes in metabolic cooperation and generation of cardiac arrhythmias.

It is known that cell swelling occurs during hypoxia/ischemia, hyponatremia, activation of the renin angiotensin system [28,30], hypothermia, which inhibits the Na^{+}-K^{+}-ATPase, as well as increment of extracellular K concentrations and intracellular acidosis/diabetic ketoacidosis. Therefore, the reduction of cell swelling during these conditions might be critical to prevent the generation of cardiac arrhythmias and to reestablish chemical communication between cells.

6. Conclusions

Evidence is now available that cell volume is an important regulator of cell communication. This finding highly suggests that cell swelling induced by pathological conditions like myocardial ischemia or activation of the renin angiotensin system, creates the conditions for slow conduction and generation of cardiac arrhythmias. This conclusion is substantiated by the finding that hypotonic solution increased heart cell volume and generated early afterdepolarization and spontaneous rhythmicity in the failing heart [30]. Furthermore, the metabolic cooperation between cells, which depends on gap junction communication, is probably impaired in swollen cells with serious consequences for the integration of tissue function.

Acknowledgement

This work was supported in part by NIH grant GM 61838.

References

[1] Leaf A Maintenance of concentration gradients and regulation of cell volume. *Ann. N Y Acad. Sci.* 1959 ;72:396-404.

[2] Tosteson DC, Hoffman JF. Regulation of cell volume by active cation transport in high and low potassium sheep red cells. *J. Gen. Physiol.* 1960; 44: 169–194.

[3] Ussing HH. Active and passive transport of the alkali metal ions. In: *The alkali metal ions in biology*, edited by Ussing HH, Kruhöffeer P, Hess Thaysen J, and Thorn NA. Berlin: Springer-Verlag, 1960, p. 45–143.

[4] Hoffmann EK, Lambert IH, Pedersen SF. Physiology of Cell Volume Regulation in Vertebrates. *Physiol. Rev.* 2009; 89: 193-277.

[5] Lang F, Busch GL, Ritter M, Volkl H, et al. Functional significance of cell volume regulatory mechanisms. *Physiol. Rev. 1998; 78: 247–306.*

[6] Takeuchi A,Tatsumi S, Sarai N,Terashima K et al Ionic mechanisms of cardiac cell swelling induced by blocking Na+/K+ pump as revealed by experiments and simulation. *J. Gen. Physiol.* 2006 ; 128: 495-507.

[7] Sackin, H. *Stretch activated ion channels*. Kidney Int 1995; 48: 1134-47.

[8] Groulx N, Boudreault F, Oslov SN,Grygorezyk R Membrane reserves and hypotonic cell swelling. *J. Membr. Biol. 2006; 214:43-56.*

[9] Hume, J. R.,Horowitz B. A plethora of cardiac chloride conductances: molecular diversity or a related gene family? *J. Cardiovasc. Electrophysiol.*1995; 6: 325-331.

[10] Hart P, Warth JD, P. C. Levesque, M. L. Collier, Geary Y,et al. Cystic fibrosis gene encodes a cAMP-dependent chloride channel in heart. *Proc. Natl. Acad. Sci. USA* 1996; 93: 6343-6348.

[11] Duan, D.,Winter C, Cowley S, Hume JR, Horowitz B. Molecular identification of a volume-regulated chloride channel. *Nature* 1997; 390: 417-421.

[12] Du, X. Y., Sorota S. Cardiac swelling-induced chloride current depolarizes canine atrial myocytes. *Am. J. Physiol. Heart Circ. Physiol.* 1997; 272 : H1904-H1916.

[13] Carmeliet E Cardiac Ionic Currents and Acute Ischemia: From Channels to Arrhythmias *Physiological Reviews*, 1999, 79: 917-1017.

[14] Gadsby, D. C., G. Nagel G, Hwang TC. The CFTR chloride channel of mammalian heart. *Annu. Rev. Physiol.* 1995; 57: 387- 416 .

[15] Horowitz, B., Tsung SS, Hart P, Levesque PC, HUME JR. Alternative splicing of CFTR Cl− channels in heart. *Am. J. Physiol. Heart Circ. Physiol.* 1993; 264: H2214-H2220.

[16] Peters NS, Coromilas J, Severs NJ, Wit AL, Disturbed connexin43 gap junction distribution correlates with the location of reentrant circuits in the epicardial border zone of healing canine infarcts that cause ventricular tachycardia. *Circulation* ; 1997; 95:988-996.

[17] Costeas C, Peters NS, Waldecker B, Ciaccio EJ, Wit AL, Coromilas J Mechanisms causing sustained ventricular tachycardia with multiple QRS morphologies: results of mapping studies in the infarcted canine heart. *Circulation*. 1997 ; 96:3721-31.

[18] De Mello WC Effect of intracellular injection of calcium on cell communication in heart. *J. Physiol.* 1975; 250:231–236.

[19] De Mello WC The role of cAMP and Ca on the modulation of junctional conductance: an integrated hypothesis. *Cell Biol. Int. Rep.* 1983 ;7:1033-40.

[20] Burt JM, Spray DC Inotropic agents modulate gap junctional conductance between cardiomyocytes. *Am. J. Physiol.* 1988; 363 ; 254:H1206–H1210.

[21] Turner L, Warner AE Carbon dioxide reversely abolishes ionic communication between cells of early amphibian embryo. *Nature* 1978; 270:56-60.

[22] De Mello WC The influence of pH on the healing-over of mammalian cardiac muscle. *J. Physiol.* 1983; 339; 299-305.

[23] De Mello WC Renin angiotensin system and cell communication in the failing heart. *Hypertension* 1996; 27; 1267-72.

[24] De Mello WC Is an intracellular renin angiotensin system involved in the control of cell communication in heart? *J. Cardiovasc. Pharmacol.* 1994; 23: 640-46.

[25] Gilula NB,Reeves OR, Steinbach A Metabolic coupling, ionic coupling and cell contacts. *Nature* 1972; 235:262.

[26] Oviedo-Orta E, Gasque P , Evans WH Immunoglobulin and cytokine expression in mixed lymphocyte cultures is reduced by disruption of gap junction intercellular communication. *The FASEB Journal* 2001; 15:768-774.

[27] Pitts JD, Finbow ME Junctional permeability and its consequences. In *Intercellular Communication* (De Mello, WC ed),Plenum Press, New York,1977,p 61-86.

[28] De Mello, WC. Intracellular and extracellular renin have opposite effects on the regulation of heart cell volume. Implications to myocardial ischemia. *J. Renin Angiotensin Aldosterone Syst*. 2008; 9: 112-8.

[29] Baumgarten, C.M., Clemo, H.F. Swelling-activated chloride channels in cardiac physiology and pathophysiology. *Prog. Biophys. Mol. Biol.* 2003: 122: 689-70.

[30] De Mello, W.C. Cell swelling, impulse conduction and cardiac arrhythmias in the failing heart. Opposite effects of angiotensin II and angiotensin (1-7) on cell volume regulation. *Mol. Cell Biochem.* 2009; 330: 211-7.

[31] Ferrario, C., Chapell, M., Tallant, EK. et al Counterregulatory actions of angiotensin (1-7). *Hypertension* 1997; 30:535-541.

[32] Donoghue, M., Hsieh, F., Baronas, E. et al A novel angiotensin converting enzyme related to carboxypeptidase (ACE2) converts angiotensin I to angiotensin (1-9). *Circ. Res*. 2000; 87: E1-E9.

[33] De Mello, WC. Angiotensin (1-7) re-establishes impulse conduction in cardiac muscle during ischemia/reperfusion.The role of the sodium pump. *J. Renin Angiotensin Aldosterone Syst*. 2004; 5:203-208.

[34] Ferreira, AJ., Santos, RA., Almeida, AP. Angiotensin (1-7); cardioprotective effect in myocardial ischememia/reperfusion. *Hypertension* 2001; 38:665-668.

[35] De Mello WC Cell swelling impairs dye coupling in adult rat ventricular myocytes. Cell volume as a regulator of cell communication. *Mol. Cell Biochem.* 2010; 343:107-13.

[36] De Mello WC, van Loon P Influence of cyclic nucleotides on junctional permeability in atrial muscle. *J. Mol. Cell Cardiol.* 1987; 19: 83-94.

[37] Veenstra R Biophysics of Gap Junction Channels. In: *Heart Cell Coupling and Impulse Propagation in health and Disease*.(De Mello WC, Janse M eds) Kluwer Academic Publishers, Massachusetts 2002;143-83.

[38] Richter, EA, Cleland PJ, Rattigan S, Clark MG. Contraction-associated translocation of protein kinase C in rat skeletal muscle. *FEBS Lett.* 217:232-236, 1987.

[39] De Mello WC Intracellular angiotensin II regulates the inward calcium current in cardiac myocytes *Hypertension*. 1998; 32:976-82.

[40] Ismailov I, Benos DJ *Effects of phosphorylation on ion channel function.* Kidney Int. 1995; 48:1167-79.

[41] Laird DW, Puranam KL,Revel JP Turnover and phosphorylation dynamics of connexin43 gap junction protein in cultured cardiac myocytes. *Biochem. J.* 1991; 273:67-72.

[42] Viana F, de la Peña E, Pecson B, Schmidt RF, Belmonte C. Swelling-activated calcium signalling in cultured mouse primary sensory neurons. *Eur. J. Neurosci.* 2001 ; 13:722-34.

[43] Tomaselli, GF., Beuckelmann, DJ., Calkins, HG., Berger, RD. et al Sudden cardiac death in heart failure. The role of abnormal repolarization. *Circulation* 1994; 90:2534-2539.

[44] De Mello, WC. Cell coupling and impulse propagation in the failing heart. *J. Cardiovasc. Electrophysiol.* 1999; 10:1409-30.

[45] Severs, NJ. Pathophysiology of gap junctions in heart disease. *J. Cardiovasc. Electrophysiology* 1994; 5:462-75.

[46] Wang, GL., Wang, GX., Yamamoto, S., and Ye L et al Molecular mechanisms of regulation of fast-inactivating voltage-dependent transient outward K+ current in mouse heart by cell volume changes. *J. Physiol.* 2005; 568: 423-43.

[47] Chia-Chi KGK, Chen CC,Wang BW, Kuan P Angiotensin II receptor antagonist blocks the expression of connexin43 induced by cyclical mechanical stretch in cultured neonatal rat cardiac myocytes *J. Mol. Cell Cardiol.* 2001; 33: 691-698.

[48] de Boer, RA., van Geel, PP., Pinto, YM., Suurmeijer, AJ. et al Efficacy of angiotensin II type 1 receptor blockade on reperfusion-induced arrhythmias and mortality early after myocardial infarction is increased in transgenic rats with cardiac angiotensin II type 1 overexpression. *J. Cardiovasc. Pharmacol.* 2002; 39:610-9.

[49] Bosh, RF., Nattel, S. Cellular electrophysiology and atrial fibrillation. *Cardiovasc. Res.* 2002; 54:259-69.

[50] Janse, MJ., Coronel, R., Francien, JG. et al Mechanical effects on arrhythmogenesis: from the pipette to patient. *Prog. Biophys. Mol. Biol.* 2003; 82:187-95.

[51] D. R. Van, Wagoner, J. M. Nerbonne. Molecular Basis of Electrical Remodeling in Atrial Fibrillation. *J. Mol. Cell Cardiol.* 2000; 32, 1101–1117.

[52] De Mello, WC. Cardiac arrhythmias: the possible role of the renin angiotensin system. *J. Mol. Med.* 2001; 79: 103-108.

[53] Gavras, I., Gavras, H. Angiotensin II as a cardiovascular risk factor. *J. Hum. Hypertens.* 2002 May; 16 Suppl 2:S2-6.

[54] Richter, EA, Cleland PJ, Rattigan S, Clark MG. Contraction-associated translocation of protein kinase C in rat skeletal muscle. *FEBS Lett.* 1987; 217:232-236.

In: Angiotensin: New Research
Editors: S. Harada, I. Moi, pp. 205-213
ISBN: 978-1-62100-773-9

Chapter 10

DIABETIC CARDIOMYOPATHY: ROLE OF RENIN ANGIOTENSIN SYSTEM

***Kenichi Watanabe*[1], *Somasundaram Arumugam*[1], *Rajarajan A. Thandavarayan*[1], *Takashi Nakamura*[1], *Kenji Suzuki*[2] *and Makoto Kodama*[3]**

[1] Department of Clinical Pharmacology, Faculty of Pharmaceutical Sciences, Niigata University of Pharmacy and Applied Life Sciences, Niigata, Japan.

[2] Department of Gastroenterology, Niigata University Graduate School of Medical and Dental Sciences, Niigata, Japan.

[3] First Department of Medicine, Niigata University Graduate School of Medical and Dental Sciences, Niigata, Japan.

ABSTRACT

The renin angiotensin system (RAS) maintains the cardiovascular (CV) homeostasis and is involved in the pathogenesis of several disorders majorly related to heart and kidney. There are several peptides under RAS in which angiotensin (Ang) II is the major contributor. It was reported about the role of Ang II and its receptor Ang II type 1 (AT1) in mediating the CV remodeling during heart failure. Another receptor AT2 acts primarily opposite to that of AT1. Ang (1-7) is a peptide which can prevent the ventricular remodeling during cardiac complications acting via Mas receptor. Diabetes mellitus is characterized by multiple organ damage and also increases the prevalence and severity of CV diseases. Hyperglycemia activates the local RAS, resulting in the formation of Ang II and stimulation of the endogenous cell death pathway. Cardiac remodeling, including fibrosis and left ventricular hypertrophy, is found in the diabetic heart as a result of the activation of the RAS. Blockade of the AT1 receptor by Ang receptor blocker (ARB) can be effectively used to prevent the cardiac remodeling in the form of hypertrophy and fibrosis during diabetic conditions. By blocking the actions of Ang II on AT1 receptors, ARBs facilitate its action on AT2 receptors and also improves the conversion of Ang II to Ang (1-7), which upon acting on Mas receptor to counteract the activated RAS in diabetic cardiomyopathy.

Renin Angiotensin System

The RAS is a coordinated hormonal cascade that controls CV, renal, and adrenal function by governing body fluid and electrolyte balance as well as arterial pressure [1]. A single, obligate precursor protein, angiotensinogen (452 amino acids), remains the source of all Ang peptides. Circulating angiotensinogen from liver is primarily cleaved by the protease, renin from kidney, to yield a 10 amino acid peptide, Ang I, which in turn is processed by Ang converting enzyme (ACE) in lung to produce the active octapeptide, Ang II. Ang II is degraded to Ang III by angiotensinases that are located in red blood cells and the vascular beds of most tissues. Ang IV is a hexapeptide that, like Ang III, has some lesser activity. ACE2 is an exopeptidase that catalyses the conversion of Ang I to the nonapeptide Ang (1-9) or the conversion of Ang II to Ang (1-7) [2]. The former reaction is quantitatively less because of the lesser affinity of Ang I towards ACE2 whereas the latter reaction is significantly higher, which produces the Ang (1-7), another important peptide in maintenance of homeostasis [3].

Ang II and Cardiac Complications

Ang II is the principal effector peptide of the RAS. It plays an important role in the pathogenesis of a variety of clinical conditions, including atherosclerosis, hypertension, left ventricular hypertrophy, myocardial infarction and heart failure [4]. Through its binding to the Ang II type 1 (AT1) receptor, it mediates a range of processes, including vasoconstriction, aldosterone, and vasopressin release, sodium and water retention, and sympathetic activation [5]. Recent clinical and experimental studies have identified the importance of classical neurohormones such as Ang II as biological mediators and/or modifiers of left ventricular remodeling and disease progression in the failing heart [6]. Increased activity of Ang II is associated with the induction of monocyte chemoattractant protein-1 (MCP-1), in particular in the vascular wall of various hypertensive and atherosclerotic models. Ang II, in addition to its action as a potent vasoconstrictor, also promotes vascular inflammation, proliferation and hypertrophy. It was also shown to play a key role in the hypertrophic process in terms of protein synthesis and expression of the immediate early gene critical for cell proliferation [7]. The mechanisms mediating this are thought to act by activation of AT1 receptor and through oxidative stress related pathways [8]. Imbalance between nitric oxide and Ang II results in oxidative stress by stimulating NADH and NADPH oxidase to generate reactive oxygen species. This leads to endothelial dysfunction and inflammation mediated by various cytokines. Increased Ang II levels stimulate the release of endothelin-1 and various growth factors involved in the tissue remodeling. Ang II along with the releases endothelin-1 and growth factors transactivate heparin-binding epidermal growth factor-like growth factor (HB-EGF), a member of the EGF family that binds to and activates the EGF receptor to induce cardiac hypertrophy via the phospho inositol 3 kinase (PI3K)-Akt, mitogen activated protein kinase (MAPK), janus kinase-signal transducer and activator of transcription (JAK-STAT) and extracellular signal-regulated kinase5 (ERK5) pathways [9]. Apoptosis signal-regulating kinase 1 (ASK1), one of MAPK kinase kinases, plays a key role in stress-induced cellular responses and it was reported using the ASK1 deficient transgenic mouse that ASK1 is the critical signaling molecule for Ang II-induced cardiac hypertrophy and remodeling [10].

Ang II and AT2 Receptor

AT2 is another class of receptor where Ang II can act, mostly involving the opposite effects as that of AT1 receptor stimulation. Decrease in blood pressure, vasodilatation, reduced peripheral resistance are the effects produced upon activation of AT2 receptors via Ang II [11]. AT1 receptor is widely distributed in adult tissues (blood vessels, kidney, adrenal gland, heart liver, and brain) whereas the AT2 receptor is ubiquitously expressed in fetal tissues but the expression of the AT2 receptor declines rapidly after birth with very low abundance in ventricular myocytes and vascular endothelium and absence in fibroblasts. Disturbances in the action of Ang II on AT1 receptor leads to the modulation of AT2 receptor expression [12]. Still debate exists about the exact role of AT2 receptors in the physiological processes and pathological alterations during various cardiac complications. AT2 receptor knockout prevented the cardiac hypertrophic response to both aortic stenosis and chronic Ang II infusion in mice suggesting that AT2 receptor is essential for the development of cardiac hypertrophy and dysfunction [13]. Acute myocardial infarction in AT2 receptor knockout mice resulted in higher mortality rate, higher left ventricular weight/body weight, lung weight/body weight, and decreased ejection fraction versus wild type mice suggesting that AT2 receptor has antihypertrophic remodeling effects and may be important for maintaining cardiac function under certain stress [14]. Thus new transgenic mouse models that conditionally overexpress or disrupt AT2 receptor in specific cell types in addition to cardiomyocytes in the heart may be useful for studying the pathophysiological role of AT2 receptors [12].

ACE2 and Its Products

ACE2 has direct effects on cardiac function, and is expressed predominantly in vascular endothelial cells of the heart and the kidneys. In the absence of ACE2, biomechanical stress triggers activation of the myocardial NAPDH oxidase system with a critical role of the $p47^{phox}$ subunit. Increased production of superoxide, activation of matrix metalloproteinase, and pathological signaling in ACE2 knockout mice lead to severe adverse myocardial remodeling and dysfunction [15].

Ang (1–7), the major peptide formed by the action of ACE2, is an endogenous ligand for the G-protein coupled receptor Mas and the latter receptor appears to mediate most of the biological actions of Ang (1–7) [16]. Heptapeptide Ang (l-7), a member of the family of Ang peptides stimulates vasopressin secretion and facilitates neuronal activity. Furthermore, Ang (1-7) caused cultured astrocytes, vascular endothelial cells, and smooth muscle cells to release prostaglandins without increasing intracellular Ca^{++} and thus Ang (1-7) contributes the antihypertensive actions. It was reported that overexpression of Ang (1-7) improves cardiac function and attenuates left ventricular remodeling post-myocardial infarction and this appear to be mediated, at least in part, through modulation of the cardiac RAS and cytokine production [17].

DIABETIC CARDIOMYOPATHY (CM)

Diabetes mellitus is characterized by multiple organ damage (nerves, kidney and eyes) and also increases the prevalence and severity of CV diseases [18]. Diabetic CM as a clinical entity remains elusive, despite more than 3.5 decades of basic and clinical investigations [19]. Diabetic CM can be clinically defined by the presence of abnormal myocardial performance or structure in the absence of epicardial coronary artery disease, hypertension, and significant valvular disease and it has been well documented in both humans and animals [20]. The mechanism of diabetic cardiac dysfunction is complex and involves increased oxidative/nitrative stress, activation of various downstream transcription factors, proinflammatory and cell death pathways such as nuclear factor kappa B (NFκB), poly (adenosine diphosphate [ADP]-ribose) polymerase (PARP), and MAPK, inactivation of pro-survival pathways such as Akt, eventually culminating in cell death and changes in the composition of extracellular matrix (ECM) with enhanced cardiac fibrosis and increased inflammation [21]. Pathological alterations in diabetic CM include those relevant to muscle tissue and cells, such as the presence of myocardial hypertrophy and impaired contraction, those associated with ECM proteins, such as excess deposition of collagens, abnormal glycosylation/crosslinking, and alterations in diastolic compliance. Other abnormalities include those associated with the vascular compartment, such as the thickening of the endothelium basal lamina [22]. Apoptosis of cardiomyocytes appears to be of pathophysiological significance in different cardiac diseases (ischemic CM, idiopathic dilated CM, hypertrophic CM) [23, 24], but only recently the impact of cardiomyocyte apoptosis has been suggested to be related to diabetes mellitus.

RAS IN DIABETIC CM

Activation of RAS is thought to play a major role in the pathogenesis of heart failure and to contribute significantly to myocardial dysfunction and neurohumoral disturbances [25]. It is also implicated in the progression of heart failure, hypertension, and kidney disease. In the rat model of pressure overloaded hypertrophy, the local RAS was significantly upregulated at the stage of compensatory cardiac hypertrophy. Stimulation of the local RAS and apoptosis characterize the diabetic heart. Hyperglycemia activates the local RAS, resulting in the formation of Ang II and stimulation of the endogenous cell death pathway. Activation of the RAS in diabetes includes activation of new components, such as the pro-renin receptor and interaction of pro-renin with its receptor. The pro-renin receptor is a unique molecule that binds pro-renin and renin in tissues, not only leading to their activation, but also inducing intracellular signaling. As a key player in the local RAS, pro-renin receptor activation plays an important role in the development of cardiac fibrosis and proteinuria in hypertension and diabetes [26]. Although circulating renin and Ang II levels are reduced in diabetes, pro-renin levels are enhanced severalfold. Pro-renin may have dual effects, providing for generation of Ang I at tissue sites through receptor-mediated nonproteolytic activation and directly through activation of receptor-mediated signaling pathways. Ang II is then formed from Ang I via ACE. The formed Ang II stimulates superoxide production via the AT1 receptor by activation of NADPH oxidase, which is localized in many tissues, including vascular smooth muscle cells, fibroblasts, and heart tissue. Oxidative stress might be considered the common trigger for cardiac myocyte apoptosis in hypertension and diabetes. Cooperation between Ang II and reactive oxygen species may be required for cell death to occur in the diabetic heart. Enhanced levels of Ang II found in different pathophysiologic conditions such as hypertension and heart failure cause increased superoxide production concurrently with a decrease in nitric oxide activity. In experimental settings, continuous infusion of Ang II [27] stimulates cardiomyocyte apoptosis, and large cardioprotective benefits were observed when the β-adrenergic system and the RAS were blocked in patients affected by diabetes.

The change in Ang II and Ang II receptors in diabetic hearts appears to be local and independent of the circulating RAS. Up-regulation of the local RAS in diabetes may enhance oxidative damage, activating cardiac cell apoptosis and necrosis. Thus, either increased Ang II or increased Ang II receptor density enhances the effect of Ang II. Whichever the mechanism, Ang II has dose-dependent effects on collagen secretion and production in rat adult cardiac fibroblasts. Cardiac remodeling, including fibrosis and left ventricular hypertrophy, is found in the diabetic heart as a result of the activation of the RAS. Advanced hyperglycemia and increased cytoplasmic glucose concentration may lead to glycosylation of the C-terminal of the tumor suppressor p53. Activation of p53 may result in its translocation to the nucleus, where it initiates transcription of a number of p53-dependent genes including angiotensinogen and AT1 receptor [28]. Upregulation of angiotensinogen increases the synthesis of Ang II, the local release of which may trigger cell death in susceptible myocytes and promote hypertrophy in responding cells. Downregulation of p53 function decreases transcription of angiotensinogen, which is the limiting factor in the synthesis of Ang II in myocytes.

The effects of Ang II may also be promoted by the production and release of Transforming growth factor (TGF)-β1 by cardiac fibroblasts. TGF-β1 plays a critical role in organ morphogenesis, development, growth regulation, cellular differentiation, gene expression, and tissue remodeling [29]. TGF-β1 induced by metabolic abnormalities (chronic postprandial hyperglycemia, hyperinsulinemia and insulin resistance) has also been implicated in the development of diabetic CM.

Loss of ACE2 exacerbates diabetic CM characterized by worsening diastolic function and systolic dysfunction independent of changes in blood pressure. Protective role of ACE2-Ang (1-7)-Mas axis in diabetic nephropathy has been suggested by several studies. Similarly in diabetic CM, ACE2 protein synthesis is reduced in the diabetic heart indicating its importance in prevention of cardiac remodeling.

The diabetic myocardium is susceptible to higher than normal rates of myocyte death by both apoptosis and necrosis. Studies suggest that hyperglycemia results in production of reactive oxygen species, contributing to accelerated apoptosis. Some of this proapoptotic effect of hyperglycemia is triggered by glycosylation and phosphorylation of p53, and excessive synthesis of Ang II. Myocardial fibrosis and collagen deposition are the primary structural changes observed in diabetic CM. Diabetes activates locally active myocardial renin-Ang and endothelin systems, contributing to myocyte necrosis and fibrosis [19].

ARB IN DIABETIC CM

Components of RAS are well established targets for pharmacological interventions in various disorders. Many of them suggest the blockade of the actions of the vasoactive peptide Ang II on its receptors or prevention of its formation by blocking the enzyme ACE. Glucose concentrations are directly correlated with Ang II production, which increases in myocyte apoptosis [28] and oxidative stress [30]. Blockade of the AT1 receptor and its effector pathway by ARB prevented cell death and reduced the formation of Ang II in myocytes without affecting hyperglycemia. Apart from this an ARB can be effectively used to prevent the cardiac remodeling in the form of hypertrophy and fibrosis during diabetic conditions. By blocking the actions of Ang II on AT1 receptors, ARBs facilitate its action on AT2 receptors and also improves the conversion of Ang II to Ang (1-7), which upon acting on Mas receptor to counteract the activated RAS in diabetic CM.

We have recently reported the effects of losartan an AT1 antagonist on streptozotocin induced diabetes. It has added the evidences that fibrosis and oxidative stress occur in vivo in the heart of diabetic rats, and that ARB treatment could improve cardiac function by attenuating fibrosis and reversing oxidative stress, suggesting the beneficial effect of ARB treatment in the prevention of development and progression of diabetic disease [31]. Similarly another AT1 receptor blocker valsartan, protected against oxidative stress at multiple levels and enhanced insulin signaling and sensitivity in a model of type 2 diabetes mellitus [32].

CONCLUSION

Diabetic CM, a disorder of the heart muscle in people with diabetes mellitus without coronary artery disease, can lead to heart failure.

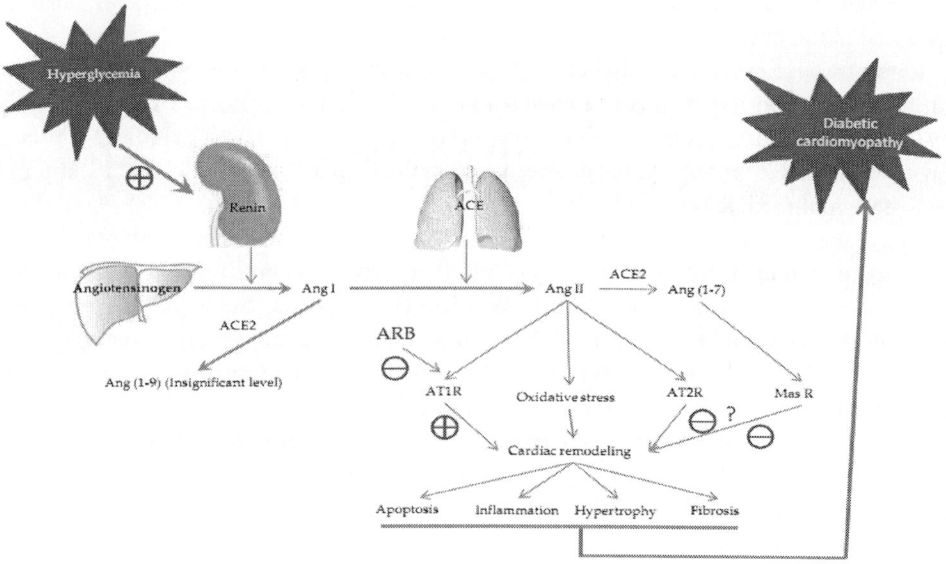

Figure 1. Role of RAS and ARB in Diabetic cardiomyopathy.

Activation of RAS, one of the major causes for the impaired cardiac function in diabetic CM, acts via several peptide members belonging to Ang family (Figure 1). ARBs, when added to conventional treatment for patients with heart failure, are associated with a reduction in morbidity and mortality as well as an improvement in quality of life. The treatment option with ARB against the cardiac complications involving Ang II has widened the area of CV research which will benefit the number of suffering population.

References

[1] Mesquita, FF; Gontijo, JA; Boer PA. Expression of renin-angiotensin system signalling compounds in maternal protein-restricted rats: effect on renal sodium excretion and blood pressure. *Nephrol. Dial. Transplant.*, 2010, 25(2), 380-388.

[2] George, AJ; Thomas, WG; Hannan, RD. The renin–angiotensin system and cancer: old dog, new tricks. *Nature Reviews Cancer*, 2010, 10, 745-759.

[3] Stewart, JA Jr; Lazartigues, E; Lucchesi, PA. The angiotensin converting enzyme 2/Ang-(1-7) axis in the heart: a role for MAS communication? *Circ. Res.*, 2008, 103(11), 1197-1199.

[4] Hoogwerf, BJ. Renin-angiotensin system blockade and cardiovascular and renal protection. *Am. J. Cardiol.*, 2010, 105(1 Suppl.), 30A-35A.

[5] Schmieder, RE. Mechanisms for the clinical benefits of angiotensin II receptor blockers. *Am. J. Hypertens.*, 2005, 18(5 Pt 1), 720-730.

[6] Mann, DL. Mechanisms and models in heart failure: A combinatorial approach. *Circulation*, 1999, 100, 999-1088.

[7] Iwanaga, Y; Kihara, Y; Inagaki, K; Onozawa, Y; Yoneda, T; Kataoka, K; Sasayama, S. Differential effects of angiotensin II versus endothelin-1 inhibitions in hypertrophic left ventricular myocardium during transition to heart failure. *Circulation*, 2001, 104(5), 606-612.

[8] Bush, E; Maeda, N; Kuziel, WA; Dawson, TC; Wilcox, JN; DeLeon, H; Taylor, WR. CC chemokine receptor 2 is required for macrophage infiltration and vascular hypertrophy in angiotensin II-induced hypertension. *Hypertension,* 2000, 36(3), 360-363.

[9] Lee, KS; Park, JH; Lim, HJ; Park, HY. HB-EGF induces cardiomyocyte hypertrophy via an ERK5-MEF2A-COX2 signaling pathway. *Cell Signal,* 2011, 23(7), 1100-1109.

[10] Izumiya, Y; Kim, S; Izumi, Y; Yoshida, K; Yoshiyama, M; Matsuzawa, A; Ichijo, H; Iwao, H. Apoptosis signal-regulating kinase 1 plays a pivotal role in angiotensin II-induced cardiac hypertrophy and remodeling. *Circ. Res.*, 2003, 93(9), 874-883.

[11] Katada, J; Majima, M. AT(2) receptor-dependent vasodilation is mediated by activation of vascular kinin generation under flow conditions. *Br. J. Pharmacol.*, 2002, 136(4), 484-491.

[12] Avila, MD; Morgan, JP; Yan, X. Genetically modified mouse models used for studying the role of the AT2 receptor in cardiac hypertrophy and heart failure. *J. Biomed. Biotechnol.,* 2011, 141039. Epub 2011 Apr 27.

[13] Ichihara, S; Senbonmatsu, T; Price, E Jr; Ichiki, T; Gaffney, FA; Inagami, T. Angiotensin II type 2 receptor is essential for left ventricular hypertrophy and cardiac

fibrosis in chronic angiotensin II-induced hypertension. *Circulation*, 2001, 104(3), 346-351.

[14] Akishita, M; Iwai, M; Wu, L; Zhang, L; Ouchi, Y; Dzau, VJ; Horiuchi, M. Inhibitory effect of angiotensin II type 2 receptor on coronary arterial remodeling after aortic banding in mice. *Circulation*, 2000, 102(14), 1684-1689.

[15] Bodiga, S; Zhong, JC; Wang, W; Basu, R; Lo, J; Liu, GC; Guo, D; Holland, SM; Scholey, JW; Penninger, JM; Kassiri, Z; Oudit, GY. Enhanced susceptibility to biomechanical stress in ACE2 null mice is prevented by loss of the p47phox NADPH oxidase subunit. *Cardiovasc. Res.*, 2011, 91(1), 151-161.

[16] Santos, RAS; Simoes e Silva, AC; Maric, C; Silva, DMR; Machado, RP; Buhr, I, et al. Angiotensin-(1–7) is an endogenous ligand for the G-protein coupled receptor Mas. *Proc. Natl. Acad. Sci. USA*, 2003, 100, 8258–8263.

[17] Qi, Y; Shenoy, V; Wong, F; Li, H; Afzal, A; Mocco, J; Sumners, C; Raizada, MK; Katovich, MJ. Lentiviral mediated overexpression of Angiotensin-(1-7) attenuated ischemia-induced cardiac pathophysiology. *Exp. Physiol.*, 2011, Jun 17. [Epub ahead of print].

[18] Fiordaliso, F; De Angelis, N; Bai, A; Cuccovillo, I; Salio, M; Serra, DM; Bianchi, R; Razzetti, R; Latini, R; Masson, S. Effect of beta-adrenergic and renin-angiotensin system blockade on myocyte apoptosis and oxidative stress in diabetic hypertensive rats. *Life Sci.*, 2007, 81(12), 951-959.

[19] Aneja, A; Tang, WH; Bansilal, S; Garcia, MJ; Farkouh, ME. Diabetic cardiomyopathy: insights into pathogenesis, diagnostic challenges, and therapeutic options. *Am. J. Med.*, 2008, 121(9), 748-757.

[20] Tarquini, R; Lazzeri, C; Pala, L; Rotella, CM; Gensini, GF. The diabetic cardiomyopathy. *Acta Diabetol.*, Mar 2010 [Epub ahead of print].

[21] Rajesh, M; Mukhopadhyay, P; Batkai, S; Patel, V; Saito, K; Matsumoto, S; Kashiwaya, Y; Horváth, B; Mukhopadhyay, B; Becker, L; Hasko, G; Liaudet, L; Wink, DA; Veves, A; Mechoulam, R; Pacher, P. Cannabidiol attenuates cardiac dysfunction, oxidative stress, fibrosis, and inflammatory and cell death signaling pathways in diabetic cardiomyopathy. *J. Am. Coll. Cardiol.*, 2010, 56(25), 2115-2125.

[22] Asbun, J; Villarreal, FJ. The pathogenesis of myocardial fibrosis in the setting of diabetic cardiomyopathy. *J. Am. Coll. Cardiol.*, 2006, 47(4), 693-700.

[23] Kavantzas, NG; Lazaris, AC; Agapitos, EV; Nanas, J; Davaris, PS. Histological assessment of apoptotic cell death in cardiomyopathies. *Pathology*, 2000, 32, 176–180.

[24] Narula, J; Pandey, P; Arbustini, E; Haider, N; Narula, N; Kolodgie, FD; Dal Bello, B; Semigran, MJ; Bielsa-Masdeu, A; Dec, GW; Israels, S; Ballester, M; Virmani, R; Saxena, S; Kharbanda, S. Apoptosis in heart failure: release of cytochrome c from mitochondria and activation of caspase-3 in human cardiomyopathy. *Proc. Nat. Acad. Sci. USA*, 1999, 96 (14), 8144–8149.

[25] Yamazaki, T; Komuro, I; Yazaki, Y. Role of the renin-angiotensin system in cardiac hypertrophy. Am J Cardiol, 1999, 83(12A), 53H-57H.

[26] Kinouchi, K; Ichihara, A; Itoh, H. Functional characterization of (pro)renin receptor in association with V-ATPase. *Front Biosci.*, 2011, 17, 3216-3223.

[27] De Angelis, N; Fiordaliso, F; Latini, R; Calvillo, L; Funicello, M; Gobbi, M; Mennini, T; Masson, S. Appraisal of the role of angiotensin II and aldosterone in ventricular

myocyte apoptosis in adult normotensive rat. *J. Mol. Cell Cardiol.*, 2002, 34(12), 1655-1665.

[28] Fiordaliso, F; Leri, A; Cesselli, D; Limana, F; Safai, B; Nadal-Ginard, B; Anversa, P; Kajstura, J. Hyperglycemia activates p53 and p53- regulated genes leading to myocyte cell death. *Diabetes*, 2001, 50 (10), 2363–2375.

[29] Beers, MF; Solarin, KO; Guttentag, SH; Rosenbloom, J; Kormilli, A; Gonzales, LW; Ballard, PL. TGF-beta1 inhibits surfactant component expression and epithelial cell maturation in cultured human fetal lung. *Am. J. Physiol.,* 1998, 275(5 Pt 1), L950-960.

[30] Kajstura, J; Fiordaliso, F; Andreoli, AM; Li, B; Chimenti, S; Medow, MS; Limana, F; Nadal-Ginard, B; Leri, A; Anversa, P. IGF-1 overexpression inhibits the development of diabetic cardiomyopathy and angiotensin-II-mediated oxidative stress. *Diabetes,* 2001, 50, 1414–1424.

[31] Arozal, W; Watanabe, K; Veeraveedu, PT; Ma, M; Thandavarayan, RA; Suzuki, K; Tachikawa, H; Kodama, M; Aizawa, Y. Effects of angiotensin receptor blocker on oxidative stress and cardio-renal function in streptozotocin-induced diabetic rats. *Biol. Pharm. Bull.*, 2009, 32(8), 1411-1416.

[32] Shiuchi, T; Iwai, M; Li, HS; Wu, L; Min, LJ; Li, JM; Okumura, M; Cui, TX; Horiuchi, M. Angiotensin II type-1 receptor blocker valsartan enhances insulin sensitivity in skeletal muscles of diabetic mice. *Hypertension,* 2004, 43(5), 1003-1010.

In: Angiotensin: New Research
Editors: S. Harada, I. Moi, pp. 215-271

ISBN: 978-1-62100-773-9

Chapter 11

HYPERTENSION A RISK FACTOR FOR AGE-RELATED MACULAR DEGENERATION: ROLE OF ANGIOTENSIN II

Maria E. Marin-Castaño*

From the Department of Ophthalmology, Bascom Palmer Eye institute,
University of Miami, Miami, FL, U.S.A.

1. ABSTRACT

The goal of this chapter is to review the most relevant scientific evidence supporting the role of Angiotensin II (Ang II), the major hormone associated with hypertension, in the pathogenesis of dry age-related macular degeneration (AMD), a leading cause of blindness among the elderly and to highlight the importance of hypertension treatment to reduce the risk for developing AMD. AMD is a late onset (after age 50), progressive degeneration of the retina associated with vision loss coupled with a spectrum of specific clinical, physiological and histopathological features. The early or dry stage of AMD is characterized by the accumulation of drusen, specific lipid rich deposits under the retina whereas the late or wet stage is characterized by growth of abnormal new vessels under the retinal pigment epithelium (RPE) from the subjacent choroid, termed choroidal neovascularization (CNV). Extracellular matrix turnover (ECM) and inflammation are key cellular processes that play a central role in the pathogenesis of AMD. The scientific evidence to support the proposed role of Ang II-mediated RPE effects on subretinal deposits formation and inflammation is reviewed in depth.

Keywords: Age-related Macular Degeneration, system renin-angiotensin, hypertension, Angiotensin II, Angiotensin II receptors, response to injury, blebbing, extracellular matrix turnover, sub-RPE deposits, inflammation, animal model.

---

* Reprint requests: Maria E. Marin-Castaño, M.D., PhD, William L. McKnight Vision Research Center, 1638 N.W. 10th Avenue, Miami, FL 33136, Tel.: (305) 482-5142, E-mail: mcastano@med.miami.edu

2. The System Renin Angiotensin

Knowledge of the renin–angiotensin system (RAS) has advanced remarkably over recent years from that of a classical endocrine system that explained homeostasis for maintenance of circulating intravascular volume and thereby restoration of arterial pressure to a newer concept including a number of local RASs that operate independently within several organs. Classically, the systemic RAS basically depends upon its rate-limiting enzyme renin which is produced in the juxtaglomerular apparatus of the kidney. Thus, with the release of renin from the juxtaglomerular apparatus, it gains access to the circulation where it acts on its protein substrate angiotensinogen (an alpha-2 globulin synthesized by the liver) to generate the decapeptide angiotensin I. In turn, angiotensin I is converted by the angiotensin converting enzyme 1 (ACE1), which is predominantly expressed in high concentrations on the surface of endothelial cells in the pulmonary circulation [1], into the octapeptide angiotensin II (Ang II) by cleavage of the terminal dipeptide from the parent decapeptide. The result is freely circulating Ang II, the most important hormone associated with hypertension (Figure 1). Ang II effects are mediated by the type 1 (AT1) a type 2 (AT2) Ang II cell surface receptors which belong to a group of seven-transmembrane domain G-protein coupled receptors and have a 30% sequence similarity and different functional properties and signal transduction mechanisms [2, 3]. In rodents, AT1 receptors can be subdivided into AT1a and AT1b subtypes [4, 5], which share 95% sequence homology and exhibit similar ligand binding affinities and signal-transduction properties, but differ in their tissue expression.

RAS acts as a feedback system, in which Ang II is traditionally considered the main regulatory peptide and ACE1, the main regulatory enzyme and AT1 receptor, the main regulatory receptor. In view of controlling blood pressure, the most important actions of Ang II are vasoconstriction, sympathetic nervous stimulation, increased aldosterone biosynthesis and renal actions [6]. These Ang II effects elicit tissue responses mainly via AT1 receptors. In fact, according to recent evidence, the circulating RAS is not thought to be directly responsible for the rise in blood pressure especially in essential hypertension in elderly people, but there are more important non-circulating "local" renin-angiotensin autocrine or paracrine systems, which have important roles in adjusting blood pressure and regional blood flow [7].

As mentioned above, in addition to the circulatory RAS, there is a tissue-localized system which has been known for some time and which is known to regulate long-term changes in a variety of organs like kidneys, adrenals, brain, reproductive organs and vasculature [8-10]. In tissues, Ang II is derived either from the circulation or from local production. Local Ang II formation can also be catalyzed by enzymes other than the classical ACE. These actions are called renin-independent or ACE-independent pathways for Ang II production e.g. via chymase or cathepsin G, but they may have a minor role and evidence-based studies are warranted [10]. By blocking the activity of these enzymes, Ang II production can be reduced. In addition to these ACE-independent enzymes, there is an important, recently found RAS component: angiotensin-converting enzyme 2 (ACE2). ACE2 can degrade Ang I to Ang [2-10] and Ang II to form the biologically active Ang [1-7], which in turn and in many respects acts oppositely to Ang II [11]. Ang [1-7] mainly acts via a novel angiotensin receptor type, Mas receptor. Mas receptor is a G-protein-coupled receptor encoded by the Mas protooncogene found first in the mouse kidney [12]. The activation of Mas receptor causes effects opposite to the AT1 receptor activation, such as vasodilatation, antiproliferation, antifibrosis and it plays a role in fluid volume homeostasis [13]. All of these alternative pathways for Ang II production and for degradation are important both physiologically and pathophysiologically. In addition to these above-mentioned alternative pathways of local RAS activatory and inhibitory components, there is an interesting receptor type, a tissue (pro)renin receptor (PRR) which seems to act in the kidney, the heart and in the retina [14, 15]. PRR-bound renin and prorenin display increased enzymatic activity, and binding activates intracellular signalling, up-regulating the expression of profibrotic proteins. According to experimental studies, it is involved (independently of renin) in adult and embryonic stem cell biology, embryonic development and diseases including diabetic retinopathy [14, 15].

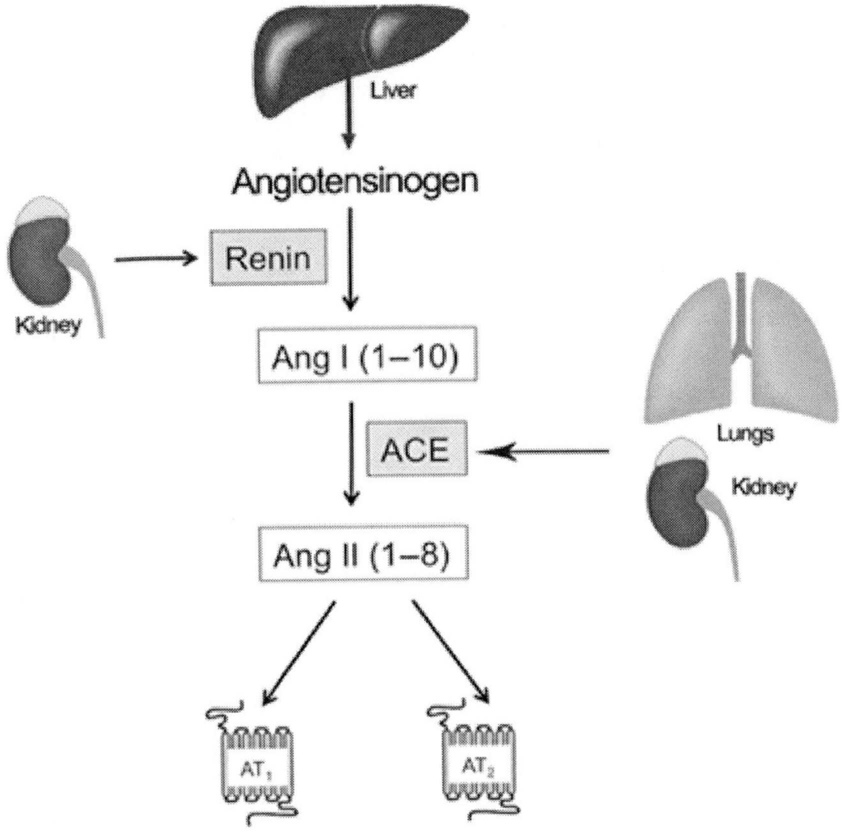

Figure 1. The renin–angiotensin system (RAS). The juxtaglomerular apparatus of the kidney produces renin. Renin cleaves its protein substrate angiotensinogen, which is synthesized by the liver, generating the decapeptide Ang I. In turn, Ang I is converted by the ACE in the pulmonary circulation and renal endothelium into the octapeptide Ang II by cleavage of the terminal dipeptide from the parent decapeptide. ACE, angiotensin-converting enzyme; Ang, angiotensin; AT1, angiotensin receptor type 1; AT2, angiotensin receptor type 2.

3. Effects of Angiotensin II

Ang II, a major effector of RAS, is know as a vasoconstrictor, however, recent studies have shown its role as a potent mediator in the regulation of blood pressure and volume, thirst, sympathetic nervous activity, vascular remodeling, cell growth and differentiation, apoptosis, and inflammatory mechanisms among others. These universal paracrine and autocrine actions may be important in many organ systems and can mediate important physiological stimuli becoming increasingly important in the study of organ physiology but also for a fresh look at the implications of these findings for organ pathophysiology.

Blood Pressure and Sodium–Volume Homeostasis

Ang II, increases arterial blood pressure through Ang II type AT1 receptor-dependent arterial vasoconstriction and by decreasing renal salt and water excretion through extrarenal and intrarenal mechanisms. AT2 receptors are assumed to oppose these responses mediated by AT1 receptors, thereby attenuating the pressor effects of Ang II.

Ang II causes the kidneys to retain salt and water through extrarenal and intrarenal mechanisms [16]. Ang II increases sympathetic nerve stimulation, which increases renal tubular sodium reabsorption directly or indirectly through renal vasoconstriction. Moreover, Ang II stimulates the synthesis and secretion of aldosterone from the adrenal cortex, and aldosterone in turn increases salt and water reabsorption by the distal tubule [17, 18]. Within the kidney, Ang II increases predominantly proximal tubular sodium reabsorption. It also induces renal microvascular constriction, in particular of the efferent arterioles. This helps maintaining the glomerular filtration rate and tends to increase sodium reabsorption by altering peritubular capillary physical forces [19]. During hypovolemia (for example, hemorrhagic shock) and in sodium-deficient states, intrarenal Ang II levels are elevated and, in turn, increase both renal sodium and water reabsorption, thereby playing an important physiological role in maintaining circulating volume and blood pressure [16, 20].

Intracardiac Effects

The existence and function of a specific cardiac RAS has been a matter of debate since it has been difficult to differentiate the effects of intracardiac Ang II generation from actions by plasma-borne Ang II. Nevertheless, it has become quite clear that cardiac actions of drugs inhibiting Ang II actions such as ACE inhibitors and Ang II receptor blockers are in part explained by local effects at the cellular level.The predominant physiological role of the cardiac RAS appears to be the maintenance of an appropriate cellular milieu balancing stimuli inducing and inhibiting cell growth and proliferation as well as mediating adaptive responses to myocardial stress.

a) Inotropic Effects

It was suggested that supraphysiological concentration of Ang II acts as an inotropic agent [21]. Direct effects by Ang II have been verified [22], which are thought to be mediated by intracellular calcium influx and changes of the plateau phase of the cardiac action potential. In vitro studies in human preparations carried out physiological conditions in right atrial and right and left ventricular myocardial preparations of patients with a variety of cardiac diseases suggested that Ang II exerts positive inotropic effects only in atrial preparations [23]. However, transgenic overexpression of the human AT1 receptor on cardiac myocytes in a transgenic rat model has supported the early findings since transgenic AT1 upregulation led to an enhanced intracellular calcium response after Ang II stimulation [24].

b) Hypertrophic Effects

Ang II mediates myocyte hypertrophy due to activation of the AT1 receptor as an adaptive response to increased myocardial stress. Left ventricular hypertrophy due to enhanced Ang II production in the heart has also been described in transgenic rat models with overexpression of RAS components such as mouse renin [25], human AT1 receptor [24, 26], human ACE [27, 28], and double transgenic rats expressing human renin and human angiotensinogen [29]. In some of these models it has been clearly shown that the Ang II effects occur independently from its effects on blood pressure, suggesting a functional role of the local cardiac RAS in mediating these changes. Hypertrophic changes induced by Ang II are mediated by several distinct intracellular pathways such as the activation of tyrosine kinase and RhoA cascades which include activation of mitogen activated protein kinase MAPK and JAK/STAT pathways [30-33]. While the AT2 receptor has been initially associated with antihypertrophic effects [34], some studies in AT2-deficient mice indicated that AT2 has a significant effect on cardiac hypertrophy induced by aortic banding [35] or Ang II infusion [36].

c) Apoptosis

Whereas earlier studies carried out in a rat pheochromocytoma cell line have suggested that programmed cell death is mediated by the AT2 receptor [37], it is generally accepted that apoptosis of cardiac myocytes is mediated via the AT1 receptor [38]. The process is thought to be involved in cardiac remodeling, for example, after myocardial infarction [39], hypertensive cardiomyopathy [40], and diabetic cardiomyopathy [41]. It can be effectively blocked by AT1 antagonists [42], which suggest that the beneficial effects of RAS blockade in heart failure could be due in part to this intracardiac mechanism.

Vascular effects

The vascular wall is the effector organ for the hormonal or plasma RAS where AT1 receptors localized on vascular smooth muscle cells mediate vasoconstriction. The concept of a vascular RAS was generated when it became evident that Ang II can differentially affect growth properties of vascular cells and those RAS components can be formed intracellularly in the vasculature.

a) Vascular Tone and Endothelial Function

In response to either systemically or locally generated Ang II, the AT1 receptor mediates the contractile response by phospholipase C-dependent mechanisms leading to an increase in intracellular calcium [30, 43]. It also acts indirectly, by stimulating the synthesis of other vasoconstrictors such as endothelin-1 [44-46]. In contrast, activation of AT2 receptors results in activation of protein phosphatases, thereby reversing the effects mediated by Ang II binding to AT1 receptors [47]. Thus the AT2 receptor appears to mediate mechanisms that are counterregulatory and prevent the occurrence of pathological vascular changes [48, 49]. The functional role of the AT_2 receptor was primarily seen during fetal development during which AT2 is highly expressed [50, 51]. Subsequently, reappearance of AT2 in the adult organism was associated with pathological events that can be viewed as fetal-reprogramming. This, however, does not rule out the possibility that AT2 plays an important role for the regulation of vascular tone and blood pressure under physiological conditions [52]. Indeed, a large body of evidence obtained primarily in animals supports a role for AT2 receptor-mediated vasodilation [52-54]. Importantly, however, this vasodilatory role of AT2 has been also clearly demonstrated in human coronary microarteries [52, 55], while the effects in larger human coronary arteries [52] and human forearm resistance vessels [56] were not significant [52, 55]. Collectively, the vasodilatory effect mediated by AT2 receptors appears to be predominantly attributable to direct activation of the nitric oxide (NO)-cGMP pathway, while indirect activation of NO via bradykinin and B2 receptors as mediators of AT2-induced vasodilation is less well established [52]. However, recent experimental work in hypertensive rats clearly demonstrates that AT2 receptor-mediated vasodilatation in vivo depends on the blood pressure status [57]. In addition to the modulation of vascular tone by Ang II via the NO-cGMP pathway, research carried out during the last decade has clearly shown that the effects of Ang II in the vasculature are mediated at least in part by the modification of the redox milieu of its target cells [58]. Ang II has been shown to activate the vascular nicotinamide adenine dinucleotide phosphate (NADPH) oxidase(s) resulting in the production of reactive oxygen species (ROS), namely, superoxide and hydrogen peroxide [58-64]. Consequently, Ang II is capable of increasing NO bioavailability by activation NO-cGMP pathway via AT2 and decreasing NO bioavailability by promoting oxidative stress via the AT1 receptor [58, 59, 65]. In this regard, Ang II plays an important role in modulating the balance between NO and ROS in the endothelium and thereby maintaining homeostasis of the vascular wall. Oxidative stress has been shown to play a critical role in the development of endothelial dysfunction and hypertension and atherosclerosis [58, 65, 66]. Nevertheless, the relative contribution of redox-independent hemodynamic mechanisms and oxidative stress in maintaining vascular function and their modulation by Ang II via AT1 and AT2 receptors needs further in-depth analysis.

b) Tissue Remodeling

In addition to the well-established long-term effects of the RAS on vascular remodeling that are mediated by proliferative effects on vascular smooth muscle cells and fibroblast [67-71], the production of ROS by NAD(P)H oxidase in response to Ang II has been demonstrated as an important mechanism linking activation of the RAS to events such as inflammation, atherosclerosis, hypertrophy, remodeling, and angiogenesis [58, 59, 65].

The production of ROS by NAD(P)H oxidase in response to Ang II stimulation in endothelial and vascular smooth muscle cells activates signal pathways such as MAP kinases, tyrosine kinases, and transcription factors that lead to these events [58, 59, 60, 65]. In the Ang II/AT1-driven processes leading to vascular damage and chronic atherosclerosis by increased production of ROS by Ang II, additional mechanisms such as low-density lipoprotein (LDL) oxidation and uptake, increased LDL-receptor expression [72, 73], increased expression of molecular mediators of inflammation such as nuclear factor-kappaB (NFκB) or cell adhesion molecules such as vascular cell adhesion molecule (VCAM)-1 or intercellular adhesion molecule (ICAM)-1 is involved [74-77]. In addition, chemokines and proinflammatory cytokines are activated [74,76]. Moreover, apoptotic changes in response to Ang II in the vascular wall have been described [78]. This, in addition to Ang II-induced modulation of extracellular matrix (ECM) components by matrix metalloproteinases (MMPs) and tissue inhibitors of MMPs (TIMPs), may play a role in vascular remodeling [79, 80] including processes such as the disruption of the normal endothelial layer in early atherosclerosis or plaque rupture in more advanced atherosclerosis [81]. Moreover, AT1 and AT2 receptors have been shown to induce opposing effects on vascular smooth muscle cell growth [82]. The AT2 receptor may again be considered as a balancing principle that counteracts many of the mechanisms indicated above that are mediated by the AT1 receptor.

c) Angiogenesis

It was demonstrated that Ang II stimulates angiogenesis, acting via AT1 receptors within the subcutaneous sponge granuloma model in the rat and that AT1 and AT2 receptors and ACE develop sequentially during microvascular maturation [83]. Studies in AT2-deficient mice and wild-type mice using the surgically induced hindlimb ischemia model indicated that AT2 confers an antiangiogenic effect that is associated with activation of apoptosis [84]. This experiment would question the beneficial role of AT2 stimulation in the context of pharmacological AT1 blockade in ischemic tissues. Interestingly, Ac-SDKP, a mediator of angiogenesis, which is inactivated by ACE, has been shown to promote neovascularization in the cornea and capillary density in the heart [85].

Central Nervous System

The postulation of an independent brain RAS was one of the first indications of the presence of local Ang formation in tissues. Specific central Ang II actions were shown by Bickerton and Buckley [86]. Moreover, several authors [35, 87] could demonstrate an interaction between Ang II and the autonomous nervous system. These data soon led to the identification of RAS components in the brain.

a) Central Neurons

Ang II activates the AT1 receptors to induce a cascade of intra-neuronal signaling events that ultimately leads to changes in membrane potential and an increase in neuronal firing [88]. Activation of neurons in cardiovascular control brain regions, such as the subfornical organ, paraventricular nucleus and rostral ventral lateral medulla, results in stimulation of the sympathetic nervous system, which mediates, at least partly, the cardiovascular complications associated with hypertension and heart failure [89, 90]. Accumulating evidence over the past 8–10 years has established that Ang II increases levels of ROS by NADPH oxidase activation, particularly $O_2{\bullet}^-$, in neurons that contribute to the increase in neuronal activation [91-97] thus, identifying $O_2{\bullet}^-$ as an important Ang II intra-neuronal signaling intermediate that leads to an increase in neuronal activity and elevated sympathetic output.

Reproductive Tract

a) Ovary

Ang II is able to induce estrogen release by in vitro pregnant mare serum gonadotrophin stimulated immature rat ovaries, suggesting that Ang II promotes follicular maturation [98]. In contrast, Morris et al. [99] suggested that Ang II inhibited estradiol (tonic inhibition by endogenous Ang II), increased progesterone formation in human cultured luteinized granulosa cells, and also increased testosterone in cultured rabbit theca cells [100].

Ovulation induced by pregnant mare serum gonadotropin in either immature rats or a perfused rat ovary system was inhibited in the presence of an Ang II receptor antagonist [101, 102]. In gonadotropin-treated rabbits, the nonselective Ang II receptor antagonist saralasin is able to inhibit ovulation [103]. This effect could not be shown by inhibition of ACE [104]. Kuji et al. [105] reported that Ang II facilitates follicular development and ovulation in the rabbit via the AT2 receptor, since an AT2 receptor antagonist (PD123319) inhibited Ang II-induced ovulation and oocyte maturation in vitro, as well as Ang II-induced estrogen and prostaglandin formation. But others [101, 106] using the same Ang II receptor antagonist, or an ACE inhibitor were unable to fully replicate the inhibition of ovulation. Steele et al. [107] also saw no impairment of ovulation in rats that were systemically administered an Ang II antagonist or an ACE inhibitor. The treatment of women of child-bearing age for hypertension with the ACE inhibitor enalapril did not affect normal cyclicity of plasma gonadotrophins, gonadal steroids, or plasma prorenin [108]. Life-long application of ACE inhibitors to rats did not impair fertility [109]. In contrast to this local situation, there was a profoundly reduced ovulation by administration of Ang II receptor antagonist or ACE inhibitor [107].

b) Uterus

It was suggested that the local function of Ang II on the uterus may be to control uterine blood flow during pregnancy [110]. As might be expected, the contractile actions of Ang II in the human uterus are mediated by AT1 receptors [111, 112]. The contractile response of the rat uterus to Ang II and both AT1 and AT2 receptor density vary considerably over the estrous cycle [113].

Skin

a) Wound Healing and REPAIR

Previous studies described a proliferative and antiproliferative effect of Ang II in the skin which appears to be mediated by AT1 and AT2 receptors [114-118].

Quantitative autoradiography demonstrated that the expression of Ang II receptors was significantly enhanced during experimental wound healing. Young rat skin normally contains mainly AT1 receptors, but during experimental wound healing a selective and localized increase in expression of AT2 receptors occurs [119]. This study suggested skin fibroblasts as the primary target cells for Ang II. Other investigators [120] have found significant decreases in the number of AT1 receptors and a modest but not statistically significant appearance of AT2 receptors in adult rat skin during wound healing. This is not necessarily a contradiction and could be an indication for the importance of the proportion or balance of these two receptors. Abiko et al. [121] have shown that an immediate and transient reduction in Ang II receptor expression occurred after wounding rat skin, followed by an increase in the number of the receptors that was maintained for 5–7 days, and that the receptors were predominantly of the AT1 receptor subtype. In a cutaneous repair model, Sun et al. [122] have shown that the appearance of myofibroblasts is associated with Ang II generation which regulates fibrogenesis by AT1 receptor binding. In rat skin slices, Ang II binding to AT1 receptors increases inositol phosphate production, while binding to AT2 decreases inositol phosphate production; thus both receptors play opposite roles [123]. It has to be noted that it was unclear in the two former studies in which cell type the Ang II receptor regulation and signal transduction occurred [122, 123]. Further investigation has suggested a mitogenic effect of Ang II of keratinocytes via a non-AT1, non-AT2 receptor [117].

Digestive Organs

a) Pancreas

The pancreatic RAS appears to regulate secretion of pancreatic hormones. There is a growing body of clinical evidence implicating the RAS in islet function. In this aspect, Ang II suppressed glucose-dependent insulin release in islets [124, 125]. In concordance, islet blood flow was decreased by local Ang II and this effect could be attenuated with a RAS blocker [126, 127]. AT1 receptor expression in β-cells is upregulated in obesity-induced animal model of diabetes type 2, i.e., db/db mice, and giving these mice with the AT1 blocker losartan decreased their blood glucose levels while improving their glucose tolerance and increasing their insulin secretion and pro-insulin biosynthesis [128]. Similar effects were also found in other diabetes type 2 animal model, such as the Zucker diabetic fatty rat [129, 130].

Continued islet functionality depends on maintenance of β-cell mass, which is determined by a balance between apoptosis and proliferation. Islet β-cell areas were reduced in db/db mice, but this deficit could be reversed by treatment with the AT1 blocker valsartan [131]. The decreased β-cell area in db/db mice may due to an imbalance between islet cell apoptosis and proliferation, islet oxidative stress, and/or inflammation-related islet fibrosis [132]. On the other hand, AT2 receptors appear not to play a direct role in glucose-induced insulin secretion, though they can stimulate somatostatin expression in a dose-dependent manner [133].

In summary, islet RAS, notably by activation of the AT1 receptors, regulates pancreatic islet insulin and somatostatin secretion, influences islet function, and thus regulates the body's glucose homeostasis. The AT1 receptor is expressed at abnormally high levels under diabetic conditions [128], and AT1 receptor antagonism can enhance insulin secretion, pro-insulin biosynthesis, islet blood flow, β-cell mass, and glucose homeostasis [126, 128, 134]. Moreover, Ang II has been implicated in a number of pathophysiologic processes with the potential to indirectly or directly influence the pathogenesis of insulin resistance and type 2 diabetes [135].

b) Intestine

Ang II causes a contractile response in the rat ileum but not in the duodenum [136], pointing to a role in inducing peristaltic waves. In the ileum, the contraction is caused by the longitudinal smooth muscle and is mediated by the AT1. Jaszewski et al. [137] have reported that mucosal levels of Ang I and II were elevated in patients with Crohn's colitis versus normal subjects and other forms of colitis and that mucosal levels of Ang I and Ang II correlated well with the degree of macroscopic inflammation in Crohn's disease.

Table 1. Localization of RAS components in ocular tissues in different species

RAS molecule	Eye part	Species	References
Prorenin	Retina	Human	Sramek et al., 1988
	Ciliary body	Human	Danser et al., 1989
	Vitreous body	Human	
Renin	Retina	Human, rabbit	Danser et al., 1989
	Ciliary body	Rabbit	Wagner et al., 1996
	Choroid	Human, rabbit	Ramirez et al., 1996
	Iris	Rabbit	
	Vitreous body	Human, rabbit	
	Aqueous humor	Rabbit	
Angiotensinogen	Retina	Human, rabbit	Sramek et al., 1992
	Ciliary body	Human, rabbit	Ramirez et al., 1996
	Choroid	Human, rabbit	Wagner et al., 1996
	Iris	Human, rabbit	
	Vitreous body	Human, rabbi	
	Aqueous humor	Rabbit	
ACE1	Retina	Dog, monkey, human	Vita et al., 1981
		Rabbit, porcine	Weinreb et al., 1985
	Ciliary body	Human, rabbit, porcine	Immonen et al.1987
	Choroid	Dog, monkey, human	Ramirez et al., 1996
		Rabbit, porcine	Wagner et al., 1996
	Sclera	Dog, monkey	Shiota et al., 1997
	Iris	Rabbit, porcine	Geng et al., 2003
	Cornea	Human	Savaskan et al., 2004
	Vitreous body	Dog, monkey, rabbit	
	Aqueous humor	Human, dog, monkey, rabbit	
	Tear fluid	Human, rabbit	
ACE2	Retina	Rodent	Tikellis et al., 2004
		Human	Senanayake et al., 2007
Chymase	Choroid	Dog	Shiota et al., 1997
	Sclera	Dog	Maruichi et al., 2004
	Vitreous body	Human	
AT1 receptor	Retina	Human	Savaskan et al., 2004
	Cornea	Human	Senanayake et al., 2007
	RPE	Human	Striker et al., 2008
	RPE	Rodent	Praddaude et al., 2009
AT2 receptor	Retina	Human	Senanayake et al., 2007
	RPE	Human	Striker et al., 2008
	RPE	Rodent	Praddaude et al., 2009
Ang I	Retina	Porcine	Danser et al., 1994
	Choroid	Porcine	
	Vitreous body	Porcine, human	
	Aqueous humor	Human	
Ang II	Retina	Human, porcine, rabbit	Danser et al., 1994
	Ciliary body	Human, rabbit	Ramirez et al., 1996
	Choroid	Porcine, human, rabbit	Savaskan et al., 2004
	Iris	Rabbit	Senanayake et al., 2007
	Cornea	Human	
	Vitreous body	Porcine, human, rabbit	
	Aqueous humor	Human, rabbit	
Ang 1-7	RPE	Rodent	Praddaude et al., 2009
	Retina	Human	Senanayake et al., 2007

c) Colon

It has been demonstrated that Ang II stimulated fluid transfer and sodium transport in segments of isolated rat proximal colon. Further investigation suggested that Ang II stimulated a coupled NaCl transport [138]. In rat distal colon, Ang II can stimulate intestinal water transport via an electroneutral mechanism already at subpressor doses; this is a specific effect and in contrast to aldosterone which stimulates intestinal sodium and water transport by electrogenic mechanisms [139] involving the epithelial sodium channel [140].

4. Local Ocular Renin Angiotensin System

Ophthalmic literature concerning the RAS started in 1977 with a study by Igic and coworkers [141] on the detection of ACE activity in homogenates of the retina. Since then, expression and localization of all components of the RAS have been well determined in adult eye tissues including the retinal pigment epithelium (RPE) (Table I), where the mediators of the RAS are locally released, conferring the molecular basis for a biological function of Ang II in the eye [142-145]. However, whether intraocular Ang II is originated from local production or from the blood compartment has been debated. It has been shown that neither Ang I, Ang II nor angiotensinogen are able to pass the blood-brain barrier and the barriers between eye and circulating blood are comparable to this [146, 147]. On the other hand, Ang II levels in the eye are higher than in plasma, indicating that there is a local production of Ang II in the eye [147, 148]. Therefore, increased local or tissue Ang II formation in the retina in the absence of elevated circulating Ang II may indeed be deleterious.

5. Age-Related Macular Degeneration and Hypertension

Age-related macular degeneration (AMD), a degenerative disease of the retina, is the leading cause of blindness in the elderly worldwide and has devastating consequences on an individual's quality of life [149-152]. As older people make up the fastest growing segment of the population, AMD is becoming a serious *public health* issue. AMD affects more than 1.75 million individuals in the United States and it is estimated that more than 300,000 new cases are diagnosed annually [149, 151]. Unless better *preventive* treatments emerge, this number is expected to climb and even reach epidemic proportions with the overall aging demographics [153]. Currently, there is no cure for AMD, and treatments are very limited. As a result, the development of preventive strategies is an area of great importance.

AMD occurs in *two* main *forms*: dry (early) and neovascular or wet (late) [154]. Early AMD is characterized by accumulation of drusen and other lipid rich extracellular deposits under the RPE [154-156]. During aging, deposits initially accumulate between the RPE and its basement membrane (called basal laminar deposit or BLD), but progression into AMD requires additional deposit formation within Bruch's membrane (BrM), (called basal linear deposit (BLiD) and "nodular" drusen). Ultimately, early AMD can progress into late or severe atrophic AMD characterized by death of RPE and photoreceptors (called geographic atrophy) [154, 155]. Late AMD is characterized by endothelial invasion and pathological CNV [154, 156]. Wet AMD is always preceded by early disease [154]. Death or dysfunction of retinal photoreceptors is the ultimate cause of vision loss [157]. However, the initial pathogenic target of AMD is the RPE, its ECM (called BrM), and the subjacent vascular bed (called choriocapillaris), the blood supply for the outer retina [158]. Atrophic AMD is the most common form, affecting approximately 85% of persons with AMD. As outlined above the accumulation of specific deposits under the RPE is a very prominent histopathologic feature of eyes with AMD [159-162] (Figure 2B). The formation of drusen is an active process with distinct biological pathways. However, lack of scientific consensus exists regarding the origin of drusen. Research from different groups has been based on the conceptually innovative RPE injury hypothesis which proposes that deposit formation and accumulation is secondary to chronic, repetitive but nonlethal RPE injury [163-169]. Irrespective of the injury, this model proposes that all stimuli result in a final common pathway of cellular responses that cause the actual deposits. Repetitive injury ultimately can kill RPE leading to late dry AMD [158]. More recently, inflammatory-derived injury stimuli have also been implicated, including oxidants, complement, immune complexes and factors produced by macrophages [164, 170, 171]. Inflammatory cells might be responsible for drusen progression into CNV by secretion of growth factors and cytokines that will damage the choriocapillaris and stimulate the invasion of neovessels into the subretinal space [172-174] (Figure 2C). To date, little is known about the pathogenesis of dry AMD and events or factors that convert the dry form of the disease to its wet form.

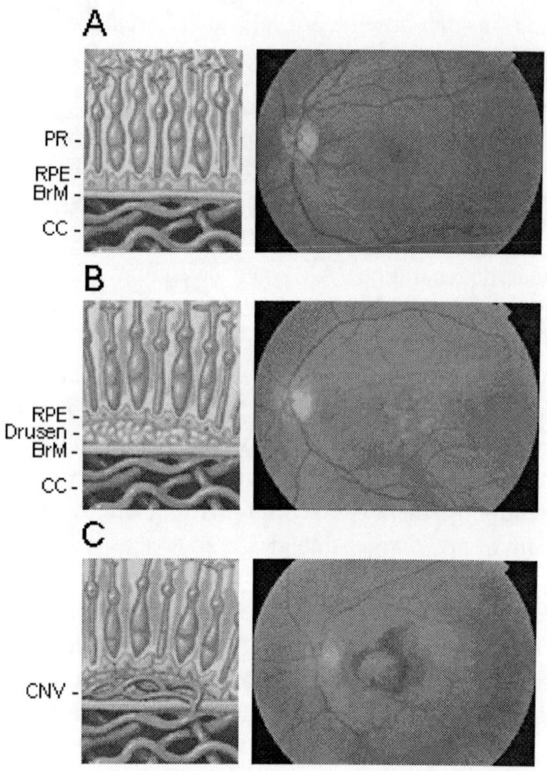

Figure 2. The pathologic changes to the macula, retina and choroidal blood vessels typical of dry AMD (B) and early wet AMD (C) respectively. Right panels; color fundus photographs of a normal macula (A), extensive solf, confluent drusen throughout the macula with subtle RPE drop-out (B), and acute sub-retinal blood (red lesions) in the macular area with subtle sub-retinal fluids and CNV (C). PR, *photoreceptors*; *RPE*, retinal pigment epithelium; BrM, Brusch's membrane; CC, choriocapillaries; CNV, choroidal neovascularization.

AMD pathogenesis is clearly multifactorial with genetic, systemic health and environmental factors. Epidemiologic studies have suggested a correlation between AMD and aging and hypertension [152, 175]. These studies indicate that aging is the risk factor with the greatest correlation with incidence, prevalence and severity of AMD, but the age-related susceptibility factors remain completely unknown [152, 175]. However, increased sensitivity to the injurious effects of hypertension and to oxidant-injury are all more severe in the elderly than in the young [176-178]. For exemple, the interaction of Ang II with AT1 receptors, produces ROS, and with advancing age, oxidative alterations accumulate in cellular components, including those in the antioxidative defense systems, due to disrupted redox regulation during aging can influence the gene transcription and signal transduction pathways.

Systemic vascular disease, especially hypertension, has long been suspected as a risk factor for AMD [152, 175, 179, 180]. In several cross sectional and case control studies, systemic hypertension was associated with increased prevalence and progression of AMD. Population based studies have also demonstrated an association between hypertension and AMD, but the magnitude of the association was relatively modest or not statistically significant. However, limitations with all of the epidemiologic studies may underestimate the importance of hypertension. The potential high importance of hypertension and drusen formation was demonstrated in a primate model of AMD. Jonas and coworkers induced renovascular hypertension in a subhuman primate model with or without high fat diet, and observed a dramatic increase in the severity and incidence of drusen [181]. No specific mechanism was determined by the investigators, but their observation is directly relevant to the pathogenesis of AMD. Moreover, a study by Nagai and colleagues suggests that Ang II is involved in the development of CNV in wet AMD through AT1 receptor activation, indicating the possibility of AT1 receptor blockade as a novel therapeutic strategy to inhibit CNV [182]. However, there is a complete lack of information regarding the contribution of Ang II signaling in the pathogenesis of dry AMD.

Traditionally, hypertension is believed to contribute to chronic diseases by at least two distinct mechanisms: hemodynamic injury and humoral factors [183-185]. Hemodynamic injury refers to mechanical damage induced by flow turbulence in large vessels or stretching of capillaries induced by increased blood pressure. Humoral factors refer to cellular activities induced by hormones or growth factors associated with hypertension [183, 184]. Among the most important is Ang II, which is upregulated in hypertension, present in the blood of many hypertensive patients and has been demonstrated to activate specific receptors to induce various cellular functions. Ang II as the molecular surrogate for the effects of hypertension in AMD, and its properties will be described below.

6. Subretinal Deposit Formation: Pathogenic Mechanisms

Drusen were first described nearly 160 years ago. However, the cellular and molecular events involved in their formation have not been fully elucidated. Lack of scientific consensus exists regarding the origin of drusen, but at least five different paradigms are currently proposed to explain deposit formation in AMD; a) genetic hypothesis, b) lysosomal failure/lipofuscin hypothesis, c) choroidal hypoperfusion hypothesis, d) barrier hypothesis, and e) RPE injury hypothesis. Because our research is based on the RPE injury hypothesis, in this section this theory is reviewed in light of the more recent finding.

As mentioned above, systemic hypertension is a systemic health factor associated with AMD severity [152, 175, 179, 180]. The interaction of Ang II with AT1 receptor produces ROS, and although no specific mechanism(s) have been determined, we believe that using Ang II as a surrogate for hypertension might directly contribute to the formation of drusen and late forms of AMD by an increase in oxidative stressors. Furthermore, based on receptor functions in other cells, we hypothesize that Ang II might damage RPE contributing to drusen pathogenesis.

There are a number of direct and/or indirect lines of evidence supporting a role for the RPE in drusen biogenesis. According to traditional models of drusen formation, any cellular material residing within drusen is predicted to be of RPE origin. Indeed, RPE-derived basal laminae, organelles and cellular fragments, and even entire cells can be detected in early "drusen". Some authors have described the appearance of RPE "debris" blebbing into drusen or pre-drusen sites [186]. RPE constituents, such as basal laminae, as well as lipofuscin and melanin granules, are observed within early drusen, where they likely contribute to drusen volume and formation.

The theory that drusen were derived from damaged RPE was originally postulated by Donders, who first described drusen in a post-mortem eye, believed that drusen were derived from RPE nuclei, based on the supposition that the latter are relatively resistant to degradation [187]. Donders' theory was later modified by De Vicentis (1887) who proposed that degenerative change in the RPE cytoplasm, rather than in the nucleus, was the precipitating event. On the other hand, Muller (1856) proposed that drusen result from aberrant secretion of basement membrane components by the aged RPE [188].With the advent of electron microscopy, the substructural features of drusen were revealed, and new variants of the earlier theories were advanced. Some investigators have concluded, that drusen are formed when the RPE expels portions of its basal cytoplasm into BrM [186], possibly as a mechanism for removing damaged cytosol [189] or as a product of phagocytic degradation [190]. Others have postulated that drusen are formed by autolysis of the RPE, due to aberrant lysosomal enzyme activity [191], although enzyme histochemical studies failed to demonstrate the presence of lysosomal enzymes in drusen [192]. Additional mechanisms for drusen formation, including lipoidal degeneration of the RPE [193, 194], have been proposed.

In the modern version, the RPE injury hypothesis proposes that deposit formation is secondary to chronic, repetitive but nonlethal RPE injury [165, 166]. Two separate phenomena must be distinguished: the injury stimulus and the cellular response. The most widely implicated injury stimuli are various oxidants, especially those induced by RPE exposure to visible light or those derived from endogenous metabolism [167, 168]. More recently, inflammatory-derived injury stimuli have also become implicated, including oxidants, complement, immune complexes and factors produced by macrophages or monocyte [171, 173, 174]. Inflammatory cells might be responsible for drusen progression into CNV by secretion of growth factors and cytokines that will damage the choriocapillaris and stimulate the invasion of neovessels into the subretinal space [172-174].

Irrespective of the injury, this model proposes that all stimuli result in a final common pathway of cellular responses that cause the actual deposits. Cellular responses that can lead to deposit formation include RPE cell membrane blebbing and dysregulation of ECM production and breakdown. Accumulation of sub-RPE blebbed material in the setting of imbalanced breakdown and resynthesis of basement membrane and BrM ECM is proposed to produce the various deposits of AMD. Repetitive injury ultimately can kill RPE, leading to late dry AMD [158].

7. Hypothetical Model for Dry AMD and its Progression to Wet

As mentioned above, our research is based on the RPE injury hypothesis. Oxidative injury-mediated non lethal RPE membrane blebbing, dysregulation of ECM turnover and inflammation are important in the formation of sub-RPE deposits. Our central hypothesis is that formation and progression of sub-RPE deposits requires three sequential processes: (1) initial RPE oxidative injury causing extrusion of blebs, which accumulate under the RPE as BLD; (2) subsequent dysregulation of RPE-derived molecules responsible for ECM turnover, leading to admixture of blebs into BrM as BLiD; and (3) altered macrophages recruitment. We postulate that the interaction of Ang II with AT1 receptor, one of the most important oxidative stress inducer: a) induces blebs formation through ROS production by activation of NADPH promoting bleb accumulation under the RPE as BLD and b) increases MMP-2 activity, MMP-14, and basigin, major mediator of *ECM* turnover through MAPK phosphorylation, and pro-inflammatory monocyte chemoattractant protein-1 (MCP-1) production through NF-kB activation by RPE stimulating RPE basement membrane breakdown and infiltration of pro-inflammatory macrophages to sub-RPE deposit areas, where they will scavenge, release inflammatory mediators, growth factors or other substances, which may promote complications and progression to CNV [172-174]. As discussed below, the effect of Ang II in the mentioned stages will be reviewed in depth.

8. Cell Membrane Blebbing: Role of Angiotensin Ii

We embrace the pathogenic paradigm based on the response-to-injury hypothesis which proposes that sub-RPE deposits originate from RPE-derived cell membrane blebs and dysregulation of ECM turnover induced by chronic nonlethal injury to the RPE in response to oxidative damage.We also propose that Ang II, one of the most important inducer of oxidative stress, contributes to the pathogeneis of AMD by causing oxidative damage to the RPE.

Nonlethal Blebbing

Membrane blebs can be described as spherical plasma membrane protrusions and can be associated with normal physiological responses induced by receptor activation such as cell movement, cytokinesis, and cell spreading [194]. The appearance of blebs on endothelial cells was introduced as a general manifestation of cellular injury by Chiang et al. in 1968 [195]. Nonlethal blebbing has been demonstrated to especially affect endothelial cells in carotid artery and lung [195, 196], epithelial cells in liver, embryonic kidney cells, and eye [197-200].

Blebbing was first introduced as a possible pathogenic mechanism in drusen formation by Feeney-Burns, who observed bleb-like structures in human drusen [186]. Subsequently Ryan's laboratory demonstrated RPE blebbing in monkeys with drusen, and in different rabbit models of RPE injury [189, 201, 202]. These observations demonstrated the occurrence of RPE blebbing in vivo. Our laboratory hypothesizes that nonlethal cell membrane blebbing is the primary cause for the accumulation of BLD that become BLinD and drusen. Blebbing is an early morphologic sign of cell injury which occurs immediately after exposure to a wide variety of toxic agents. However this process is different from lethal blebbing and apoptosis [203-205]. Several injury stimuli induce blebbing in nonocular cells, especially drugs, oxidants, physical membrane damage and certain cytokines [203, 206-211].

Membrane blebbing occurs through different cellular signaling cascades and is closely interrelated with the actin cytoskeleton [206, 212-219]. Cytoskeletal turnover is mediated by actin polymerizing protein system, which is a large system of interacting proteins.

The identity of these proteins is a rapidly growing field, and includes kinases, phosphatases, cleavage proteins, and elongating proteins. Their individual specific function and regulatory interactions remain essentially unknown and little information is available regarding the molecules that regulate the actin polymerizing protein system and disease pathogenesis. Interestingly, oxidant injury is an effective activator of increased cytoskeleton turnover, presumably secondary to direct oxidative changes of disulfide bonds within actin filaments [206, 220-223]. One of the best characterized inhibitor/ stabilizer of cytoskeleton turnover is heat shock protein 25/27 (Hsp25/27). This molecule belongs to the family of small heat shock proteins (which includes α-β crystallins) and serves a dual role as cytoskeleton stabilizer and chaperone protein [222-226].

Oxidant injury can induce a rapid upregulation and phosphorylation of Hsp25/27 protein [215-220]. Upon phosphorylation, Hsp25/27 acts as an F-actin cap-binding protein, binding to the active edge of a growing microfilament, causing a transient delay in actin cytoskeleton reassembly and repair [206, 212-229]. Transient delay in reassembly allows the unsupported plasma membrane to be forced outward by the hydrostatic forces of the cytoplasm, and a vesicle or bleb forms if cortical cytoskeleton and microfilaments do not completely reform within the outpouched membrane. Phosphorylation of Hsp25/27 is mediated through the MAPK cascade, but is directly phosphorylated by MAPKAP 2 kinase (MK2), which in turn is phosphorylated by p38 kinase [206, 230]. Thus, oxidative stress induces profound rearrangements of the actin cytoskeleton [220, 230] leading to membrane blebbing through the activation of p38 MAPK/Hsp27 pathway [221, 231]. We have reported that the RPE constitutively express phosphorylated Hsp27, and that its expression is increased in patients with dry AMD [232] providing novel evidence that phosphorylated Hsp27 may play a major role in the pathogenesis of AMD. Moreover, we showed that exposure of RPE cells to non lethal oxidative injury induces the transcriptional activation of Hsp27, accumulation of Hsp27 dimers and a rapid phosphorylation of Hsp27 as well as actin rearrangements into aggregates and membrane blebbing [232]. Our results not only showed that kinetics of p38 and ERK phosphorylation correlated well with that of Hsp27, but also that Hsp27 phosphorylation and F-actin aggregates formation were decreased after inhibition of either p38 or ERK signaling cascades. These observations suggest that p38 as well as ERK MAPK pathways are required for the optimal activation of Hsp27 leading to F-actin rearrangement and bleb formation in

RPE cells in response to oxidative stress [232]. Therefore, Hsp27 is an important mediator of RPE response to oxidative damage, which may contribute to injury-induced actin rearrangement and blebbing.

In addition to Hsp27/Hsp25, other important molecules such as small GTPases protein superfamily (RAS and Ral) have been involved in the regulation of the actin polymerizing protein system and oxidative stress [195, 233]. Membrane blebbing is RhoA-, Rho kinase (ROCK)-, and myosin light chain kinase (MLCK)-dependent, and blebs are devoid of actin, mDia1 and Arp2/3 [194]. Rals are small G proteins that cycle between an active GTP-bound state and an inactive GDP-bound state [234]. Ral GDP dissociation stimulator (RalGDS) was found to be an effector of Ras [235-237] and highly specific for RalA and RalB, whereby it facilitates the exchange of GDP for GTP on Rals [235, 238, 239]. Moreover, it has been demonstrated that RalGDS forms a cytosolic complex with β-arrestin, and that in response to formyl-Met-Leu-Phe (fMLP) receptor stimulation, RalGDS is released from β-arrestin and translocates to the plasma membrane.

RhoA is an additional small G protein that is implicated in regulating plasma membrane dynamics. RhoA is activated by Ang II and is necessary for AT1 receptor-induced stress fiber formation [240]. The proteins ROCK and mDia1 are both RhoA effectors and have been shown to play a role in changes in actin cytoskeletal reorganization. RhoA acts through ROCK to form stress fibers [240], and ROCK has been shown to be involved in cell contraction induced by Ang II [241]. mDia1 is a member of the ubiquitous formin protein family. These proteins are activated by interaction with Rho GTPases and are then able to mediate actin polymerization [242]. Overexpression of the GTP-Rho binding domain of mDia1 causes spontaneous membrane blebbing [243].

Ang II-stimulated membrane bleb formation involves RhoA. Furthermore, membrane blebbing activated by Ang II through AT1 receptor activation is attenuated in the presence of the β-arrestin amino-terminal domain, Ral GDP dissociation stimulator (RalGDS) β-arrestin binding domain, and short interfering RNA (siRNA) depletion of β-arrestin2 [197]. In addition, the inhibition of the downstream RhoA effectors ROCK and MLCK effectively attenuated AT1 receptor-mediated membrane blebbing. Thus, membrane blebbing in response to AT1 receptor signaling was dependent on β-arrestin2 and was mediated by a RhoA/ROCK/MLCK-dependent pathway providing evidence that agonist stimulation of AT1 receptor leads to plasma membrane blebbing responses by activation of RhoA and subsequent coupling to the ROCK/MLCK pathway [197].

We have used a genetically modified human RPE cell line containing green fluorescent protein anchored to the inner leaflet of the plasma membrane to demonstrate nonlethal blebbing in response to oxidative stress. Bebbing can be induced by oxidant injury with blue light, myeloperoxidase (MPO), hydroquinone (Monroy D., et al., IOVS, 2001, 42(4), ARVO Abstract, 4060; Suner I.J., et al. IOVS 2004; ARVO E-Abstract 1810) [163, 164], or Ang II (Figure 3). Cytoplasmic actin aggregates were observed after nonlethal blebbing, but not with lethal oxidant injury. Interestingly, activation of the AT1 receptor with Ang II resulted in the rapid formation of ROS and membrane blebs at early time points of Ang II stimulation that cease within 60 min of Ang II stimulation (Figure 3) (Marin-Castano., et al., IOVS, 2001, 42(4), ARVO Abstract, 4060). Further, Ang II-enhanced ROS production and blebbing was prevented by pre-treatment of RPE with the AT1 receptor blocker, which attenuates oxidative stress [244]. However, RPE derived blebs after Ang II were bigger than those seem when RPE cells were exposed to blue light, MPO, or hydroquinone. Moreover, formation of RPE-membrane blebs induced by Ang II occurred earlier than with the other oxidants we studied. Therefore, we believe that Rho-kinase pathway could be implicated as an important mediator of RPE response to Ang II-induced oxidative damage instead of Hsp27/Hsp25/p38/ERK pathway.

In conclusion, characterization of the molecular mechanism(s) by which the AT1 receptor regulates the actin cytoskeleton and plasma membrane dynamics will be essential for modulating the degree of blebbing in vitro and deposit formation in vivo for potential therapeutic strategies.

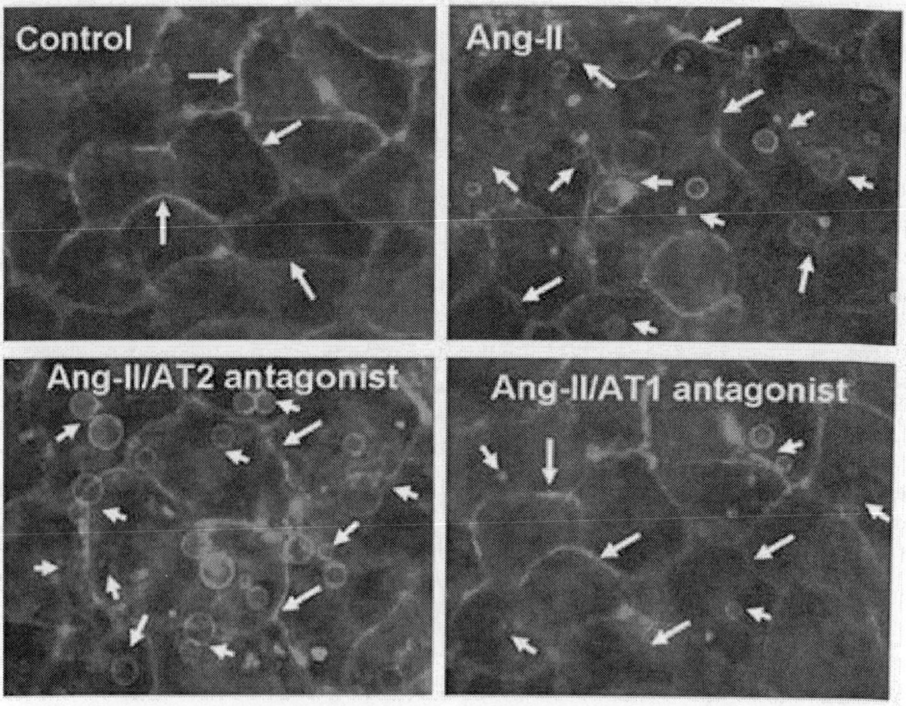

Figure 3. Induction of cellular changes in ARPE-19 cells by Ang II. Fluorescent GFP-ARPE-19 derived blebs before and after exposure to Ang II (100 nM) alone or in combination with a specific Ang II receptor antagonists AT1 (CD, 100 nM) or AT2 (PD 123319, 100 nM) for 24 hours. Cells were treated and observed immediately under epifluorescent microscope. White arrows show GFP localized to the membrane. White arrowheads show the presence of membrane blebs.

9. Extracellular Matrix Turnover: Role of Angiotensin II

Extracellular Matrix Turnover

Another injury response relevant to early AMD is imbalance in ECM turnover. The normal anatomy and physiology of ECM in most tissues requires continuous turnover of matrix components by a tightly regulated balance in the production of matrix molecules like collagen, laminin, MMPs, and TIMPs [245, 246]. It has been shown that relatively small dysregulation in the relative production of MMPs, TIMPs, and collagen types I and IV [245,

246] may lead to net changes in the ECM, including thickening and deposit formation [246, 247]. Accordingly, dysregulated turnover of ECM is a major mechanism of disease pathogenesis in many tissue sites, including renal disease, atherosclerosis, lung disease, and others [246-249]. Unfortunately, minimal information is available concerning normal turnover in healthy BrM or imbalanced turnover in AMD.

Numerous biochemical and anatomical changes occur in BrM as part of aging retina in the absence of apparent disease, including collagenous thickening, calcification and lipid infiltration [154]. However, the accumulation of specific deposits composed by blebbing from the basolateral RPE surface and other debris between the RPE basement membrane and BrM is a very prominent histopathologic feature of eyes with AMD [154, 186, 189, 203]. In addition, recent studies performed on AMD patient eyes examined by electron microscopy have reported that blebbing from the basolateral RPE surface traversed the RPE basement membrane and deposited in the inner and outer collagenous layers of BrM [250]. However, the mechanism(s) by which these sub-RPE deposits accumulate and traverse the RPE basement membrane remains unexplored. In this regard, ample evidence supports the idea that MMPs and their TIMPs play an important role in AMD. The RPE is capable of producing many ECM components such as MMP-2, MMP-14, Basigin, also known as EMMPRIN (extracellular matrix metalloproteinase inducer) or CD147, collagen types I and IV, and TIMP-2 [163, 164, 251, 252]. MMP-14 and basigin proteins are of special relevance to the AMD pathology as they promote MMP-2 activation. MMP-2 and MMP-14 are the major RPE enzymes synthesized for the degradation of matrix type IV and I collagens, laminin, and fibronectin, which are components found in BrM [251, 253]. MMP-2 is the key enzyme for ECM turnover in BrM and is synthesized as an inactive zymogen pro form (pro-MMP-2) [245]. The transmembrane metalloproteinase MMP-14 is well known to activate MMP-2 in a specific manner [253]. On the other hand, TIMP-2 may inhibit the cleavage of pro-MMP-2 into MMP-2 [246]. Based on these data our research focuses on MMP-2, MMP-14, and basigin, and propose that dysregulation of MMP-2 is the primary cause for the accumulation of sub-RPE deposits that become BLD and drusen. Thus, we propose that the progression of the sub-RPE deposits into BrM requires degradation of ECM proteins such as type IV and I collagens and laminin, which are critical components of RPE basement membrane and adjacent BrM [254, 255], and that ECM turnover upregulation via MMP-2 activation and MMP-14 is necessary for the breakdown of these physical barriers.

As mentioned previously, hypertension is of special interest as a potential link between cardiovascular pathologies and AMD [178, 181, 256, 257] and Ang II is the most important hormone associated to hypertension which plays a pivotal role in pathological complications [184, 258]. Expression of Ang II, as well as other components of the RAS, has been demonstrated in the RPE and other eye tissues [142, 259-261]. Aside from the evidence supporting the existence of a local RAS in the adult eye, the expression of Ang II receptor types AT1 and AT2 has been demonstrated in the retina and the RPE [142-145] which provides the molecular basis for a biological function of Ang II in the eye.

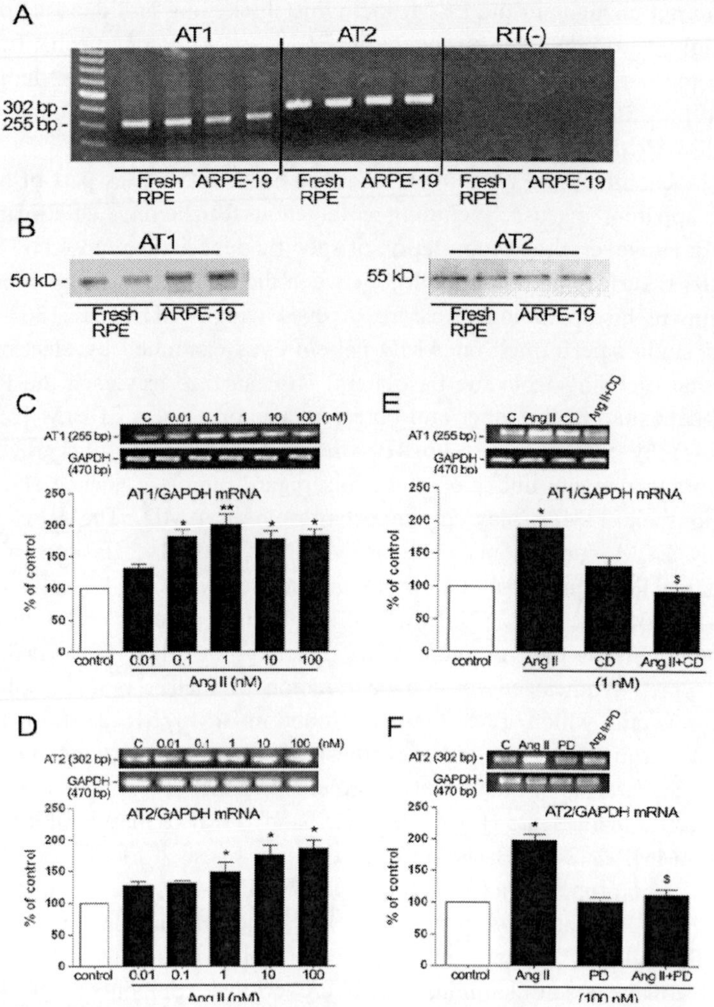

Figure 4. Human retinal pigment epithelium expresses both Ang II receptors at the mRNA and protein levels. Total RNA and protein were collected from freshly dissected human RPE and cultured ARPE-19 cells. (A): agarose gel from a representative experiment. AT1 and AT2 receptor transcription was analyzed by RT-PCR; representative amplicons of AT1, 302 bp; AT2, 255 bp, minus (-) RT, and molecular weight standard were run in parallel. (B): ARPE-19-derived AT1 and AT2 protein expression evaluated by Western blot using AT1 (N-10) antiserum (*left*) and AT2 (N-19) antiserum (*right*). (C-F): Levels of AT1 and AT2 Ang II receptor mRNA regulation by Ang II in cultured ARPE-19 cells. Cells were incubated with different concentrations of Ang II alone for 24 hours (C, D) or in combination with candesartan (CD, 1 nM), an AT1 receptor antagonist, or PD123319 (PD, 100 nM) an Ang II type 2 receptor antagonist for 30 min before Ang II stimulation (E, F), then washed with PBS and incubated in assay medium (0.1% FBS) for 24 hours. Expression of AT1, AT2, and GAPDH mRNAs was analyzed by semi-quantitative RT-PCR. AT1 and AT2 mRNA expression was normalized to GAPDH. *Top*: agarose gel from a representative experiment. The number on the left represents the molecular weight of PCR product. *Bottom*: average of results of four independent experiments. Data are expressed as percentage of control, and shown are mean results ± SEM of four independent experiments run in triplicate on cultured cells. Statistical significance is indicated by $*P < 0.05$ and $**P < 0.01$ for comparison to the control and by $^{\$}P < 0.01$ for the comparison to the 1 nM or 100 nM Ang II effects.

Ang II-mediated regulation of genes, which are expressed in RPE and are important for the ECM turnover, might contribute to subRPE deposit formation and provide a pathogenic mechanism to explain the link between hypertension and AMD. Among its many actions, Ang II promotes interstitial ECM turnover by regulation of the ECM proteins [262-269]. For example, Ang II has been shown to stimulate synthesis of fibronectin, collagen, TIMP-2, and MMP-2 in mesangial and proximal tubule cells through activation of transforming growth factor-ß secretion (TGF-β) [270, 271]. Ang II also activates TGF-β-mediated MMP-2 release in endothelial cells [272]. In addition, Ang II increases collagen type I and III production via NADPH oxidase complex in cardiac fibroblasts [273], MMP-14, MMP-2 and MMP-9 expression and activity in MKN-28 cells, arteries, and aorta [266, 267, 274], as well as TIMP-1 expression and concentration in smooth muscle cells and coronary endothelial cells [264, 275]. The RPE actively contributes to maintain a normal turnover of ECM components. However, until now, the regulatory effects of Ang II on ECM proteins expression in the RPE were unknown. Therefore, our work aimed at characterizing the expression and function of Ang II receptors in the RPE and at investigating Ang II contribution to the development of early AMD. Our study confirmed that both Ang II receptor subtypes were expressed and upregulated by Ang II in human RPE (Figure 4) and showed that stimulation of the AT1 receptor by Ang II is transduced into an intracellular signal, in particular an increase in the levels of intracellular calcium (Figure 5) [145]. This result constitutes clear evidence that the AT1 receptor expressed in human RPE is functionally active and might be efficiently coupled to the PLC-transduction pathway. Compared to these results, stimulation of the AT2 receptor by Ang II was not accompanied by mobilization of intracellular calcium. These data suggest differences in AT2 receptor coupling in human RPE cells. AT2 receptor could be specifically coupled to the cytosolic phospholipase A2 (cPLA2) as it has been shown recently in renal mesangial and proximal tubular epithelium cells and not to the PLC pathway [276]. Therefore, selective up or down-regulation of only AT2 receptor transduction pathway remains a possibility to be investigated.

Ang II also increased MMP-2 activity (Figure 6), MMP-14 (Figure 7), and basigin (Figure 8) as well as type IV collagen degradation (Figure 9) [145, 277]. These Ang II effects were abolished in the presence of the AT1 receptor antagonist candesartan (Figures 6-8). In contrast, Ang II decreased type IV collagen via both AT1 and AT2 receptors, suggesting a synergistic effect of the two receptor subtypes (Figure 9). As proposed in our hypothetical model fro dry AMD, Ang II through MMP-2, MMP-14, and basigin regulation could stimulate RPE basement membrane breakdown allowing the migration of BLD and buildup of BLiD or drusen.

The majority of intracellular actions of Ang II in most tissues are mediated by the activation of MAPKs, which are a group of serine/threonine kinases [278-280] which can be divided into three major groups: ERK, p38, and Jun N-terminus kinase (JNK) and participate in a wide array of cellular responses including proliferation, differentiation, migration, and stress responses among others [281-283]. We explored the involvement of MAPK signaling pathways as a potential key intracellular modulator of Ang II-induced increase in MMP-2 activity, MMP-14 and basigin protein expression in the RPE. We found that Ang II stimulates phosphorylation of ERK and p38 MAPK in RPE cells (Figure 10) [277]. These effects were mediated by AT1 receptors. Blockade of ERK or p38 MAPK abrogated the increase in MMP-2 activity and MMP-14 and basigin proteins in RPE cells. Given that MMP-14 and basigin are major inducers of MMP-2, our results lead us to speculate that MMP-14 and basigin might regulate Ang II-induced MMP-2 activity through MAPKs- and AT1 receptor-dependent signaling pathways in the RPE. These original observations highlight the potential importance of this *signaling pathway as a potential mediator* of RPE response to Ang II-induced ECM dysregulation and breakdown of the RPE basement membrane believed to be involved in sub-RPE deposits progression in the pathogenesis of AMD. Based on our observations, MAPKs inhibitors and AT1 receptor blockers may prevent these ECM changes essential in early AMD development and provide a potential future clinical tool for the prevention of this disease that causes a great deal of discomfort and disability.

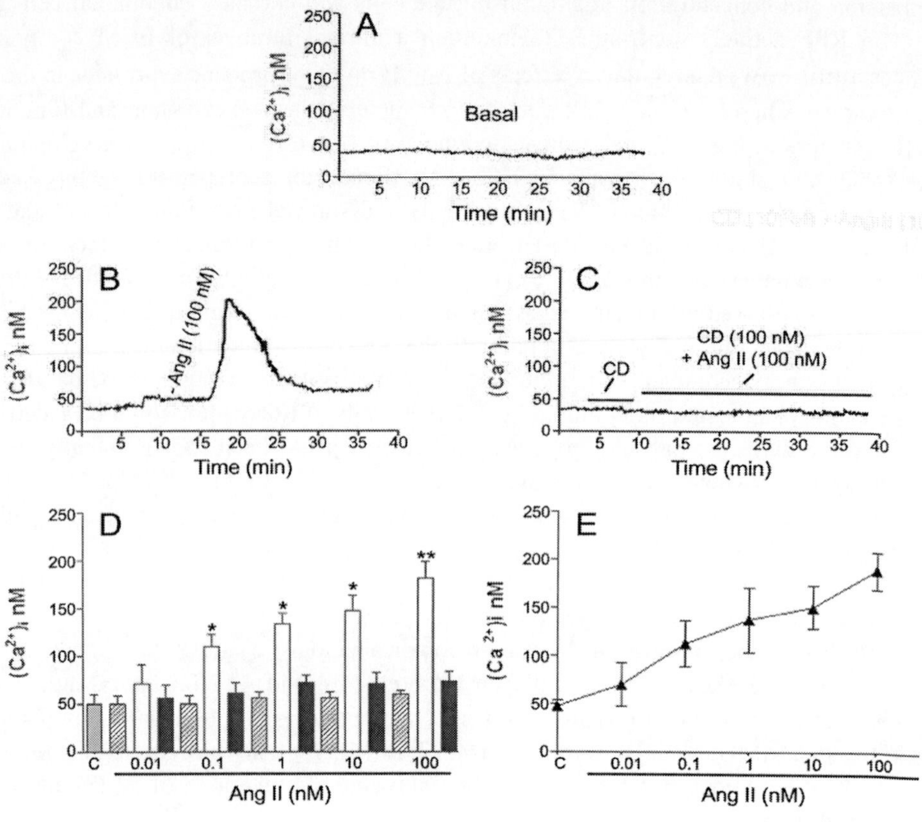

Figures 5. Ang II increases intracellular calcium. Fluorescence measurement shows intracellular calcium [Ca2+]i responses in ARPE-19 cells under basal conditions and during Ang II (100 nM) stimulation with or without candesartan (CD, 100 nM), a selective AT1 receptor antagonist added 5 min before and during Ang II stimulation. Representative recordings of intracellular calcium mobilization in response to Ang II show traces under basal conditions (A), stimulated with Ang II (100 nM) alone (B) and stimulated with Ang II (100 nM) in combination with 100 nM CD (C), added 5 min before and during Ang II stimulation antagonist. D: averaged [Ca2+]i levels during Ang II stimulation at different concentrations; baseline (hatched bars), [Ca2+]i peaks (open bars), and 25 minutes after stimulation (solid bars). Bars represent mean ± SEM (n = 4). *P<0.05, **P<0.01, and ***P<0.001 vs. control. E: dose response of Ang II-elicited peak.

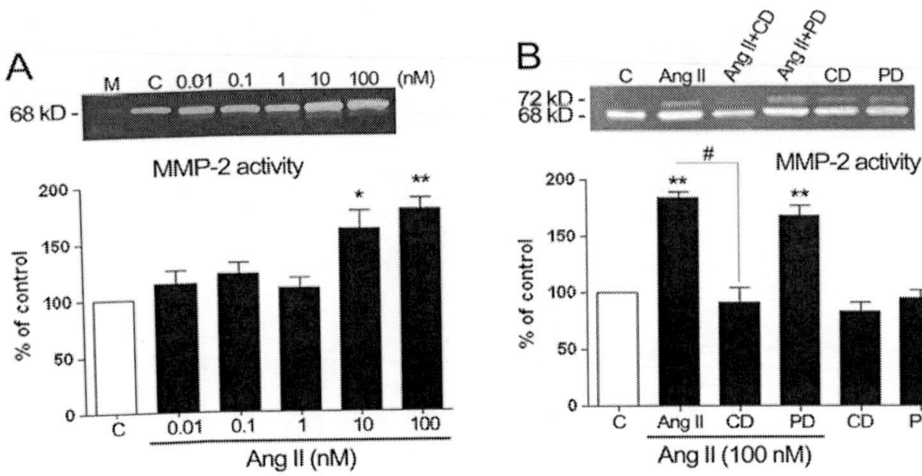

Figures 6. Exposure to Ang II up-regulated MMP-2 protein activity in the supernatant. (A): ARPE-19-derived MMP-2 protein activity evaluated by zymography in the presence of various concentrations of Ang II for 24 hours. (B): effect of candesartan (CD, 100 nM) and PD 123319 (PD, 100 nM) on Ang II induced MMP-2 protein activity. ARPE-19 cells were exposed to the AT1 or AT2 receptor blocker alone or in combination with Ang II (100 nM). CD abolished ARPE-19-derived MMP-2 protein activity increase induced by Ang II. Top: gelatin zymogram in the supernatant from a representative experiment. Lane M: marker. Lane C: control. Number on the left represents protein molecular weight in kilodaltons. Bottom: average results of four independent experiments run in triplicate on cultured cells. Data represent the relative amount of the 68 kDa form. *P< 0.05 and **P< 0.01, statistically significant difference compared with the control. #P< 0.05, statistically significant difference compared with the Ang II (100 nM).

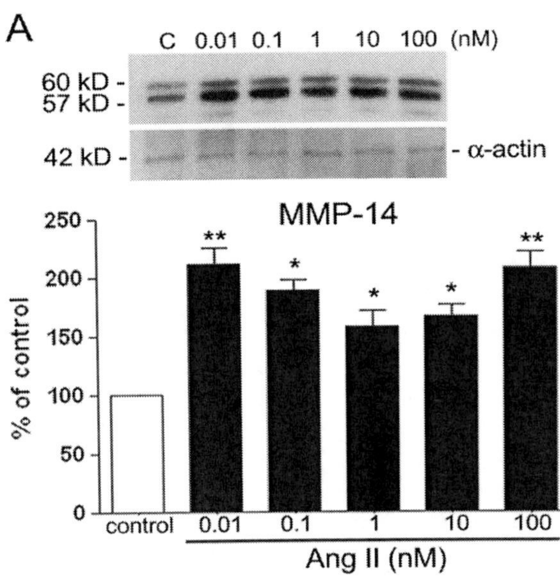

Figure 7. (Continued).

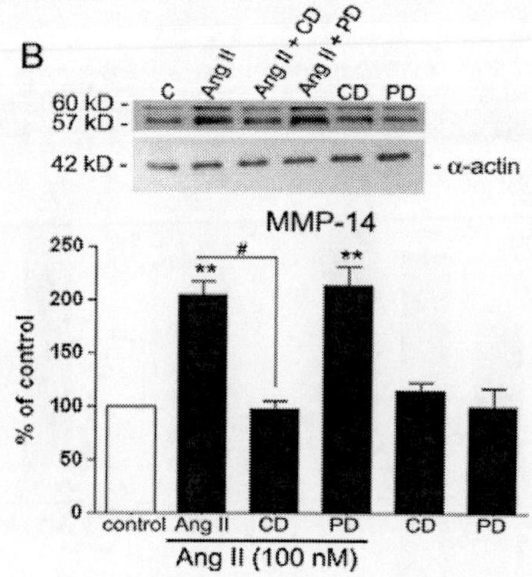

Figure 7. Angiotensin II up-regulated MMP-14 protein in the cellular lysate and this effect was abolished by candesartan (CD). A: ARPE-19-derived MMP-14 protein evaluated by Western blot in the presence of various concentrations of Ang II for 24 hours. B: effect of candesartan (CD, 100 nM) and PD 123319 (PD, 100 nM) on Ang II-induced MMP-14 protein expression. ARPE-19 cells were exposed to the AT1 or AT2 receptor blocker alone or in combination with Ang II (100 nM). Top: Immunoblotting from a representative experiment, showing change in protein expression. Lane C: control. Number on the left represents protein molecular weight in kilodaltons. Bottom: average results of four independent experiments run in triplicate on cultured cells. MMP-14 protein expression was normalized to alpha-actin. Data represent the relative amount of the 57 and 66 kDa forms. *P<0.05 and **P<0.01, statistically significant difference compared with the control. #P< 0.05 statistically significant difference compared with the Ang II (100 nM).

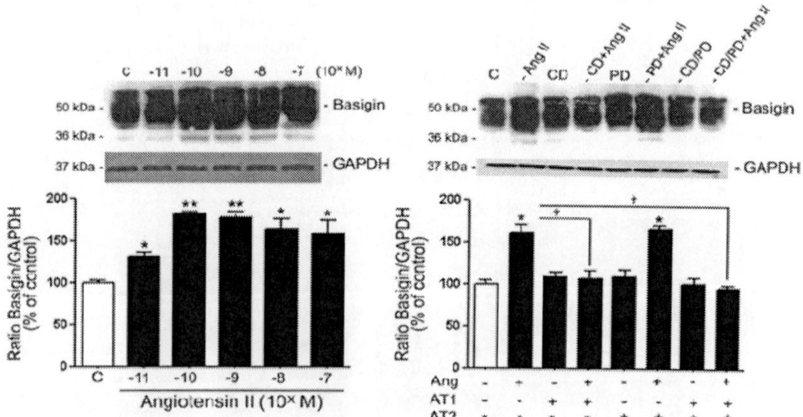

Figure 8. Ang II upregulated basigin protein expression through Ang II receptor 1 (AT1) activation in RPE-19 cells. A: RPE-derived basigin protein expression in the presence of various concentrations of Ang II for 24 hours. B: Basigin protein expression in presence of candesartan (CD) alone, PD123319 (PD) alone, or combination of both Ang II receptor blockers before treatment with Ang II. Top: Representative Western blot for basigin. Number on the left represents protein molecular weight in kilodaltons (kDa). Bottom: Ratio of basigin/GAPDH. Data are expressed as percentage of control and are mean ± SE of three independent experiments run in duplicate. *P< 0.05 and**P< 0.01 versus control. † p<0.05 versus Ang II alone.

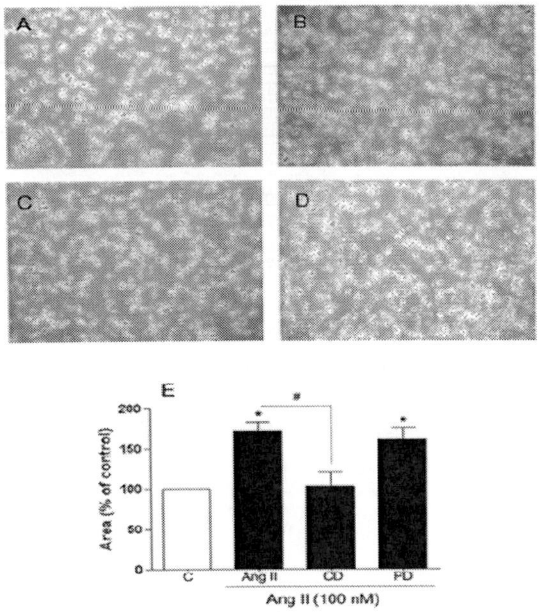

Figure 9. Collagen type IV matrix inserts stained with Coomassie blue after exposure for 24 hrs to medium of ARPE-19 cells treated with Ang II (100 nM) alone (B) or in presence of AT1 or AT2 receptor blockers (C, D). E: average results of three independent experiments run in triplicate. Results are expressed as mean±SEM. *P<0.05, statistically significant difference compared with the control (c). #P< 0.01 statistically significant difference compared with the Ang II (100 nM). Magnifications, x40.

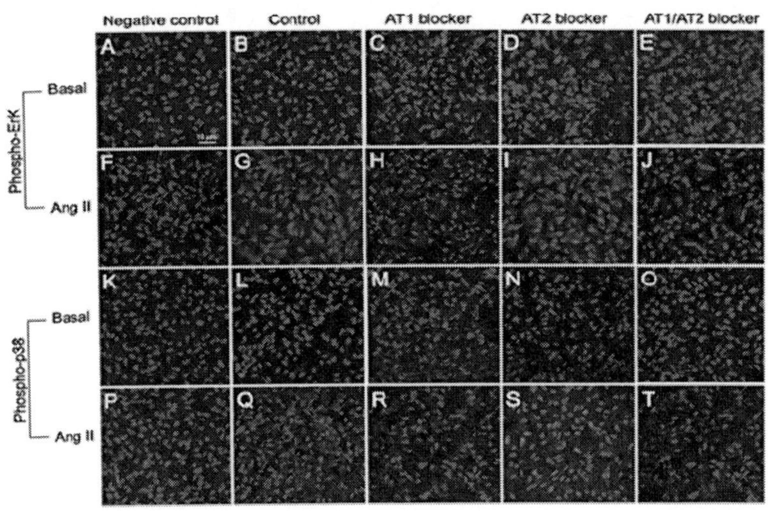

Figure 10. Representative immunofluorescent double staining of phosphorylated Erk(1/2) and p38 MAPK (green) and nuclei (blue) in Ang II-stimulated ARPE-19 cells in the presence of Ang II receptor antagonists. The figure is a composite image showing the immunostaining of non-treated ("Basal") (A-E and K-O) and treated ("Ang II") (F-J and P-T) cells in the absence ("Control") (B, G, L, Q) or presence of candesartan ("AT1 blocker") (C, H, M, R) or PD123319 ("AT2 blocker") (D, I, N, S) , or the combination of both ("AT1/2 Blockers") (E, J, O, T). Negative controls were generated by omission of the primary antibody. Sections were analyzed using confocal microscopy (magnification x40).

10. Inflammation: Role of Angiotensin II

The mechanism of how drusen might elicit CNV remains undefined. However, a growing collection of evidence suggests that inflammation is an important component in the pathogenesis of both dry and wet AMD [284-288].

While it is largely recognized that macrophages accumulate in AMD lesion [289-295], there is ambiguity surrounding their role in the disease process with conflicting evidence regarding whether they might be helpful by scavenging accumulated debris and therefore protecting against CNV or harmful by stimulating CNV [296]. This might be due to the largely observational nature of human samples but also probably reflects different functions macrophages serve during distinct phases of the disease.

Inflammation is a complex process that involves local secretion of pro-inflammatory cytokines (leukocyte adhesion molecules, ICAM-1 and VCAM-1) [297, 298], MCP-1 [299-303] NFκB [304-306], and growth factors (tumour necrosis factor, TNF-α, TGF-β). The key inflammatory molecule in initiating inflammatory responses may be MCP-1 [299-305] a powerful chemokine, expressed at sites of injury. Indeed, the importance of MCP-1 in inflammatory diseases is highlighted by a careful MEDLINE search for MCP-1, which readily returns more than 3000 citations following its characterization in the late 1980s.

NFκB appears to control expression of MCP-1 [304-306]. After release, it activates the CCR2 chemotactic receptor to induce chemotactic responses that mediate monocyte and macrophage migration into sites of active inflammation in various diseases [307, 308]. MCP-1 is postulated to be responsible for the recruitment of macrophages early in repair processes. The RPE plays a pivotal role in the maintenance of the outer retina by secreting several cytokines including MCP-1 [309, 310], which has been suggested to be implicated in the pathogenesis of AMD [311, 312]. RPE cells can secrete MCP-1 in the direction of choroidal blood vessels during inflammatory responses therefore suggesting that RPE cells might promote macrophage recruitment to the choroid from circulating monocytes [160]. Thus, we have speculated that MCP-1 produced by the RPE is a relevant molecule in dry AMD and its progression.

Previous observations made using mouse animal models suggest that MCP-1 and chemokine receptor–2 might be involved in the etiology of AMD and that macrophage dysfunction may have a central role in the early stage of AMD development [311, 312]. Indeed, it has been proposed that the spontaneous disappearance of drusen in patients with AMD may be explained by phagocytosis of debris thereby indicating a beneficial role of macrophages [160]. However, on the other hand, macrophages recruited into the choriocapillaris, which upon scavenging debris and blebs, could release additional cytokines and mediators to amplify matrix turnover and deposit formation, induce RPE cytotoxicity or damage the choriocapillaris promoting complications, especially CNV formation.

Ang II, is known as a vasoconstrictor, however, several studies have shown its role as a potent mediator in the activation of inflammatory mechanisms involved in age-related diseases [313, 314]. Ang II plays a critical role in the pathogenesis of a wide spectrum of diseases [297, 298, 305, 315-319]. At physiological levels (fentomoles), Ang II is an important physiological regulator of blood pressure, cardiac function and body salt and fluid homeostasis [315]. However, increased local or tissue Ang II formation in target organs may indeed be very deleterious [297, 315-318]. Ang II is not only a potent vasoconstrictor which elevates arterial blood pressure, but also a powerful pro-inflammatory cytokine, chemokine and growth factor [297, 304-306, 320], which mediates the activation of inflammatory mechanisms involved in age-related diseases [313, 314]. There is accumulating evidence that Ang II can cause target organ damage by facilitating inflammatory and growth responses through activation of NFκB [297, 304-306], the key nuclear transcription factor in inflammatory and fibrotic diseases. Activation of NFκB by Ang II may stimulate transcription of numerous inflammatory genes, including MCP-1, RANTES (Regulated on Active Normal T cell Expressed and Secreted) and interleukin (IL)-6, TNF-α and TGF-β [297, 304-306]. The view that MCP-1 is one of the most important chemokines in Ang II-induced inflammatory responses is supported by numerous studies, although the mechanisms by which Ang II increases MCP-1 expression and production are still not well understood [297, 304-306]. In a rabbit model of atherosclerosis, ACE1 inhibitor quinapril inhibited NFκB activity, expression and production of MCP-1 and neointimal macrophage infiltration at the injured sites [304]. In Ang II-induced hypertensive rats, vascular MCP-1 mRNA expression increased almost four-fold, which was significantly reduced by normalization of hypertension by the non-specific vasodilator hydralazine, but the effects of AT1 receptor blockade were not studied [301]. However, in a different study, Ang II enhanced expression of MCP-1 mRNA and protein production in rat vascular smooth muscle cells in a dose- and time-dependent fashion, and these effects were mediated by AT1 receptors involving the Rho-kinase pathway [321]. In mice, Wu et al. [322] showed that the AT1 receptor antagonist valsartan, at a dose that did not influence systolic blood pressure, significantly reduced the expression of MCP-1 along with other inflammatory genes such as TNF-α, IL-6, IL-1β and monocyte/macrophage infiltration in injured vessels. Interestingly, the effects of valsartan on MCP-1 expression were attenuated in AT2 receptor-deficient mice, suggesting that both AT1 and AT2 receptors are involved.The advantage of using a lower dose of AT1 receptor blockers is that the treatment does not reduce systolic blood pressure to the normotensive level, but retains clinical efficacy in inhibiting MCP-1 expression and improving cardiac function and mortality. Accordingly, the beneficial effects of the AT1 receptor blockers may be explained by a mechanism other than high blood pressure. A direct effect of Ang II on MCP-1 expression and production may be implicated [320].

Finally, the signalling mechanisms by which Ang II increases MCP-1 expression and production and induces end-organ damage remain to be elucidated. As mentioned previously, there is mounting evidence that NFκB may be one of the most important nuclear transcription factors that mediates Ang II-stimulated MCP-1 expression and production [297, 304-306]. However, the signalling pathways by which Ang II directly or indirectly activates NFκB, which is then translocated into the nucleus to mediate MCP-1 transcription and synthesis, remain largely unknown. A local RAS may be activated in most, if not all, diseases with consequently increased tissue or intracellular Ang II. Binding of extracellular Ang II to cell surface AT1 receptors may stimulate MCP-1 mRNA expression through activation of different intracellular signalling cascades, likely involving protein kinase C-activated intracellular calcium mobilization [323], tyrosine kinase and MAPK [324], phospholipase A_2 [325] and redox-sensitive NADH/NAD(P)H oxidase [324]. Future studies further addressing these important issues could improve our understanding of the potential role of pro-inflammatory cytokines and chemokines in mediating Ang II-induced target organ damage and assist in further development of novel drugs to prevent and treat these diseases.

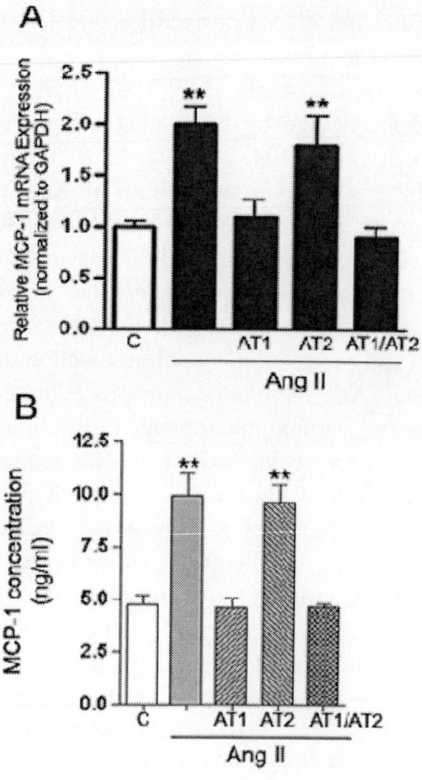

Figure 11. Ang II upregulated MCP-1 protein expression (A) and secretion (B) through Ang II receptor 1 (AT1) activation in RPE cells. Human ARPE-19 cells were incubated with Ang II alone (100 nM) for 24 hours or in combination with candesartan (CD, 100 nM), an AT1 receptor antagonist, or PD123319 (PD, 100 nM) an Ang II type 2 receptor antagonist for 30 min before Ang II stimulation, then washed with PBS and incubated in assay medium (0.1% FBS) for 24 hours. Supernatants and cell homogenates were collected to assess MCP-1 mRNA expression by real-time PCR and protein secretion by ELISA. Results are expressed as mean±SEM. **$P<0.01$, statistically significant difference compared with the control.

Even if it has been suggested that increased MCP-1 expression may be a key mediator between Ang II and retinal damage in hypertensive patients, MCP-1 expression has not been investigated in RPE from hypertensive patients with AMD nor has been the regulation of RPE-derived MCP-1 expression following Ang II-mediated injury.

On the basis of our preliminary data and those of others, we have proposed a molecular inflammatory hypothesis for AMD that describes a central role for the redox-sensitive NF-κB in modulating the gene expression of MCP-1. Many studies have provided experimental evidence indicating that NF-κB can be activated by oxidative stress [326-329] and that the anti-oxidant may have beneficial effects on vascular inflammation that occurs in other age-related diseases [330, 331]. Thus, we proposed that Ang II will active RPE MCP-1 production leading to recruitment of macrophages to sub-RPE deposit areas, where they will scavenge, release more cytokines and mediators, and amplify the process promoting complications, especially CNV formation. Our preliminary data indicate that expression of MCP-1, key mediators pertinent to inflammation is markedly increased *in cultured human RPE cells in response to Ang II (Figure 11)*. Moreover, our data indicate that the increase in MCP-1 mRNA and protein secretion by RPE was through AT1 receptors activation (Figure 11), highlighting such pro-inflammatory role of Ang II and their mechanism. These observations may have strong implications for the drusen progression to CNV in hypertensive patients with dry AMD. Future studies addressing whether or not Ang II directly or indirectly activates NFκB and the signalling pathways could improve our understanding of the potential role of Ang II in the progression of dry AMD to CNV.

Because hypertension has been unequivocally linked to the pathogenesis of AMD, it can be speculated that increase in RPE-derived MCP-1 production resulting from exposure to Ang II may be an important factor that could accelerate and promote the progression of early AMD to CNV. This theory is put forth bearing in mind the complexity of underlying cellular and *molecular mechanisms involved* in the inflammatory response.

11. Angiotensin II-Induced Hypertension: Animal Model for Dry AMD

Animal models are extremely useful in preclinical testing of theories of disease pathogenesis and therapeutic interventions. However, until recently, no animal models for dry AMD were available. The only available model for dry AMD and hypertension was reported by Jonas et al in 2003 [181]. The purpose of this study was to evaluate whether arterial hypertension (renovascular hypertension) influence the development and severity of AMD. The authors showed that the development of macular drusen as part of AMD in rhesus monkeys may be associated with experimentally induced arterial hypertension.

Based on the idea that Ang II might contribute to drusen pathogenesis, we extended our in vitro data to a more physiological environment using the 9-month-old C57BL/6 mouse model for dry AMD published by our laboratory [165, 169, 332, 333], but providing an alternative source of oxidant stimulus by replacing exposure to blue light or hydroquinone with exposure to Ang II alone or in combination with the AT1 receptor antagonist (candesartan) or the AT2 receptor antagonist (PD123319) for 4 weeks [334, 277] or 4.5 months. We used Ang II to determine whether hypertension-associated Ang II was important for ECM regulation in RPE and the development of sub-RPE deposits. We reported that Ang II-treated mice had increased blood pressure as well as plasma and ocular levels of Ang II relative to control mice [334] (Figure 12). Ang II also regulated AT1a and AT1b receptor mRNA expression (Figure 13A), and the intracellular concentration of calcium $[Ca^{2+}]_I$ (Figure 13B,C), showing that Ang II AT1 receptor is functional. In addition, MMP-2 activity (Figure 14), and type IV collagen accumulation (Figure 15) were regulated by Ang II. Concurrent administration of Ang II with the AT1 receptor blocker prevented the increase in blood pressure and rise in ocular Ang II levels, as well as the calcium (Figure 12) and MMP-2 responses (Figure 14). In contrast, the type IV collagen response to Ang II was prevented by blockade of AT2 receptors, but not AT1 receptors (Figure 15). Plasma Ang II levels were not modified by the AT1 or AT2 receptor blockade (Figure 12B). In addition, Ang II stimulates MMP-14 (Figure 16), basigin (Figure 17), and phosphorylation of ERK, p38, and JNK in RPE sheets from mice (Figure 18). These effects were mediated by Ang II type 1 receptors (Figures 16-18).

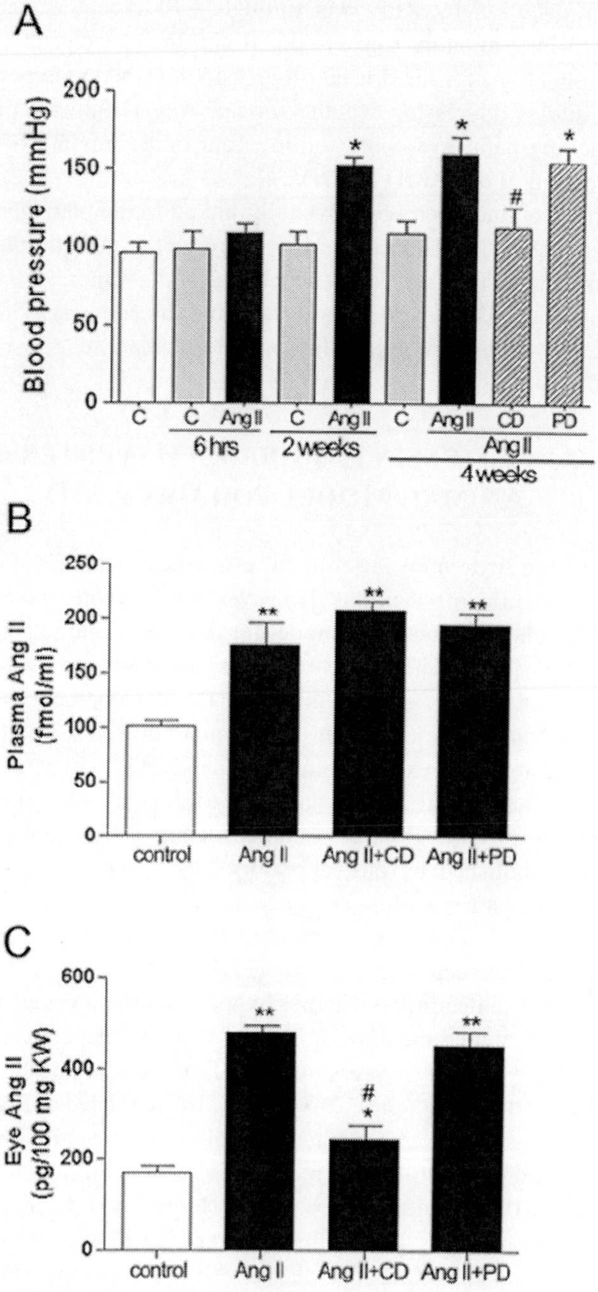

Figure 12. Systolic blood pressure (A) and circulating (B) and whole eye (C) Ang II levels Ang II levels in response to administration of Ang II (3.0 µg/ Kg/min) alone for 6 hr, 2 wk, or 4 wk and Ang II in combination with the AT1 receptor antagonist candesartan (CD, 10 mg/Kg/day) or the AT2 receptor antagonist PD123319 (PD, 50 mg/Kg/day) for 4 weeks in C57BL/6 mice. Data are expressed as percentage of control and graphed as mean ± SEM. *P <0.05 and **P <0.01 vs. control. #P <0.05 vs. Ang II treated group. n = 6 eyes/group.

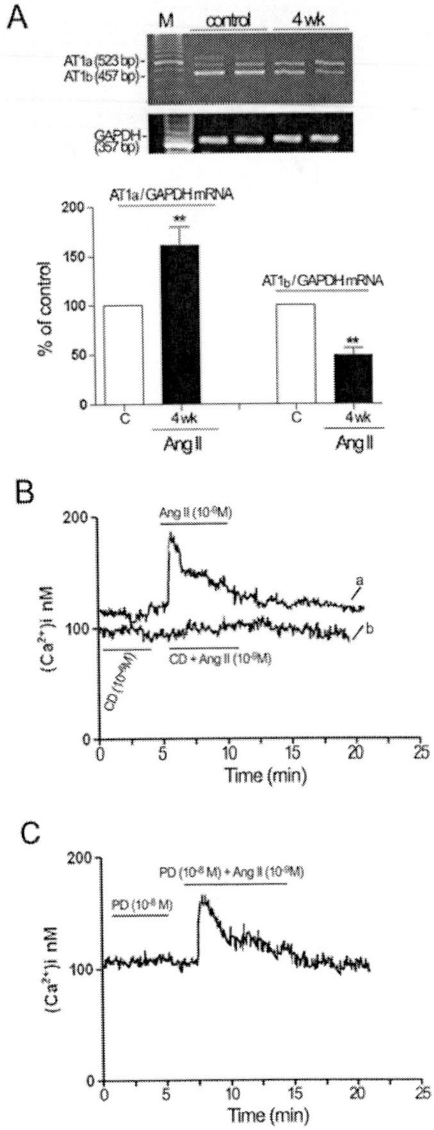

Figure 13. (A) Regulation of AT1a and AT1b mRNA in dissected RPE from mice infused with saline or Ang II (3.0 μg/Kg/min) for 4 weeks. Expression of AT1a, AT1b and GAPDH mRNA was analyzed by RT-PCR. AT1a and AT1b mRNA expression was normalized to GAPDH. Total RNA was extracted from RPE sheets (n = 6 eyes/ group). Top: agarose gel from two representative experiments. Lane M: marker. The number on the left represents the molecular weight of PCR product. Bottom: data are the average results from six eyes. Data are expressed as percentage of control, and shown are mean results ± SEM. Statistical significance is indicated by $^{**}P < 0.01$ for compared to the control group. (B,C) Representative recording of intracellular calcium [Ca2+]i mobilization in isolated RPE sheets under basal conditions and during Ang II (1 nM) stimulation with or without candesartan (CD, 10 nM), a selective AT1 receptor antagonist or PD123319 (PD, 10 nM), a selective AT2 receptor antagonist added 5 minutes before and during Ang II stimulation. (B) Stimulation with Ang II (1 nM) alone (a) and in combination with CD (b). (C) Stimulation with Ang II in combination with PD, added 5 minutes before and during Ang II stimulation. Ang II increased [Ca2+]i via AT1 receptor.

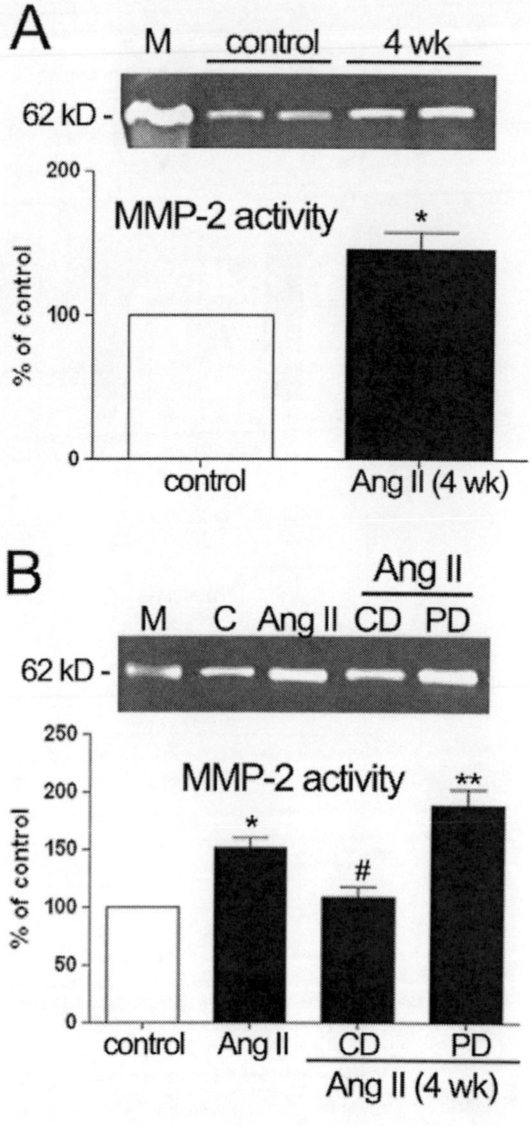

Figure 14. MMP-2 activity and protein in freshly isolated RPE sheets from control and treated mice. Elevated circulating levels of Ang II associated with HTN up-regulated MMP-2 protein activity, and did not alter MMP-2 protein expression. RPE-derived MMP-2 activity evaluated by zymography (A, B). Protein was extracted from RPE sheets (n = 6 eyes/ group). Animals were treated with saline, Ang II (3.0 μg/Kg/min) or Ang II (3.0 μg/Kg/min) in combination with candesartan (10 mg/ Kg/day) or PD123319 (50 mg/Kg/day). Top: gelatin zymogram or Western blot from two representative experiments. Bottom: data are the average results from six eyes expressed as percentage of control. Lane M: marker. Lane C: control. Number on the left represents protein molecular weight in kilodaltons. Data represent the relative amount of the 62 kDa form (A, B). Statistically significant differences (*P< 0.05 and **P< 0.01) compared with the controls. #P< 0.05, is statistically significant compared with the Ang II treated mice.

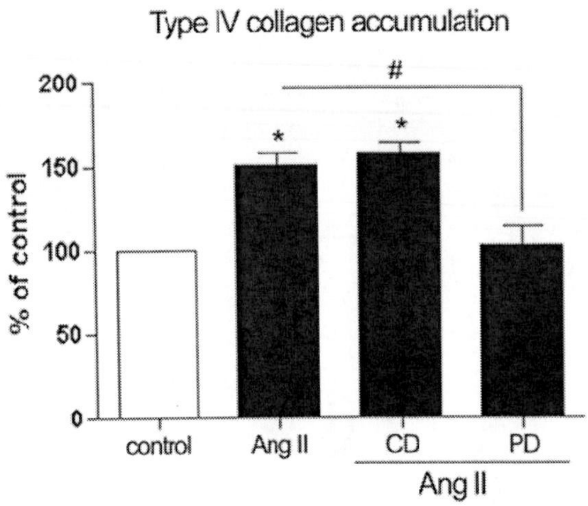

Figure 15. Quantification of type IV collagen accumulation in isolated RPE sheets by ELISA. Infusion of Ang II (3.0 μg/Kg/min) for 4 weeks upregulated type IV collagen accumulation in freshly RPE sheets from C57BL/6 mice but did not induce changes in collagen type IV accumulation in these animals during the concurrent administration of Ang II (3.0 μg/Kg/min)with the AT1 receptor blocker candesartan (CD, 10 mg/Kg/day). The effect of Ang II infusion on type IV collagen was inhibited by the AT2 receptor blocker PD123319 (PD, 50 mg/Kg/ day). Data are the average results from six eyes expressed as percentage of control, and shown are mean results ± SEM. Statistical significance (*P < 0.05) compared with the control and #P< 0.05 compared with the Ang II treated mice.

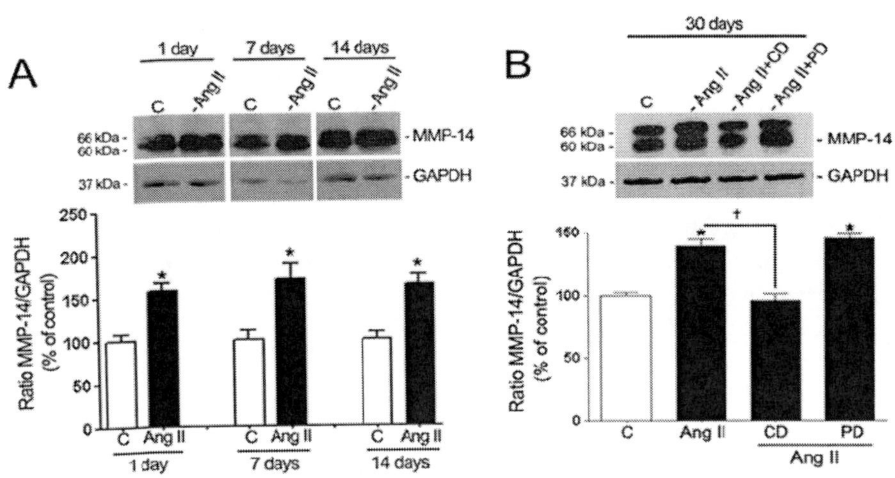

Figure 16. MMP-14 protein expression in isolated RPE sheets from control and treated mice. (A): Effect of 1, 7, and 14 days treatment with saline or Ang II on MMP-14 protein expression. (B): RPE-derived MMP-14 protein expression in mice treated with saline, Ang II or Ang II in combination with candesartan (CD) or PD123319 (PD) for 30 days. Top: Ratio MMP-14/GAPDH protein expression evaluated by Western blot from a representative experiment. Numbers on the left represent protein molecular mass in kilodaltons (kDa). Bottom: average densitometry results. Data are expressed as percentage of control and are means+ SE. * is p<0.05 versus control; †is p<0.05 versus Ang II.

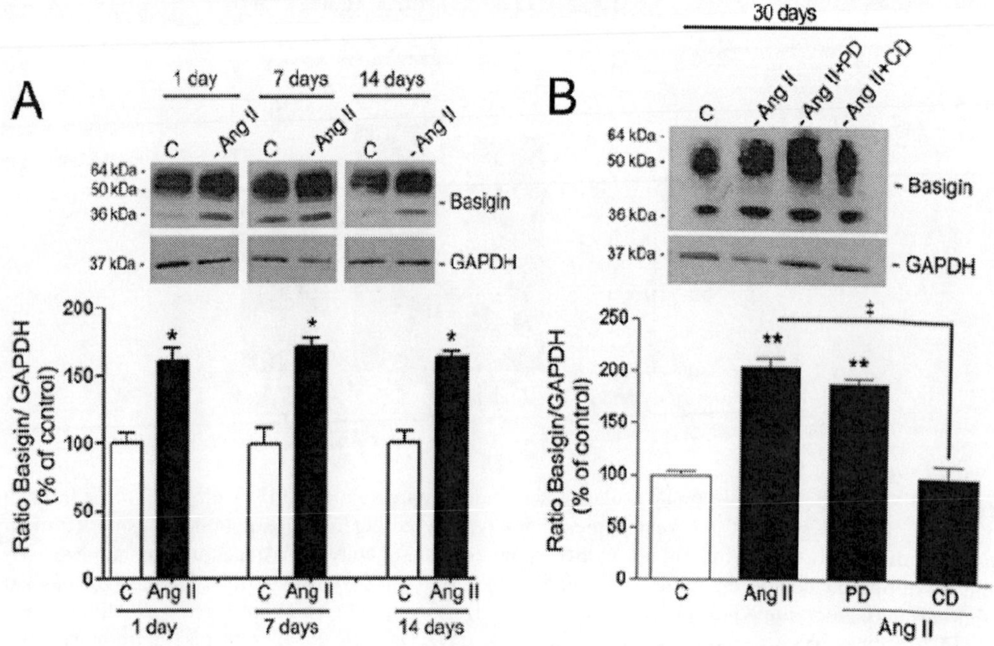

Figure 17. Basigin protein expression in isolated RPE sheets from control and treated mice. (A): RPE-basigin protein expression in mice treated with saline or Ang II for 1, 7, and 14 days. (B): Basigin protein expression in mice treated saline, Ang II or Ang II in combination with candesartan (CD) or PD123319 (PD) for 30 days.Top: Ratio basigin/GAPDH protein expression evaluated by Western blot from a representative experiment. Numbers on the left represent protein molecular mass in kilodaltons (kDa). Bottom: average densitometry results. Data are expressed as percentage of control and are means+ SE. * is $p<0.05$ and ** is p<0 01versus control; ‡ is $p<0.01$ versus Ang II.

Animals exposed to Ang II for 3.5 months revealed moderate BLD deposits (Figure 19). Sub-RPE changes were characterized by accumulation of moderately dense homogeneous material between the RPE and its basement membrane (under white line, unpublished data). Given that the Ang II receptors in rodents are similar to human Ang II receptors, our study help to elucidate the mechanism(s) by which Ang II receptor blockers may prevent these ECM changes important for early AMD development and provide a potential future clinical tool for the prevention of AMD. Moreover, our observations indicate that Ang II may induce the development of BLD. Thus, the results suggest the role for Ang II in ECM turnover and sub-RPE formation and propose Ang II-induced hypertension as an injury stimulus to the RPE, which may serve to explain the mechanisms that underlie pathologic BLD deposits in early AMD.

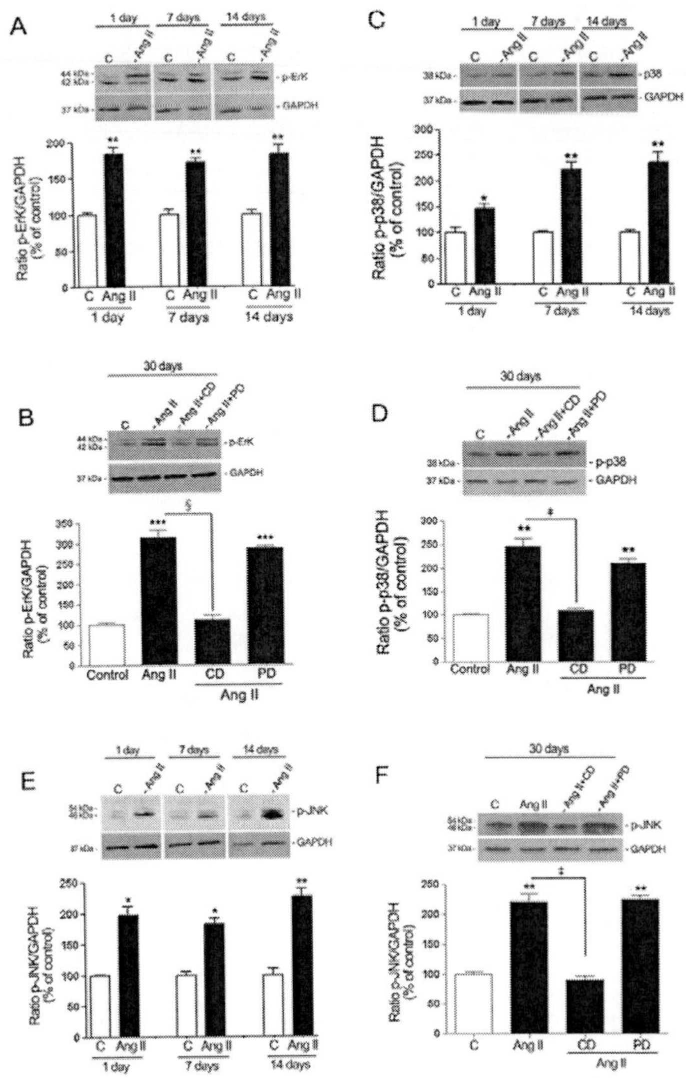

Figure 18. Regulation of phosphorylated ErK(1/2) MAPK (A, B), p38 (p-p38) (C, D), and JNK MAPK in disseted RPE sheets from mice treated with Ang II infused subcutaneously via osmotic minipumps. Proteins were extracted from RPE sheets (n = 6 eyes/group). (A): phosphorylated ErK(1/2) (p-ErK) protein expression evaluated by Western blot in RPE from mice treated with Ang II for 1, 7, and 14 days. Top: Western blot from a representative experiment. Number on the left represent protein molecular mass in kilodaltons (kDa). Bottom: Ratio of p-ErK/GAPDH. Data are the average results from six eyes expressed as percentage of control and shown are mean results ± SE. **$p<0.01$ versus control. (B): RPE-derived p-ErK protein expression evaluated by Western blot in RPE sheets from mice treated with saline, Ang II or Ang II in combination with candesartan (CD) or PD123319 (PD) for 30 days. Protein was extracted from RPE sheets (n = 6 eyes/ group). Top: Western blot from a representative experiment. Numbers on the left represent protein molecular mass in kilodaltons (kDa). Bottom: Ratio of p-ErK/GAPDH. Data are expressed as percentage of control and shown are mean results ± SE. ***$p< 0.001$ versus control. §$p< 0.001$ versus Ang II treated mice. (C): p-p38 protein expression evaluated by Western blot in RPE sheets from mice treated with Ang II for 1, 7, and 14 days. Top: Western blot from a representative experiment. Numbers on the left represent protein molecular mass in kilodaltons (kDa). Bottom: Ratio of p-p38/GAPDH protein. Data are the average

results from six eyes and were expressed as percentage of control and shown are mean results ± SE. *p< 0.05 and **p<0.01 versus control. (D): RPE-derived p-p38 protein expression evaluated by Western blot in RPE sheets from mice treated with saline, Ang II alone or Ang II in combination with candesartan (CD) or PD123319 (PD) for 30 days. Protein was extracted from RPE sheets (n = 6 eyes/ group). Top: p-p38 protein expression evaluated by Western blot from a representative experiment. Numbers on the left represent protein molecular mass in kilodaltons (kDa). Bottom: Ratio of p-p38/GAPDH protein expression. Data are expressed as percentage of control and shown are mean results ± SE. **p<0.01 versus control and ‡p< 0.01 versus Ang II treated mice. (E): Phosphorylated JNK (p-pJNK) protein expression evaluated by Western blot in RPE from mice treated with Ang II for 1, 7, and 14 days. Top: Western blot from a representative experiment. Number on the left represent protein molecular mass in kilodaltons (kDa). Bottom: Ratio of p-JNK/GAPDH. Data are the average results from six eyes expressed as percentage of control and shown are mean results ± SE. *p< 0.05 and **p< 0.01 versus control. (F): RPE-derived p-JNK protein expression evaluated by Western blot in RPE sheets from mice treated with saline, Ang II or Ang II in combination with candesartan (CD) or PD123319 (PD). Protein was extracted from RPE sheets (n = 6 eyes/ group). Top: Western blot from a representative experiment. Numbers on the left represent protein molecular mass in kilodaltons (kDa). Bottom: Ratio of p-JNK/GAPDH. Data are expressed as percentage of control and shown are mean results ± SE. **p< 0.01 versus control and ‡p< 0.01 versus Ang II treated mice.

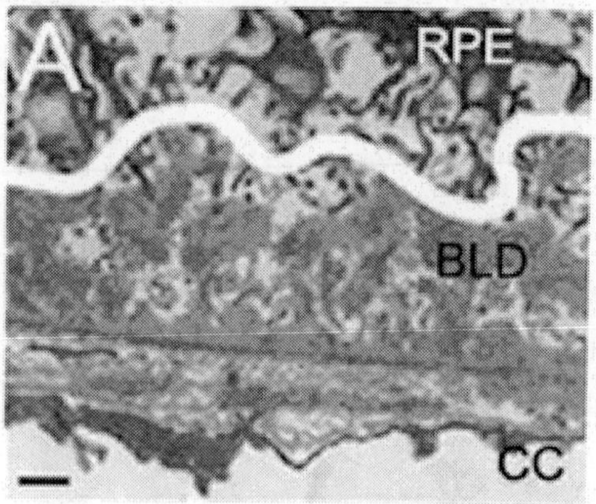

Figure 19. Transmission electron microscopy of the outer retina and choroid from a 9-month-old female mouse infused subcutaneously with Ang II for 3.5 months. Outer retina and choroid of a mouse fed a regular diet without oxidant showed a normal RPE, BrM, and choriocapillaris. The figure shows the outer retina and choroid. Mice exposed to Ang II revealed sub-RPE deposits characterized by accumulation of moderately dense homongeneous material between the RPE and its basement membrane (under white line, unpublished data).The specimen, also, shows the abnormal choriocapillaris endothelium with increased thickening and loss of fenestration. RPE, retinal pigment epithelium, BLD, basal laminar deposits, CC, choriocapillaris. Bar = 500 nm.

12. Conclusion

In summary, we postulate that Ang II plays a role in the development of dry AMD and its progression to wet AMD. Although this hypothesis remains to be proven, we have proposed new ideas and suggested different mechanisms highlighting MMP-2, basigin, MMP-14, MAPK, and MCP-1 as potential disease-related proteins as well as biochemical pathways for potential therapeutic strategies, which might result in prevention of more severe and irreversible late stages of this dreadful disease. Our goal is to intervene promptly in the early stages of the disease so that progression to the more severe late forms of AMD can be prevented. In this respect, RPE-derived MMPs are potential target due to their pivotal role in stimulating drusen formation and progression into CNV. Levels of glycosilated basigin and MMP-14, as well as, MCP-1 could be markers, which may contribute and aid to the ophthalmologic community in the management of the drusen. Moreover, AT1 receptor antagonists and p38/ERK1/2 MAPK blockers could be used successfully on the prevention of sub-RPE deposits formation in selected high-risk AMD patients.

BIBLIOGRAPHY

[1] Paul, M; Mehr, AP; Kreutz, R. Physiology of local renin-angiotensin systems. *Physiological Reviews,* 2006;86(3):747-803.

[2] Mukoyama, M. Expression cloning of type 2 angiotensin II receptor reveals a unique class of seven-transmembrane receptors. *J Biol Chem,* 1993; 268(33):24539-24542.

[3] Murphy, TJ; Wayne Alexander, R; Criendling, KK; Runge, MS; Bernstein, KE. Isolation of a cDNA encoding the vascular type-1 angiotensin II receptor. *Nature,* 1991; 351(6323):233-236.

[4] de Gasparo, M; Levens, NR. Pharmacology of Angiotensin II receptors in the kidney. *Kidney. Int,* 1994;46:1486-1491.

[5] Douglas, JG; Hopfer U. Novel aspect of angiotensin receptors and signal transduction in kidney. *Annu. Rev. Physiol,* 1994;56:649-669.

[6] Fyhrquist, F; Metsärinne, K; Tikkanen, I. Role of angiotensin II in blood pressureregulation and in the pathophysiology of cardiovascular disorders. *J Hum Hypertens,* 1995;5:19-24.

[7] Beevers, G; Lip, GY; O'Brien, E. ABC of hypertension: The pathophysiology of hypertension. *BMJ,* 2001;322:912-916.

[8] Metsärinne, KP; Helin, KH; Saijonmaa, O; Stewen, P; Sirviö, ML; Fyhrquist, FY. Tissuespecific regulation of angiotensin-converting enzyme by angiotensin II and losartan in the rat. *Blood Press,* 1996;5:363-370.

[9] Bader, M; Peters, J; Baltatu, O; Müller, DN; Luft, FC; Ganten, D. Tissue renin-angiotensin systems: new insights from experimental animal models in hypertension research. *J Mol Med,* 2001;79:76-102.

[10] Kramkowski, K; Mogielnicki, A; Buczko, W. The physiological significance of the alternative pathways of angiotensin II production. *J Physiol Pharmacol,* 2006;57:529-539.

[11] Tikellis, C; Bernardi, S; Burns, WC. Angiotensin-converting enzyme 2 is a key modulator of the renin-angiotensin system in cardiovascular and renal disease. *Curr Opin Nephrol Hypertens,* 2011;20:62-68.

[12] Santos, RA; Simoes, E; Silva, AC; Maric, C; Silva, DM; Machado, RP; de Buhr, I. Angiotensin (1-7) is an endogenous ligand for the G-protein-coupled receptor Mas. *Proc Natl Acad Sci USA,* 2003;8:825882-63.

[13] Kostenis, E; Milligan, G; Christopoulos, A; Sanchez-Ferrer, CF; Heringer-Walther, S; Sexton, PM. G-protein-coupled receptor Mas is a physiological antagonist of the angiotensin II type I receptor. *Circulation,* 2005;111:1806-1813.

[14] Nguyen G. Renin, (pro)renin and receptor: an update. *Clin Sci (Lond)*, 2011;120:169-78.

[15] Wilkinson-Berka, JL; Miller, AG; Fletcher, EL. Prorenin and the (pro)renin receptor: do they have a pathogenic role in the retina? *Front Biosci (Elite Ed)*, 2010;2:1054-1064.

[16] Ingert, C; Grima, M; Coquard, C; Barthelmebs, M; Imbs, JL. Contribution of angiotensin II internalization to intrarenal angiotensin II levels in rats. *Am J Physiol Renal Physio,l* 2002; 283: F1003–F1010.

[17] Guyton, AC (ed). *Human Physiology and Mechanisms of Disease*, 5th edn. WB Saunders: Philadelphia, PA, 1992, 157pp.

[18] Lumbers, ER. Angiotensin and aldosterone. *Regul pept,* 1999; 80: 91–100.

[19] Hall JE. Control of sodium excretion by angiotensin II: intrarenal mechanisms and blood pressure regulation. *Am J Physiol,* 1986; 250(6, Part 2): R960–R972.

[20] Daniels, D; Yee, DK; Fluharty, SJ. Angiotensin II receptor signaling. *Exp Physio,l* 2007; 92: 523–527.

[21] Koch-Weser, J. Myocardial actions of angiotensin. *Circ Res,* 1964;14:337-344.

[22] Dempsey, PJ; McCallum, ZT; Kent, KM; Cooper, T. Direct myocardial effects of angiotensin II. *Am J Physiol,* 1971;220:477–481.

[23] Holubarsch, C; Hasenfuss, G; Schmidt-Schweda, S; Knorr, A; Pieske, B; Ruf, T; Fasol, R; Just, H. Angiotensin I and II exert inotropic effects in atrial but not in ventricular human myocardium. An in vitro study under physiological experimental conditions. *Circulation,* 1993;8:1228–1237.

[24] Hoffmann, S; Krause, T; van Geel, PP; Willenbrock, R; Pagel, I; Pinto, Y; Buikema, H; van Gilst, WH; Lindschau, C; Paul, M; Inagami, T; Ganten, D; Urata, H. Overexpression of the human angiotensin II type 1 receptor in the rat heart augments load induced cardiac hypertrophy. *J Mol Med,* 2001;79:601–608.

[25] Pinto, YM; Buikema, H; van Gilst, WH; Scholtens, E; van Geel, PP; de Graeff, PA; Wagner, J; Paul, M. Cardiovascular end-organ damage in Ren-2 transgenic rat compared to spontaneously hypertensive rats. J Mol Med, *1997;*75:371–377.

[26] Hoffmann, S. Cardiac-specific overexpression of angiotensin II type 1 receptor in transgenic rats. *Methods Mol Med,* 2005;112: 389–403.

[27] Pokharel, S; van Geel, PP; Sharma, UC; Cleutjens, JP; Bohnemeier, H; Tian, XL; Schunkert, H; Crijns, HJ; Paul, M; Pinto, YM. Increased myocardial collagen content in transgenic rats overexpressing cardiac angiotensin-converting enzyme is related to enhanced breakdown of *N*-acetyl-Ser-Asp-Lys-Pro and increased phosphorylation of Smad2/3. *Circulation,* 2004;110: 3129–3135.

[28] Tian, XL; Pinto, YM; Costerousse, O; Franz, WM; Lippoldt, A; Hoffmann, S; Unger, T; Paul, M. Over-expression of angiotensin converting enzyme-1 augments cardiac hypertrophy in transgenic rats. *Hum Mol Genet,* 2004;13: 1441–1450.

[29] Muller, DN; Fischli, W; Clozel, J; Hilgers, KF; Bohlender, J; Menard, J; Busjahn, A; Ganten, D; Luft ,FC. Local angiotensin II generation in the rat heart. Role of renin uptake. *Circ Res,* 1998;82: 13–20.

[30] De Gasparo, M; Catt, KJ; Inagami, T; Unger, T. International Union of Pharmacology. XXIII. The angiotensin II receptors. *Pharmacol Rev,* 2000;52: 415–472.

[31] Marrero, MB; Schieffer, B; Paxton, WG; Heerdt, L; Berk, BC; Delafontaine, P; Bernstein, KE. Direct stimulation of Jak/STAT pathway by the angiotensin II AT_1 receptor. *Nature,* 1995;375: 247–250.

[32] Schieffer, B; Drexler, H; Ling, BN; Marrero, MB. G protein-coupled receptors control vascular smooth muscle cell proliferation via pp60c-src and p21ras. *Am J Physiol Cell Physiol,* 1997;272: C2019–C2030.

[33] Unger, T; Chung, O; Csikos, T; Culman, J; Gallinat, S; Gohlke, P; Hohle, S; Meffert, S; Stoll, M; Stroth, U; Zhu, YZ. Angiotensin receptors. *J Hypertens Suppl,* 1996;14: S95–S103.

[34] Levy, BI. Can angiotensin II type 2 receptors have deleterious effects in cardiovascular disease? Implications for therapeutic blockade of the renin-angiotensin system. *Circulation,* 2004;109: 8–13.

[35] Shenoy, U; Cassis, L. Characterization of renin activity in brown adipose tissue. *Am J Physiol Cell Physiol,* 1997;272: C989–C999.

[36] Ichihara, S; Senbonmatsu, T; Price, E Jr; Ichiki, T; Gaffney, FA; Inagami, T. Angiotensin II type 2 receptor is essential for left ventricular hypertrophy and cardiac fibrosis in chronic angiotensin II-induced hypertension. *Circulation,* 2001;104: 346–351.

[37] Yamada, T; Horiuchi, M; Dzau, VJ. Angiotensin II type 2 receptor mediates programmed cell death. *Proc Natl Acad Sci USA,* 1996;93:156–160.

[38] Cigola, E; Kajstura, J; Li, B; Meggs, LG; Anversa, P. Angiotensin II activates programmed myocyte cell death in vitro. *Exp Cell Res,* 1997;231:363–371.

[39] Anversa, P; Cheng, W; Liu, Y; Leri, A; Redaelli, G; Kajstura, J. Apoptosis and myocardial infarction. *Basic Res Cardiol,* 1998;93(3)3: 8–12.

[40] Diez, J; Panizo, A; Hernandez, M; Vega, F; Sola, I; Fortuno, MA; Pardo, J. Cardiomyocyte apoptosis and cardiac angiotensin-converting enzyme in spontaneously hypertensive rats. *Hypertension,* 1997;30: 1029–1034.

[41] Fiordaliso, F; Li, B; Latini, R; Sonnenblick, EH; Anversa, P; Leri, A; Kajstura, J. Myocyte death in streptozotocin-induced diabetes in rats is angiotensin II-dependent. *Lab Invest,* 2000;80: 513–527.

[42] Diep, QN; El Mabrouk, M; Yue, P; Schiffrin, EL. Effect of AT(1) receptor blockade on cardiac apoptosis in angiotensin II-induced hypertension. *Am J Physiol Heart Circ Physiol,* 2002;282: H1635–H1641.

[43] Sayeski, PP; Bernstein, KE. Signal transduction mechanisms of the angiotensin II type AT(1)-receptor: looking beyond the heterotrimeric G protein paradigm. *J Renin Angiotensin Aldosterone Syst,* 2001;2: 4–10.

[44] Paul, M; Zintz, M; Böcker, W; Dyer, M. Analysis and functional characterization of the rat endothelin-1 promoter. *Hypertension,* 1995;25: 683–687.

[45] Rossi, GP; Sacchetto, A; Cesari, M; Pessina, AC. Interactions between endothelin-1 and the renin-angiotensin-aldosterone system. *Cardiovasc Res,* 1999;43: 300–307.

[46] Schiffrin, EL. Vascular endothelin in hypertension. *Vasc Pharmacol,* 2005;43:19–29.

[47] Nouet, S; Nahmias, C. Signal transduction from the angiotensin II AT_2 receptor. *Trends Endocrinol Metab,* 2000;11: 1–6.

[48] Carey, RM; Jin, XH; Siragy, HM. Role of the angiotensin AT_2 receptor in blood pressure regulation and therapeutic implications. *Am J Hypertens,* 2001;14: 98S–102S.

[49] Widdop, RE; Jones, ES; Hannan, RE; Gaspari, TA. Angiotensin AT_2 receptors: cardiovascular hope or hype? *Br J Pharmacol,* 2003;140: 809–824.

[50] Shanmugam, S; Corvol, P; Gasc, JM. Ontogeny of the two angiotensin II type 1 receptor subtypes in rats. *Am J Physiol Endocrinol Metab,* 1994;267: E828–E836.

[51] Unger, T. The angiotensin type 2 receptor: variations on an enigmatic theme. *J Hypertens,* 1999;17: 1775–1786.

[52] Batenburg, WW; Tom, B; Schuijt, MP; Danser, AH. Angiotensin II type 2 receptor-mediated vasodilation. Focus on bradykinin, NO and endothelium-derived hyperpolarizing factor(s). *Vasc Pharmacol,* 2005;42: 109–118.

[53] Gohlke, P; Pees, C; Unger, T. AT_2 receptor stimulation increases aortic cyclic GMP in SHRSP by a kinin-dependent mechanism. *Hypertension,* 1998;31: 349–355.

[54] Walters, PE; Gaspari, TA; Widdop, RE. Angiotensin-(1 -7) acts as a vasodepressor agent via angiotensin II type 2 receptors in conscious rats. *Hypertension,* 2005;45:960-966.

[55] Batenburg, WW; Garrelds, IM; Bernasconi, CC; Juillerat-Jeanneret, L; van Kats, JP; Saxena, PR; Danser, AH. Angiotensin II type 2 receptor-mediated vasodilation in human coronary microarteries. *Circulation,* 2004;109: 2296–2301.

[56] Maassen Van Den Brink, A; De, VR; Saxena, PR; Schalekamp, MA; Danser, AH. Vasoconstriction by in situ formed angiotensin II: role of ACE and chymase. *Cardiovasc Res,* 1999;44: 407–415.

[57] You, D; Loufrani, L; Baron, C; Levy, BI; Widdop, RE; Henrion, D. High blood pressure reduction reverses angiotensin II type 2 receptor-mediated vasoconstriction into vasodilation in spontaneously hypertensive rats. *Circulation,* 2005;111:1006–1011.

[58] Hanna, IR; Taniyama, Y; Szocs, K; Rocic, P; Griendling, KK. NAD(P)H oxidase-derived reactive oxygen species as mediators of angiotensin II signaling. *Antioxid Redox Signal,* 2002;4: 899–914.

[59] Cai, H; Griendling, KK; Harrison, DG. The vascular NAD(P)H oxidases as therapeutic targets in cardiovascular diseases. *Trends Pharmacol Sci* , 2003;24: 471–478.

[60] Griendling, KK; Minieri, CA; Ollerenshaw, JD; Alexander, RW. Angiotensin II stimulates NADH and NADPH oxidase activity in cultured vascular smooth muscle cells. *Circ Res,*1994; 74: 1141–1148.

[61] Mollnau, H; Wendt, M; Szocs, K; Lassegue, B; Schulz, E; Oelze, M; Li, H; Bodenschatz, M; August, M; Kleschyov, AL; Tsilimingas, N; Walter, U; Forstermann, U; Meinertz, T; Griendling, K; Munzel, T. Effects of angiotensin II infusion on the expression and function of NAD(P)H oxidase and components of nitric oxide/cGMP signaling. Circ Res, *2002;* 90: E58–E65.

[62] Rajagopalan, S; Kurz, S; Munzel, T; Tarpey, M; Freeman, BA; Griendling, KK; Harrison, DG. Angiotensin II-mediated hypertension in the rat increases vascular superoxide production via membrane NADH/NADPH oxidase activation. Contribution to alterations of vasomotor tone. *J Clin Invest,* 1996; 97: 1916–1923.

[63] Seshiah, PN; Weber, DS; Rocic, P; Valppu, L; Taniyama, Y; Griendling, KK. Angiotensin II stimulation of NAD(P)H oxidase activity: upstream mediators. *Circ Res,* 2002;91: 406–413.

[64] Touyz, RM; Schiffrin, EL. Increased generation of superoxide by angiotensin II in smooth muscle cells from resistance arteries of hypertensive patients: role of phospholipase D-dependent NAD(P)H oxidase-sensitive pathways. *J Hypertens,* 2001;19: 1245–1254.

[65] Schulman, IH; Zhou, MS; Raij, L. Nitric oxide, angiotensin II, and reactive oxygen species in hypertension and atherogenesis. *Curr Hypertens Rep,* 2005;7: 61–67.

[66] Ackermann, A; Fernandez-Alfonso, M; Sanchez de Rojas, R; Ortega, T; Paul, M; Gonzalez, C. Modulation of angiotensin-converting enzyme by nitric oxide. *Br J Pharmacol,* 1998;124: 291–298.

[67] Alexander, RW; Griendling, KK. Signal transduction in vascular smooth muscle. *J Hypertens Suppl,* 1996;14: S51–S54.

[68] Campbell-Boswell, M; Robertson, AL Jr. Effects of angiotensin II and vasopressin on human smooth muscle cells in vitro. *Exp Mol Pathol,* 1981;35: 265–276.

[69] Geisterfer, AA; Peach, MJ; Owens, GK. Angiotensin II induces hypertrophy, not hyperplasia, of cultured rat aortic smooth muscle cells. *Circ Res,* 1998;62: 749–756.

[70] Gibbons, GH; Pratt, RE; Dzau, VJ. Vascular smooth muscle cell hypertrophy vs. hyperplasia. Autocrine transforming growth factor-beta 1 expression determines growth response to angiotensin II. *J Clin Invest,* 1992;90: 456–461.

[71] Schelling, P; Ganten, D; Speck, G; Fischer, H. Effects of angiotensin II and angiotensin II antagonist saralasin on cell growth and renin in 3T3 and SV3T3 cells. *J Cell Physiol,* 1979;98:503-513.

[72] Keidar, S. Angiotensin, LDL peroxidation and atherosclerosis. *Life Sci,* 1998;63:1-11.

[73] Nickenig, G; Jung, O; Strehlow, K; Zolk, O; Linz, W; Scholkens, BA; Bohm, M. Hypercholesterolemia is associated with enhanced angiotensin AT_1-receptor expression. *Am J Physiol Heart Circ Physiol,* 1997;272: H2701–H2707.

[74] Cheng, ZJ; Vapaatalo, H; Mervaala, E. Angiotensin II and vascular inflammation. *Med Sci Monit,* 2005;11: RA194–RA205.

[75] Diep, QN; El Mabrouk, M; Cohn, JS; Endemann, D; Amiri, F; Virdis, A; Neves, MF; Schiffrin, EL. Structure, endothelial function, cell growth, and inflammation in blood vessels of angiotensin II-infused rats: role of peroxisome proliferator-activated receptor-gamma. *Circulation,* 2002;105: 2296–2302.

[76] Luft, FC. Proinflammatory effects of angiotensin II and endothelin: targets for progression of cardiovascular and renal diseases. *Curr Opin Nephrol Hyperten,s* 2002;11: 59–66.

[77] Pastore, L; Tessitore, A; Martinotti, S; Toniato, E; Alesse, E; Bravi, MC; Ferri, C; Desideri, G; Gulino, A; Santucci, A. Angiotensin II stimulates intercellular adhesion molecule-1 (ICAM-1) expression by human vascular endothelial cells and increases soluble ICAM-1 release in vivo. *Circulation,* 1999;100:1646–1652.

[78] Diep, QN; Li, JS; Schiffrin, EL. In vivo study of AT(1) and AT(2) angiotensin receptors in apoptosis in rat blood vessels. *Hypertension,* 1999;34: 617–624.

[79] Bode, W; Fernandez-Catalan, C; Grams, F; Gomis-Ruth, FX; Nagase, H; Tschesche H; Maskos, K. Insights into MMP-TIMP interactions. *Ann NY Acad Sci,* 1999;878: 73–91.

[80] Jacob, MP. Extracellular matrix remodeling and matrix metalloproteinases in the vascular wall during aging and in pathological conditions. *Biomed Pharmacother,* 2003;57: 195–202.

[81] Cipollone, F; Fazia, M; Iezzi, A; Pini, B; Cuccurullo, C; Zucchelli, M de CD; Ucchino, S; Spigonardo, F; De, LM; Muraro, R; Bei, R; Bucci, M; Cuccurullo, F; Mezzetti, A. Blockade of the angiotensin II type 1 receptor stabilizes atherosclerotic plaques in humans by inhibiting prostaglandin E_2-dependent matrix metalloproteinase activity. *Circulation,* 2004;109: 1482–1488.

[82] Hutchinson, HG; Hein, L; Fujinaga, M; Pratt, RE. Modulation of vascular development and injury by angiotensin II. *Cardiovasc Res, 1999;* 41: 689-700.

[83] Walsh, DA; Hu, DE; Wharton, J; Catravas, JD; Blake, DR; Fan, TP. Sequential development of angiotensin receptors and angiotensin I converting enzyme during angiogenesis in the rat subcutaneous sponge granuloma. *Br J Pharmacol,* 1997;120: 1302-1311.

[84] Silvestre, JS; Tamarat, R; Senbonmatsu, T; Icchiki, T; Ebrahimian, T; Iglarz, M; Besnard, S; Duriez, M; Inagami, T; Levy, BI. Antiangiogenic effect of angiotensin II type 2 receptor in ischemia-induced angiogenesis in mice hindlimb. *Circ Res,* 2002;90: 1072-1079.

[85] Wang, D; Carretero, OA; Yang, XY; Rhaleb, NE; Liu, YH; Liao, TD; Yang, XP. *N*-acetyl-seryl-aspartyl-lysyl-proline stimulates angiogenesis in vitro and in vivo. *Am J Physiol Heart Circ Physiol,* 2004;287: H2099–H2105.

[86] Bickerton, R; Buckley, JP. Evidence for a central mechanism of angiotensin induced hypertension. *Proc Soc Exp Biol Med,* 1961;106: 834–837.

[87] Ferrario, CM; Dickinson, CJ; McCubbin, JW. Central vasomotor stimulation by angiotensin. *Clin Sci,* 1970;39: 239–245, 1970.

[88] Sumners, C; Fleegal, MA; Zhu, M. Angiotensin AT1 receptor signalling pathways in neurons. *Clin Exp Pharmacol Physiol,* 2002;29:483-490.

[89] Carlson, SH; Wyss, JM. Neurohormonal regulation of the sympathetic nervous system: new insights into central mechanisms of action. *Curr Hypertens Rep,* 2008;10:233-240.

[90] Zucker, IH. Novel mechanisms of sympathetic regulation in chronic heart failure. *Hypertension,* 2006;48:1005-1011.

[91] Sun, C; Sellers, KW; Sumners, C; Raizada, MK. NAD(P)H oxidase inhibition attenuates neuronal chronotropic actions of angiotensin II. *Circ Res,* 2005;96:659-666.

[92] Wang, G; Anrather, J; Huang, J; Speth, RC; Pickel, VM; Iadecola, C.NADPH oxidase contributes to angiotensin II signaling in the nucleus tractus solitarius. *J Neurosci,* 2004;24:5516-5524.

[93] Wang, G, Anrather, J;Glass, MJ; Tarsitano, MJ; Zhou, P; Frys, KA; Pickel, VM; Iadecola, C. Nox2, Ca2+, and protein kinase C play a role in angiotensin II-induced free radical production in nucleus tractus solitarius. *Hypertension,* 2006;(48):482-489.

[94] Zimmerman, MC; Lazartigues, E; Lang, JA; Sinnayah, P; Ahmad, IM; Spitz, DR; Davisson, RL. Superoxide mediates the actions of angiotensin II in the central nervous system. *Circ Res,* 2002;91:1038-1045.

[95] Zimmerman, MC; Lazartigues, E; Sharma, RV; Davisson, RL. Hypertension caused by angiotensin II infusion involves increased superoxide production in the central nervous system. *Circ Res*, 2004;95:210-216.

[96] Zimmerman, MC; Sharma, RV; Davisson, RL. Superoxide mediates angiotensin II-induced influx of extracellular calcium in neural cells. *Hypertension*, 2005;45:717-723.

[97] Okado-Matsumoto, A; Fridovich, I. Subcellular distribution of superoxide dismutases (SOD) in rat liver: Cu, Zn-SOD in mitochondria. *J Biol Chem,* 2001;276:38388-38393.

[98] Pucell, AG; Bumpus, FM; Husain, A. Rat ovarian angiotensin II receptors: characterization and coupling to estrogen secretion. *J Biol Chem,* 1987;262: 7076–7080.

[99] Morris, RS; Francis, MM; Do, YS; Hsueh, WA; Lobo, RA; Paulson, RJ. Angiotensin II (AII) modulation of steroidogenesis by luteinized granulosa cells in vitro. *J Assist Reprod Genet,* 1994;11: 117–122.

[100] Feral, C; Le Gall, S; Leymarie, P. Angiotensin II modulates steroidogenesis in granulosa and theca in the rabbit ovary: its possible involvement in atresia. *Eur J Endocrinol,* 1995;133: 747–753.

[101] Pellicer, A; Palumbo, A; DeCherney, AH; Naftolin, F. Blockage of ovulation by an angiotensin antagonist. *Science,* 1988;240: 1660–1661.

[102] Peterson, CM; Zhu, C; Mukaida, T; Butler, TA; Woessner, JF; LeMaire, WJ. The angiotensin II antagonist saralasin inhibits ovulation in the perfused rat ovary. *Am J Obstet Gynecol,* 1993;168: 242–245.

[103] Sahin, Y; Kontas, O; Muderris, II; Cankurtaran, M. Effects of angiotensin converting enzyme inhibitor cilazapril and angiotensin II antagonist saralasin in ovarian hyperstimulation syndrome in the rabbit. *Gynecol Endocrinol,* 1997;11: 231–236.

[104] Peterson, CM; Morioka, N; Zhu, C; Ryan, JW; LeMaire, WJ. Angiotensin-converting enzyme inhibitors have no effect on ovulation and ovarian steroidogenesis in the perfused rat ovary. *Reprod Toxicol,* 1993;7: 131–135.

[105] Kuji, N; Sueoka, K; Miyazaki, T; Tanaka, M; Oda, T; Kobayashi, T; Yoshimura, Y. Involvement of angiotensin II in the process of gonadotropin-induced ovulation in rabbits. *Biol Reprod,* 1996;55: 984–991.

[106] Naftolin, F; Andrade-Gordon, P; Pellicer, A; Palumbo, A; Apa, R; Zreik, T; Yoon, TK; DeCherney, A. Angiotensin II: does it have a direct obligate role in ovulation? *Science,* 1989;245: 870–871.

[107] Steele, MK; Gallo, RV; Ganong, WF. A possible role for the brain renin-angiotensin system in the regulation of LH secretion. *Am J Physiol Regul Integr Comp Physiol,* 1983;245: R805–R810.

[108] Troffa, C; Tonolo, G; Melis, MG; Manunta, P; Soro, A; Pala, F; Pazzola, A; Sabino, G; Masala, A; Maioli, M. Effect of angiotensin converting enzyme inhibition on the menstrual cycle of hypertensive women. *J Cardiovasc Pharmacol,* 1991;18: 462–467.

[109] Wu, JN; Edwards, D; Berecek, KH. Changes in renal angiotensin II receptors in spontaneously hypertensive rats by early treatment with the angiotensin-converting enzyme inhibitor captopril. *Hypertension,* 1994;23: 819–822.

[110] Hagemann, A; Nielsen, AH; Poulsen K. The uteroplacental renin-angiotensin system: a review. *Exp Clin Endocrinol,* 1994;102: 252–261.

[111] Cox, BE; Word, RA; Rosenfeld, CR. Angiotensin II receptor characteristics and subtype expression in uterine arteries and myometrium during pregnancy. *J Clin Endocrinol Metab,* 1996;81: 49–58.

[112] Schirar, A; Capponi, A; Catt, KJ. Regulation of uterine angiotensin II receptors by estrogen and progesterone. *Endocrinology,* 1980;106: 5–12.

[113] Speth, RC; Daubert, DL; Grove, KL. Angiotensin II: a reproductive hormone too? *Regul Pept,* 1999;79: 25–40.

[114] Clyne, CD; Nicol, MR; MacDonald, S; Williams, BC; Walker, SW. Angiotensin II stimulates growth and steroidogenesis in zona fasciculata/reticularis cells from bovine adrenal cortex via the AT_1 receptor subtype. *Endocrinology,* 1993;132: 2206–2212.

[115] Neuss, M; Regitz-Zagrosek, V; Hildebrandt, A; Fleck, E. Human cardiac fibroblasts express an angiotensin receptor with unusual binding characteristics which is coupled to cellular proliferation. *Biochem Biophys Res Commun,* 1994;204: 1334–1339.

[116] Paquet, JL; Baudouin-Legros, M; Brunelle, G; Meyer, P. Angiotensin II-induced proliferation of aortic myocytes in spontaneously hypertensive rats. *J Hypertens,* 1990;8: 565–572.

[117] Steckelings, UM; Artuc, M; Paul, M; Stoll, M; Henz, BM. Angiotensin II stimulates proliferation of primary human keratinocytes via a non-AT_1, non-AT_2 angiotensin receptor. *Biochem Biophys Res Commun,* 1996;229: 329–333.

[118] Stoll, M; Steckelings, UM; Paul, M; Bottari, SP; Metzger, R; Unger, T. The angiotensin AT_2-receptor mediates inhibition of cell proliferation in coronary endothelial cells. *J Clin Invest,* 1995;95: 651–657.

[119] Viswanathan, M; Saavedra, JM. Expression of angiotensin II AT_2 receptors in the rat skin during experimental wound healing. *Peptides,* 1992;13: 783–786.

[120] Kimura, B; Sumners, C; Phillips, MI. Changes in skin angiotensin II receptors in rats during wound healing. *Biochem Biophys Res Commun,* 1992;187: 1083–1090.

[121] Abiko, M; Rodgers, KE; Campeau, JD; Nakamura, RM; Dizerega, GS. Alterations of angiotensin II receptor levels in sutured wounds in rat skin. *J Invest Surg,* 1996;9: 447–453.

[122] Sun, Y; Ramires, FJ; Zhou, G; Ganjam, VK; Weber, KT. Fibrous tissue and angiotensin II. *J Mol Cell Cardiol,* 1997;29: 2001–2012.

[123] Gyurko, R; Kimura, B; Kurian, P; Crews, FT; Phillips, MI. Angiotensin II receptor subtypes play opposite roles regulating phosphatidylinositol hydrolysis in rat skin slices. *Biochem Biophys Res Commun,* 1992;186: 285–292.

[124] Fliser, D; Schaefer, F; Schmid, D; Veldhuis, JD; Ritz, E. Angiotensin II affects basal, pulsatile, and glucose-stimulated insulin secretion in humans. *Hypertension,* 1997;30:1156–1161.

[125] Dunning, BE; Moltz, JH; Fawcett, CP. Actions of neurohypophysial peptides on pancreatic hormone release. *Am J Physiol*, 1984;246:E108–114.

[126] Kampf, C; Lau, T; Olsson, R; Leung, PS; Carlsson, PO. Angiotensin II type 1 receptor inhibition markedly improves the blood perfusion, oxygen tension and first phase of glucose-stimulated insulin secretion in revascularised syngeneic mouse islet grafts. *Diabetologia*, 2005;48: 1159–1167.

[127] Carlsson, PO; Berne, C; Jansson, L. Angiotensin II and the endocrine pancreas: effects on islet blood flow and insulin secretion in rats. *Diabetologia*,1998;41:127–133.

[128] Chu, KY; Lau, T; Carlsson, PO; Leung, PS. Angiotensin II type 1 receptor blockade improves beta-cell function and glucose tolerance in a mouse model of type 2 diabetes. *Diabetes*, 2006;55:367–374.

[129] Janiak, P; Bidouard, JP; Cadrouvele, C; Poirier, B; Gouraud, L; Grataloup, Y; Pierre, F; Bruneval, P; O'Connor, SE; Herbert, JM. Long-term blockade of angiotensin AT1 receptors increases survival of obese Zucker rats. *Eur J Pharmacol,* 2006;534:271–9.

[130] Sealey, JE; Catanzaro, DF; Lavin, TN; Gahnem, F; Pitarresi, T; Hu, LF; Laragh, JH. Specific prorenin/renin binding (ProBP). Identification and characterization of a novel membrane site. *Am J Hypertens*, 1996;9:491–502.

[131] Cheng, Q; Law, PK; de Gasparo, M; Leung, PS. Combination of the dipeptidyl peptidase IV inhibitor LAF237 [(S)-1-[(3-hydroxy-1-adamantyl)ammo]acetyl-2-cyanopyrrolidine] with the angiotensin II type 1 receptor antagonist valsartan [N-(1-oxopentyl)-N-[[2'- (1H-tetrazol-5-yl)-[1,1'-biphenyl]-4-yl]methyl]-L-valine] enhances

pancreatic islet morphology and function in a mouse model of type 2 diabetes. *J Pharmacol Exp Ther*, 2008;327:683–91.

[132] Chu, KY; Leung, PS. Angiotensin II Type 1 receptor antagonism mediates uncoupling protein 2-driven oxidative stress and ameliorates pancreatic islet beta-cell function in young Type 2 diabetic mice. *Antioxid Redox Signal*, 2007;9:869–78.

[133] Wong, PF; Lee, SS; Cheung, WT. Immunohistochemical colocalization of type II angiotensin receptors with somatostatin in rat pancreas. *Regul Pept*, 2004;117:195–205.

[134] Lau, T; Carlsson, PO; Leung, PS. Evidence for a local angiotensin-generating system and dose-dependent inhibition of glucose-stimulated insulin release by angiotensin II in isolated pancreatic islets. *Diabetologia*, 2004;47:240–248.

[135] Hershon, KS. Mechanistic and clinical aspects of renin-angiotensin-aldosterone system blockade in the prevention of diabetes mellitus and cardiovascular disease. *Endocr Pract*, 2001;17(3):430-440.

[136] Schinke, M; Doods, HN; Entzeroth, M. Characterization of the angiotensin II receptor subtype in rat ileum. *Naunyn-Schmiedeberg's Arch Pharmacol,* 1991;343: 282.

[137] Jaszewski, R; Tolia, V; Ehrinpreis, MN; Bodzin, JH; Peleman, RR; Korlipara, R; Weinstock, JV. Increased colonic mucosal angiotensin I and II concentrations in Crohn's colitis. *Gastroenterology,* 1990;98: 1543–1548.

[138] De los, R; Labajos, M; Manteca, A; Morell, M; Souviron, A. Stimulatory action of angiotensin II on water and electrolyte transport by the proximal colon of the rat. *J Endocrinol,* 1980;86:35–43.

[139] Levens, NR; Peach, MJ; Carey, RM; Poat, JA; Munday, KA. Changes in an electroneutral transport process mediated by angiotensin II in the rat distal colon in vivo. *Endocrinology,* 1981;108: 1497–1504.

[140] Berger, S; Bleich, M; Schmid, W; Greger, R; Schutz, G. Mineralocorticoid receptor knockout mice: lessons on Na^+ metabolism. *Kidney Int,* 2000;57: 1295–1298.

[141] Igić, R; Robinson, CJ; Milosević, Z; Wilson, CM; Erdös, EG. Activity of renin and angiotensin I converting enzyme in retina and ciliary body. *Lijec Vjesn,* 1977;99(8):482-484.

[142] Wheeler-Schilling, TH; Kohler, K; Sautter, M; Guenther, E. Angiotensin II receptor subtype gene expression and cellular localization in the retina and non-neuronal ocular tissues of the rat. *Eur J Neurosci*, 1999. 11;3387-3394

[143] Savaskan, E; Loffler, KU; Meier, F; Muller-Spahn, F; Flammer, J; Meyer, P. Immunohistochemical localization of angiotensin-converting enzyme, angiotensin II and AT1 receptor in human ocular tissues. *Ophthalmic Res*, 2004. 36;312-320

[144] Senanayake, P; Drazba, J; Shadrach, K; Milsted, A; Rungger-Brandle, E; Nishiyama, K; Miura, S; Karnik, S; Sears, JE; Hollyfield, JG. Angiotensin II and its receptor subtypes in the human retina, *Invest Ophthalmol Vis Sci*, 2007, 48: 3301-3311

[145] Striker, GE; Praddaude, F; Alcazar, O; Cousins, SW; Marin-Castano, ME. Regulation of angiotensin II receptors and extracellular matrix turnover in human retinal pigment epithelium: role of angiotensin II. *Am J Physiol Cell Physiol*, 2008. 295; C1633-1646

[146] Cunha-Vaz, J. The blood-ocular barriers. *Surv Ophthalmol*, 1979. 23;279-296.

[147] Danser, AHJ; Derkx, FHM; Admiraal, PJJ; Deinum, J; de Jong, PTVM; Schalekamp, MADH. Angiotensin levels in the eye. *Invest Ophthalmol Vis Sci*, 1994. 35;1008-1018

[148] Otani, A; Takagi, H; Suzuma, K; Honda, Y. Angiotensin II potentiates endothelial growth factor-induced angiogenic activity in retinal microcapillary endothelial cells. *Circ Res,*1998. 82;619-628.

[149] Augood, CA; Vingerling, JR; de Jong, PT. Prevalence of age-related maculopathy in older Europeans: the European Eye Study (EUREYE). *Arch Ophthalmol,* 2006.124;529-535.

[150] Evans, JR. Risk factors for age-related macular degeneration. *Prog Retin Eye Res,* 2001. 20;227-253.

[151] Javitt, JC; Zhou, Z; Maguire, MG; Fine, SL; Willke, RJ. Incidence of exudative age-related macular degeneration among elderly Americans. *Ophthalmology,* 2003. 110:1534-1539.

[152] Klein, R; Peto, T; Bird, A; Vannewkirk, MR. The epidemiology of age-related macular degeneration. *Am J Ophthalmol,* 2004. 137;486-495.

[153] Rein, DB; Wittenborn, JS; Zhang, X; Honeycutt, AA; Lesesne, SB; Saaddine, J. Forecasting age-related macular degeneration through the year 2050: the potential impact of new treatments. *Arch Ophthalmol,* 2009. 127;533-540.

[154] Green, WR. Histopathology of age-related macular degeneration. *Mol Vis,* 1999, 5:27.

[155] Bird, AC; Bressler, NM; Bressler, SB; Chisholm, IH; Coscas, G; Davis, MD. An international classification and grading system for age-related maculopathy and age-related macular degeneration. The International ARM Epidemiological Study Group. *Surv Ophthalmol*, 1995; 39(5):367-374.

[156] Gass, JD. Drusen and disciform macular detachment and degeneration. *Trans Am Ophthalmol Soc*, 1972; 70:409-436.

[157] Curcio, CA; Medeiros, NE; Millican, CL. Photoreceptor loss in age-related macular degeneration. *Invest Ophthalmol Vis Sci*, 1996; 37(7):1236-1249.

[158] Zarbin, MA. Current concepts in the pathogenesis of age-related macular degeneration. *Arch Ophthalmol*, 2004; 122(4):598-614.

[159] Hageman, GS; Luthert, PJ; Victor Chong, NH; Johnson, LV; Anderson, DH; Mullins, RF. An integrated hypothesis that considers drusen as biomarkers of immune-mediated processes at the RPE-Bruch's membrane interface in aging and age-related macular degeneration. *Prog Retin Eye Res*, 2001; 20(6):705-732.

[160] Penfold, PL; Madigan, MC; Gillies, MC; Provis, JM. Immunological and aetiological aspects of macular degeneration. *Prog Retin Eye Res*, 2001; 20(3):385-414.

[161] Hageman, GS; Mullins, RF. Molecular composition of drusen as related to substructural phenotype. *Mol Vis*, 1999;5:28. Review.

[162] Anderson, DH; Mullins, RF; Hageman, GS; Johnson, LV. A role for local inflammation in the formation of drusen in the aging eye. *Am J Ophthalmol*, 2002; 134(3):411-431.

[163] Marin-Castaño, ME; Csaky, KG; Cousins, SW. Nonlethal oxidant injury to human retinal pigment epithelium cells causes cell membrane blebbing but decreased MMP-2 activity. *Invest Ophthalmol Vis Sci*, 2005;46(9):3331-3340.

[164] Marin-Castaño, ME; Striker, GE; Alcazar, O; Catanuto, P; Espinosa-Heidmann, DG; Cousins, SW. Repetitive nonlethal oxidant injury to retinal pigment epithelium decreased extracellular matrix turnover in vitro and induced sub-RPE deposits in vivo. *Invest Ophthalmol Vis Sci*, 2006;47(9):4098-4112.

[165] Cousins, SW; Espinosa-Heidmann, DG; Alexandridou, A; Sall, J; Dubovy, S; Csaky, K. The role of aging, high fat diet and blue light exposure in an experimental mouse model for basal laminar deposit formation. *Exp Eye Res*, 2002; 75(5):543-553.

[166] Strunnikova, N; Zhang, C; Teichberg, D; Cousins, SW; Baffi, J; Becker, KG; Csaky, KG. Survival of retinal pigment epithelium after exposure to prolonged oxidative injury: a detailed gene expression and cellular analysis. *Invest Ophthalmol Vis Sci*, 2004;45(10):3767-3777.

[167] Beatty, S; Koh, H; Phil, M; Henson, D; Boulton, M. The role of oxidative stress in the pathogenesis of age-related macular degeneration. *Surv Ophthalmol*, 2000; 45(2):115-134.

[168] Winkler, BS; Boulton, ME; Gottsch, JD; Sternberg, P. Oxidative damage and age-related macular degeneration. *Mol Vis*, 1999; 5:32.

[169] Espinosa-Heidmann, DG; Suner, IJ; Catanuto, P; Hernandez, EP; Marin-Castano, ME; Cousins, SW. Cigarette smoke-related oxidants and the development of sub-RPE deposits in an experimental animal model of dry AMD. *Invest Ophthalmol Vis Sci*, 2006;47(2):729-737.

[170] Rodrigues, EB. Inflammation in dry age-related macular degeneration. *Ophthalmologica*, 2007;221;143-152.

[171] Chisolm, GM III; Hazen, SL; Fox, PL; Cathcart, MK. The oxidation of lipoproteins by monocytes-macrophages. Biochemical and biological mechanisms. *J Biol Chem*, 1999; 274(37):25959-25962.

[172] Grossniklaus, HE; Ling, JX; Wallace, TM; Dithmar, S; Lawson, DH; Cohen, C et al. Macrophage and retinal pigment epithelium expression of angiogenic cytokines in choroidal neovascularization. *Mol Vis*, 2002; 8:119-126.

[173] Cousins, SW; Espinosa-Heidmann, DG; Csaky, KG. Monocyte activation in patients with age-related macular degeneration: a biomarker of risk for choroidal neovascularization? *Arch Ophthalmo*l, 2004; 122(7):1013-1018.

[174] Espinosa-Heidmann, DG; Suner, IJ; Hernandez, EP; Monroy, D; Csaky, KG; Cousins, SW. Macrophage depletion diminishes lesion size and severity in experimental choroidal neovascularization. *Invest Ophthalmol Vis Sci*, 2003; 44(8):3586-3592.

[175] Vingerling, JR; Klaver, CC; Hofman, A. Epidemiology of age-related maculopathy. *Epidemiol.Rev*, 1995;17:347-360.

[176] Bilato, C; Crow, MT. Atherosclerosis and the vascular biology of aging. *Aging* (Milano), 1996;8:221-234.

[177] Hariri, RJ; Alonso, DR; Hajjar, DP. Aging and arteriosclerosis. I. Development of myointimal hyperplasia after endothelial injury. *J Exp.Med*, 1986;164:1171-1178.

[178] Spagnoli, LG; Sambuy, Y; Palmieri, G. Age-related modulation of vascular smooth muscle cells proliferation following arterial wall damage. *Artery*, 1985;13:187-198.

[179] Klein, R; Klein, BE; Jensen, SC. The relation of cardiovascular disease and its risk factors to the 5- year incidence of age-related maculopathy: the Beaver Dam Eye Study. *Ophthalmology*, 1997;104:1804-1812.

[180] Smith, W; Mitchell, P; Leeder, SR. Plasma fibrinogen levels, other cardiovascular risk factors, and age- related maculopathy: the Blue Mountains Eye Study. *Arch.Ophthalmol*, 1998;116:583-587.

[181] Jonas, JB; Hayreh, SS; Martus, P. Influence of arterial hypertension and diet-induced atherosclerosis on macular drusen. *Graefes Arch Clin Exp Ophthalmol*, 2003;24(2):125-134.

[182] Nagai, N; Oike, Y; Izumi-Nagai, K; Urano, T; Kubota, Y; Noda, K; Ozawa, Y; Inoue, M; Tsubota, K; Suda, T; Ishida, S. Angiotensin II type 1 receptor-mediated inflammation is required for choroidal neovascularization. *Arterioscler Thromb Vasc Biol*, 2006;26(10):2252-2259.

[183] Ruiz-Ortega, M; Ruperez, M; Esteban, V. Molecular Mechanisms of Angiotensin II-induced Vascular Injury. *Curr Hypertens.Rep*, 2003;5:73-79.

[184] Taylor, WR. Hypertensive vascular disease and inflammation: mechanical and humoral mechanisms. *Curr Hypertens.Rep*, 1999;1:96-101.

[185] Dorey, CK; Wu, G; Ebenstein, D. Cell loss in the aging retina. Relationship to lipofuscin accumulation and macular degeneration. *Invest Ophthalmol Vis Sci,* 1989;30:1691-1699.

[186] Ishibashi, T; Patterson, R; Ohnishi, Y; Inomata, H; Ryan, S. Formation of drusen in the human eye. *Am. J. Ophthalmol*, 1986;101:342–353.

[187] Donders, F. Beitrage zur pathologischen Anatomie des Auges. Graefe's Arch. *Clin. Exp. Ophthalmol*, 1854;1:106–118.

[188] Muller, H. Anatomische beitrage zur ophthalmologie. Albrecht von Graefe Arch *Ophthalmol*, 1856; 2:1–69.

[189] Burns, R; Feeney Burns, L. Clinico-morphologic correlations of drusen of Bruch's membrane. *Trans Am Ophthalmol Soc*, 1980;78:206–225.

[190] Young, RW. Pathophysiology of age-related macular degeneration. *Surv Ophthalmol*, 1987; 31(5):291-306.

[191] Farkas, T; Sylvester, V; Archer, D. The ultrastructure of drusen. *Am J Ophthalmol*, 1971;71:1196–1205.

[192] Feeney-Burns, L; Gao, C; Tidwell, M. Lysosomal enzyme cytochemistry of human RPE, Bruch's membrane and drusen. *Invest. Ophthalmol Visual Sci*, 1987;28:1138–1147.

[193] El Baba, F; Green, W; Fleischmann, J; Finkelstein, D; de la Cruz, Z. Clinicopathologic correlation of lipidization and detachment of the retinal pigment epithelium. *Am J Ophthalmol*, 1986;101:576–583.

[194] Charras, GT. A short history of blebbing. J Microsc, 2008; 231:466–478.

[195] Chiang, J; Kowada, M; Ames III, A; Wright RL; Majino, G. Cerebral isquenia III. Vascular changes. *Am. J. Path*, 1968;52:437-447.

[196] Molteni, A; Moulder, JE; Cohen, EF; Ward, WF, Fish, BL; Taylor, JM;, Wolfe, LF, Brizio-Molteni, L; Veno, P. Control ofe radiation-induced pneumopathy and lung fibrosis by angiotensin-converting enzyme inhibitors and an angiotensin II type 1 receptor blocker. *Int J Radiat Biol*, 2000;76(4):523-532.

[197] Godin, CM; Ferguson, SS. The angiotensin II type 1 receptor induces membrane blebbing by coupling to Rho A, Rho kinase, and myosin light chain kinase. *Mol Pharmacol*, 2010;77(6):903-911).

[198] Strunnikova N, Baffi J, Gonzalez A, Silk W, Cousins SW, Csaky KG. Regulated heat shock protein 27 expression in human retinal pigment epithelium. Invest Ophthalmol Vis Sci 2001; 42(9):2130-2138.

[199] Zhang C, Baffi J, Cousins SW, Csaky KG. Oxidant-induced cell death in retinal pigment epithelium cells mediated through the release of apoptosis-inducing factor. J Cell Sci 2003; 116(Pt 10):1915-1923.

[200] Khan SA, Ghosh S, Wickstrom M, Miller LA, Hess R, Haschek WM et al. Comparative pathology of microcystin-LR in cultured hepatocytes, fibroblasts, and renal epithelial cells. Nat Toxins 1995; 3(3):119-128.

[201] van der Schaft, TL; de Bruijn, BC; Mooy, GM; Ketelaars, DAM; Jong, PTVM. Is basal laminar deposit unique for age-related macular degeneration? *Arch Ophthalmol*, 1991;109:420–425.

[202] Ishibashi, T; Sorgente, N; Patterson, R; Ryan, SJ. Pathogenesis of drusen in the primate. *Invest Ophthalmol Vis Sci*, 1986;27:184-193.

[203] Zhu, ZR; Goodnight, R; Nishimura, T; Sorgente, N; Ogden, TE; Ryan, SJ. Experimental changes resembling the pathology of drusen in Bruch's membrane in the rabbit. *Curr Eye Res*,1988;7:581-592.

[204] Malorni, W; Iosi, F; Mirabelli, F; Bellomo, G. Cytoskeleton as a target in menadione-induced oxidative stress in cultured mammalian cells: alterations underlying surface bleb formation. *Chem Biol Interact*, 1991;80:217-236.

[205] Gerthoffer, WT; Gunst, SJ. Invited review: focal adhesion and small heat shock proteins in the regulation of actin remodeling and contractility in smooth muscle. *J Appl Physiol*, 2001;91:963-972.

[206] Dalle-Donne, I; Rossi, R; Milzani, A; Di Simplicio, P; Colombo, R. The actin cytoskeleton response to oxidants: from small heat shock protein phosphorylation to changes in the redox state of actin itself. *Free Radic Biol Med*, 2001; 31(12):1624-1632.

[207] Chen, WP; Tan, SK; Chen, A; Lin, CY. Intrarenal infusion of supernatant from cytokine-activated human mesangial cells may cause glomerular damage. *Zhonghua Yi Xue Za Zhi (Taipei,)* 1999; 62(10):657-665.

[208] Okamoto, K; Mizuno, M; Nakahara, N; Natsume, A; Yoshida J, Mori, T. Process of apoptosis induced by TNF-alpha in murine fibroblast Ltk-cells: continous observations with video enhanced contrats microscopy. *Apoptosis*, 2002;7(1):77-86.

[209] Ashwood-Smith, MJ; Morris, GW; Fowler, R; Appleton, TC; Ashorn, R. Physical factors are involved in the destruction of embryos and oocytes during freezing and thawing procedures. *Hum Reprod*, 1988; 3(6):795-802.

[210] Hinshaw, DB; Sklar, LA; Bohl, B; Schraufstatter, IU; Hyslop, PA; Rossi, MW. Cytoskeletal and morphologic impact of cellular oxidant injury. *Am J Pathol*, 1986; 123(3):454-464.

[211] Malorni, W; Donelli, G; Straface, E; Santini, MT; Paradisi, S; Giacomoni, PU. Both UVA and UVB induce cytoskeleton-dependent surface blebbing in epidermoid cells. *J Photochem Photobiol B*, 1994; 26(3):265-270.

[212] Lanzetti, L; Di Fiore, PP; Scita, G. Pathways linking endocytosis and actin cytoskeleton in mammalian cells. *Exp Cell Res*, 2001; 271(1):45-56.

[213] Taunton, J. Actin filament nucleation by endosomes, lysosomes and secretory vesicles. *Curr Opin Cell Biol*, 2001; 13(1):85-91.

[214] Rao, A; Craig, AM. Signaling between the actin cytoskeleton and the postsynaptic density of dendritic spines. *Hippocampus*, 2000; 10(5):527-541.

[215] Kaibuchi, K; Kuroda, S; Amano, M. Regulation of the cytoskeleton and cell adhesion by the Rho family GTPases in mammalian cells. *Annu Rev Biochem*, 1999; 68:459-486.

[216] Valentijn, K; Valentijn, JA; Jamieson, JD. Role of actin in regulated exocytosis and compensatory membrane retrieval: insights from an old acquaintance. *Biochem Biophys Res Commun*, 1999;266(3):652-661.

[217] Downey, GP. Mechanisms of leukocyte motility and chemotaxis. *Curr Opin Immunol*, 1994;6(1):113-124.

[218] Hirokawa, N. Axonal transport and the cytoskeleton. *Curr Opin Neurobiol*, 1993; 3(5):724-731.

[219] Weed, SA; Parsons, JT. Cortactin: coupling membrane dynamics to cortical actin assembly. *Oncogene*, 2001; 20(44):6418-6434.

[220] Milzani, A; DalleDonne, I; Colombo, R; Rodriguez OC. Prolonged oxidative stress on actin. *Arch Biochem Biophys*, 1997;339(2):267-274.

[221] Huot, J; Houle, F; Rousseau, S; Deschesnes, RG; Shah, GM; Landry, J. SAPK2/p38-dependent F-actin reorganization regulates early membrane blebbing during stress-induced apoptosis. *J Cell Biol*, 1998;143(5):1361-1373.

[222] Concannon, CG; Gorman, AM; Samali, A. On the role of Hsp27 in regulating apoptosis. *Apoptosis*. 2003;8(1):61-70.

[223] Delogu, G; Signore, M; Mechelli, A; Famularo, G. Heat shock proteins and their role in heart injury. *Curr Opin Crit Care*, 2002;8(5):411-416

[224] Haslbeck, M. sHsps and their role in the chaperone network. *Cell Mol Life Sci*, 2002;59(10):1649-1657.

[225] Constantin, B; Meerschaert, K; Vandekerckhove, J; Gettemans, J. Disruption of the actin cytoskeleton of mammalian cells by the capping complex actin-fragmin is inhibited by actin phosphorylation and regulated by Ca2+ ions. *J Cell Sci*, 1998;111(Pt 12):1695-1706.

[226] Schneider, GB; Hamano, H; Cooper, LF. In vivo evaluation of hsp27 as an inhibitor of actin polymerization: hsp27 limits actin stress fiber and focal adhesion formation after heat shock. *J Cell Physiol*, 1998;177(4):575-584.

[227] Ganea, E. Chaperone-like activity of alpha-crystallin and other small heat shock proteins. *Curr Protein Pept Sci.* 2001;2(3):205-225.

[228] de Lanerolle, P; Cole, AB. Cytoskeletal proteins and gene regulation: form, function, and signal transduction in the nucleus. *Sci STKE*, 2002;2002(139):E30.

[229] Landry, J; Huot, J. Modulation of actin dynamics during stress and physiological stimulation by a signaling pathway involving p38 MAP kinase and heat-shock protein 27. *Biochem Cell Biol*, 1995;73(9-10):703-707.

[230] Stokoe, D; Engel, K; Campbell, DG; Cohen, P; Gaestel, M. Identification of MAPKAP kinase 2 as a major enzyme responsible for the phosphorylation of the small mammalian heat shock proteins. *FEBS Lett*, 1992;313(3):307-313.

[231] Huot, J; Houle, F; Marceau, F; Landry, J. Oxidative stress-induced actin reorganization mediated by the p38 mitogen-activated protein kinase/heat shock protein 27 pathway in vascular endothelial cells. *Circ Res*, 1997;80:383-392

[232] Pons, M; Cousins, SW; Csaky, KG; Striker, G; Marin-Castaño, ME. Cigarette smoke-related hydroquinone induces filamentous actin reorganization and heat shock protein 27 phosphorylation through p38 and extracellular signal-regulated kinase 1/2 in retinal

pigment epithelium: implications for age-related macular degeneration. *Am J Pathol*, 2010;177(3):1198-11213.

[233] Feig, LA. Ral-GTPases: approaching their 15 minutes of fame. Trends Cell Biol, 2003; 13:419–425.

[234] Takai, Y; Sasaki, T; Matozaki, T. Small GTP-binding proteins. Physiol Rev, 2001; 81:153–208

[235] Albright, CF; Giddings, BW; Liu, J; Vito, M; Weinberg, RA. Characterization of a guanine nucleotide dissociation stimulator for a ras-related GTPase. EMBO J, 1993; 12:339–347.

[236] Hofer, F; Fields, S; Schneider, C; Martin, GS. Activated Ras interacts with the Ral guanine nucleotide dissociation stimulator. Proc Natl Acad Sci USA, 1994; 91:11089–11093.

[237] Kikuchi, A; Williams, LT. Regulation of interaction of ras p21 with RalGDS and Raf-1 by cyclic AMP-dependent protein kinase. J Biol Chem, 1996; 271:588–594.

[238] Matsubara, K; Kishida, S; Matsuura, Y; Kitayama, H; Noda, M; Kikuchi, A. Plasma membrane recruitment of RalGDS is critical for Ras-dependent Ral activation. Oncogene, 1999; 18:1303–1312.

[239] Wolthuis, RM; Bos, JL. Ras caught in another affair: the exchange factors for Ral. Curr Opin Genet Dev, 1999; 9:112–117.

[240] Barnes, WG; Reiter, E; Violin, JD; Ren, XR; Milligan, G; Lefkowitz, RJ. beta-Arrestin 1 and Galphaq/11 coordinately activate RhoA and stress fiber formation following receptor stimulation. J Biol Chem, 2005; 280:8041–8050.

[241] Matrougui, K; Tankó, LB; Loufrani, L; Gorny, D; Levy, BI; Tedgui, A; Henrion, D. Involvement of Rho-kinase and the actin filament network in angiotensin II-induced contraction and extracellular signal-regulated kinase activity in intact rat mesenteric resistance arteries. Arterioscler Thromb Vasc Biol, 2001; 21:1288–1293.

[242] Lammers, M; Meyer, S; Kühlmann, D; Wittinghofer, A. Specificity of interactions between mDia isoforms and Rho proteins. J Biol Chem, 2008; 283:35236–35246.

[243] Krebs, A; Rothkegel, M; Klar, M; Jockusch, BM. Characterization of functional domains of mDia1, a link between the small GTPase Rho and the actin cytoskeleton. J Cell Sci, 2001; 114:3663–3672.

[244] Min Kim, J; Uehara, Y; Ja Choi, Y; Mi Ha, Y; Hyeok Ye, B, Pal Yu, B; Young Chung, H. Mecahnism of attenuation of pro-inflammatory Ang II-induced NF-kB activation by genistein in the kidneys of male rats during aging. Biogerontology, 2011 (DOI 10.1007/s10522-011-9345-4).

[245] Aumailley, M; Gayraud, B. Structure and biological activity of the extracellular matrix. *J Mol Med*,1998;76:253-265.

[246] Kugler, A. Matrix metalloproteinases and their inhibitors. *Anticancer Res*, 1999;19:1589-1592.

[247] Jacot, TA; Striker, GE; Stetler-Stevenson, M. Mesangial cells from transgenic mice with progressive glomerulosclerosis exhibit stable, phenotypic changes including undetectable MMP-9 and increased type IV collagen. *Lab Invest*, 1996;75:791-799.

[248] Peten, EP; Garcia-Perez, A; Terada, Y. Age-related changes in alpha 1- and alpha 2-chain type IV collagen mRNAs in adult mouse glomeruli: competitive PCR. *Am J Physiol*, 1992;263:F951-F957.

[249] Belkhiri, A; Richards, C; Whaley, M. Increased expression of activated matrix metalloproteinase-2 by human endothelial cells after sublethal H2O2 exposure. *Lab Invest*, 1997;77:533-539.

[250] Sarks, S; Cherepanoff, S; Killingsworth, M; Sarks, J. Relationship of basal laminar deposit and membranous debris to the clinical presentation of early Age-related macular degeneration. *Invest Ophthalmol Vis Sci*, 2007; 48:968-977.

[251] Alcazar, O; Cousins, SW; Marin-Castaño, ME. MMP-14 and TIMP-2 overexpression protects against hydroquinone-induced oxidant injury in RPE: implications for extracellular matrix turnover. *Invest Ophthalmol Vis Sci*, 2007;48(12):5662-70.

[252] Alcazar, O; Hawkridge, AM; Collier, TS; Cousins, SW; Bhattacharya, SK; Muddiman, DC; Marin-Castano, ME. Proteomics characterization of cell membrane blebs in human retinal pigment epithelium cells. *Mol Cell Proteomics*, 2009;8(10):2201-2211.

[253] Wiesner, C; Faix, J; Himmel, M; Bentzien, F; Linder, S. KIF5B and KIF3A/KIF3B kinesins drive MT1-MMP surface exposure, CD44 shedding, and extracellular matrix degradation in primary macrophages. *Blood*, 2010;116(9):1559-69.

[254] Deryugina, EI; Bourdon, MA; Reisfeld, RA; Strongin, A. Remodeling of collagen matrix by human tumor cells requires activation and cell surface association of matrix metalloproteinase-2. *Cancer Res,* 1989; 58:3743-3750.

[255] Atkison, SJ; Petterson, ML; Butler, MJ; Murphy, G. Membrane type 1 matrix metalloproteinase and gelatinase A synergistically degrade type I collagen in a cell model. *FEBS Lett,* 2001; 491:222-226.

[256] Hayreh, SS; Servais, GE; Virdi, PS. Macular lesions in malignant arterial hypertension. *Ophthalmologica*, 1989;198:230-246.

[257] Hyman, L; Schachat, AP; He, Q; Leske, MC. Hypertension, cardiovascular disease, and age-related macular degeneration. Age-Related Macular Degeneration Risk Factors Study Group. *Arch Ophthalmol*, 2000;118:351-358.

[258] Lee, MA; Bohm, M; Paul, M; Ganten, D. Tissue renin-angiotensin systems. Their role in cardiovascular disease. *Circulation*, 1993;87:IV7-13.

[259] Berka, JL; Stubbs; AJ; Wang, DZ; DiNicolantonio, R; Alcorn, D; Campbell, DJ; Skinner, SL. Renin-containing Muller cells of the retina display endocrine features. *Invest Ophthalmol Vis Sci*, 1995; 36:1450-1458.

[260] . Kohler, K; Wheeler-Schilling, T; Jurklies, B; Guenther, E. Angiotensin II in the rabbit retina. *Vis Neurosci*, 1997;14:63-71.

[261] Wagner, J; Jan Danser, AH; Derkx, FH; de Jong, TV; Paul, M; Mullins, JJ; Schalekamp, MA; Ganten, D. Demonstration of renin mRNA, angiotensinogen mRNA, and angiotensin converting enzyme mRNA expression in the human eye: evidence for an intraocular renin-angiotensin system. *Br J Ophthalmol*, 1996;80: 159-163.

[262] Castoldi, G; Di Gioia, CR; Pieruzzi, F; d'Orlando, C; Van de Greef, WM; Busca, G; Sperti, G; Stella, A. ANG II increases TIMP-1 expression in rat aortic smooth muscle cells in vivo. *Am J Physiol Heart Circ Physiol,* 2003;284:H635-643.

[263] Eagleton, MJ; Ballard, N; Lynch, E; Srivastava, SD; Upchurch, GR Jr; Stanley, JC. Early increased MT1-MMP expression and late MMP-2 and MMP-9 activity during Angiotensin II induced aneurysm formation. *J Surg Res,* 2006;135:345-51.

[264] Huang, W; Yu, LF; Zhong, J; Qizo, MM; Jiang, FX; Du, F; Tian, XL; Wu, YL. Angiotensin II Type 1 Receptor Expression in Human Gastric Cancer and Induces MMP2 and MMP9 Expression in MKN-28 Cells. *Dig Dis Sci*, 2008; 53(1):163-168.

[265] Seeger, H; Lippert, C; Wallwiener, D; Mueck, AO. Valsartan and candesartan can inhibit deteriorating effects of angiotensin II on coronary endothelial function. *J Renin Angiotensin Aldosterone Syst*, 2001;2:141-143.

[266] Uchiyama-Tanaka, Y; Matsubara, H; Nozawa, Y; Murasawa, S; Mori, Y; Kosaki, A; Maruyama, K; Masaki, H; Shibasaki, Y; Fujiyama, S; Nose, A; Iba, O; Hasagawa, T; Tateishi, E; Higashiyama, S; Iwasaka, I. Angiotensin II signaling and HB-EGF shedding via metalloproteinase in glomerular mesangial cells. *Kidney Int*, 2001;60:2153-2163.

267. Wang, M; Zhang, J; Spinetti, G; Jiang, LQ; Monticone, R; Zhao, D; Cheng, L; Krawczyk, M; Talan, M; Pintu, SG; Lakatta, EG. Angiotensin II activates matrix metalloproteinase type II and mimics age-associated carotid arterial remodeling in young rats. *Am J Pathol*, 2005;167:1429-1442.

[267] Weiss, RH; Ramirez, A.TGF-beta- and angiotensin-II-induced mesangial matrix protein secretion is mediated by protein kinase C. *Nephrol Dial Transplant*, 1998;13:2804-2813.

[268] Wolf, G; Ziyadeh, NF. Renal tubular hypertrophy induced by angitensin II. *Semin Nephrol,* 1997;17:448-454.

[269] Sarlos, S; Rizkalla, B; Moravski, CJ; Cao, Z; Cooper, ME; Wilkinson-Berka, JL. Retinal angiogenesis is mediated by an interaction between the angiotensin type 2 receptor, VEGF and angiopoietin. *Am J Pathol*, 2003;879-887.

[270] Han SY, Jee YH, Han KH, Kang YS, Kim HK, Han JY, Kim YS, Cha DR. An imbalance between MMP-2 and tissue inhibitor of matrix metalloproteinase-2 contributes to the development of early nephropathy. *Nephrol Dal Transplant*, 2006;21:2406-2416.

[271] Arenas, IA; xu, Y; Lopez-Jaramillo, P; Davidge, ST. Angiotensin II-induced MMP-2 release from endothelial cells is mediated by TNF-alpha. *Am J Physiol Cell Physio,* 2004; 286:779-7784.

[272] Lijnen, P; Papparella, I; Petrov, V; Semplicini, A; Fagard, R. Angiotensin II-stimulated collagen production in cardiac fibroblasts is mediated by reactive oxygen species. *J Hypertens,* 2006;24:757-766.

[273] Flamant, M; Placier, S; Dubroca, C; Esposito, B; Lopes, I; Chatziantoniou, C; tedgui, A; Dussaule, JC; Lehoux, S. Role of Matrix Metalloproteinases in early hypertensive vascular remodeling. *Hypertension*, 2007;50:213-218.

[274] Wolf, G. Angiotensin II and tubular development. *Nephol Dial Transplant*, 2002;17:48-51.

[275] Cui, XL; Ding, Y; Alexander, LD; Bao, C; Al-Khalili, OK; Simonson, M; Eaton, DC; Douglas, JG. Oxidative signaling in renal epithelium: Critical role of cytosolic phospholipase A2 and p38(SAPK). *Free Radical Biology and Medicine*, 2006;41:190-192.

[276] Pons, M; Cousins, SW; Alcazar, O; Striker, GE; Marin-Castaño, ME. Angiotensin II-induced MMP-2 activity and MMP-14 and basigin protein expression are mediated via the angiotensin II receptor type 1-mitogen-activated protein kinase 1 pathway in retinal

pigment epithelium implications for age-related macular degeneration. *Am J Pathol*, 2011 ;178(6):2665-81.

[277] Ichijo, H; Nishida, E; Irie, K; ten Dijke, P; Saitoh, M; Moriguchi, T; Takagi, M; Matsumoto, K; Miyazono, G; Gotoh, Y. Induction of apoptosis by ASK1, a mammalian MAPKKK that activates SAPK/JNK and p38 signaling pathways. *Science*, 1997, 275:90-94.

[278] Sugden, PH; Clerk, A. Regulation of the ERK subgroup of MAP kinase cascades through G protein-coupled receptors. *Cell Signal*, 1997;9: 337-351.

[279] Taniyama, Y; Ushio-Fukai, M; Hitomi, H; Rocic, P; Kingsley, MJ; Pfahnl, C; Weber, DS; Alexander, RW; Griendling, KK. Role of p38 MAPK and MAPKAPK-2 in angiotensin II-induced Akt activation in vascular smooth muscle cells. Am J Physiol Cell Physiol, 2004, 287:C494-499.

[280] Chen, Z; Gibson, TB; Robinson, F; Silvestro, L; Pearson, G; Xu, B; Wright, A; Vanderbilt, C; Cobb, MH. MAP kinases. *Chem Rev*, 2001;101:2449-2476.

[281] Lewis, TS; Shapiro, PS; Ahn, NG. Signal transduction through MAP kinase cascades. *Adv Cancer Res*, 1998;74:49-139.

[282] Pearson, G; Robinson, F; Beers-Gibson, T; Xu, BE; Karandikar, M; Berman, K; Cobb, MH. Mitogen-activated protein (MAP) kinase pathways: regulation and physiological functions. *Endocr Rev*, 2001;22:153-183.

[283] Patel, M; Chan, CC. Immunopathological aspects of age-related macular degeneration. Semin Immunopathol, 2008;30: 97-110.

[284] Victor Chong, NH; Johnson, LV; Anderson, DH. An integrated hypothesis that considers drusen as biomarkers of immune-mediated processes at the RPE-Bruch's membrane interface in aging and age-related macular degeneration. *Prog Retin Eye* Res, 2001; 20: 705-732.

[285] . Donoso, LA; Kim, D; Frost, A; Callahan, A; Hageman, G. The role of inflammation in the pathogenesis of age-related macular degeneration. *Surv Ophthalmol*, 2006; 51: 137-152.

[286] Haines, JL; Hauser, MA; Schmidt, S; Scott, WK; Olson, LM. Complement factor H variant increases the risk of age-related macular degeneration. *Science*, 2005; 308: 419-421.

[287] . Lommatzsch, A; Hermans, P; Muller, KD; Bornfeld, N; Bird, AC. Are low inflammatory reactions involved in exudative age-related macular degeneration? Morphological and immunhistochemical analysis of AMD associated with basal deposits. *Graefes Arch Clin Exp Ophthalmol*, 2008; 246: 803-810.

[288] . Penfold, PL; Madigan, MC; Gillies, MC; Provis, JM. Immunological and aetiological aspects of macular degeneration. *Prog Retin Eye Res*, 2001; 20: 385-414.

[289] Killingsworth, MC; Sarks, JP; Sarks, SH. Macrophages related to Bruch's membrane in age-related macular degeneration. *Eye* (Lond), 1999; 4 (Pt 4): 613-621.

[290] Dastgheib, K; Green WR. Granulomatous reaction to Bruch's membrane in age-related macular degeneration. *Arch Ophthalmol*, 1994; 112: 813-818.

[291] Grossniklaus, HE; Ling, JX; Wallace, TM; Dithmar, S; Lawson, DH.Macrophage and retinal pigment epithelium expression of angiogenic cytokines in choroidal neovascularization. *Mol Vis*, 2002; 8: 119-126.

[292] . Lopez, PF; Grossniklaus, HE; Lambert, HM; Aaberg, TM; Capone, A. Pathologic features of surgically excised subretinal neovascular membranes in age-related macular degeneration. *Am J Ophthalmol*, 1991; 112: 647-656.

[293] . Oh, H; Takagi, H; Takagi, C; Suzuma, K; Otani, A. The potential angiogenic role of macrophages in the formation of choroidal neovascular membranes. *Invest Ophthalmol Vis Sci*, 1999; 40: 1891-1898.

[294] Yi, X; Takahashi, K; Ogata, N; Uyama, M. Immunohistochemical proof of origin of macrophages in laser photocoagulation lesion in the retina. *Jpn J Ophthalmol,* 1996; 40: 192-201.

[295] Ding, X; Patel, M; Chan, CC. Molecular pathology of age-related macular degeneration. *Prog Retin Eye Res*, 2009; 28: 1-18.

[296] 297. Luft FC, Mervaala E, Muller DN, Gross V, Schmidt F, Joon KP, et al. Hypertension-induced end-organ damage: a new transgenic approach to an old problem. *Hypertension.* 1999;33:212–218.

[297] Alexander RW. Hypertension and the pathogenesis of atherosclerosis: oxidative stress and the mediation of arterial inflammatory response, a new perspective. *Hypertension.* 1995;25:155–161.

[298] Yla-Herttuala, S; Lipton, BA; Rosenfeld, ME; Srakioja, T; Yoshimura, T; Leonard, EJ. Expression of monocyte chemoattractant protein-1 in macrophage-rich areas of human and rabbit atherosclerotic lesions. *Proc Natl Acad Sci USA,*1991;88:5252–5256.

[299] Yu, X; Dluz, S; Graves, DT; Zhang, L; Antoniades, HN; Hollander, W. Elevated expression of monocyte chemoattractant protein-1 by vascular smooth muscle cells in hypercholesterolemic primates. *Proc Natl Acad Sci USA, 1*992;89:6953–6957.

[300] Capers, Q; Alexander, RW; Lou, P; De Leon, H; Wilcox, JN; Ishizaka, N. Monocyte chemoattractant protein-1 expression in aortic tissues of hypertensive rats. *Hypertension, 1*997;30:1397–1402.

[301] Behr, TM; Wang, XK; Aijar, N; Coatney, RW; Li, X; Koster, P. Monocyte chemoattractant protein-1 is upregulated in rats with volume overloaded congestive heart failure. *Circulation,* 2000;102:1315–1322.

[302] Hilgers, KF; Hartner, A; Porst, M; Mai, M; Wittmann, M; Hugo, C. Monocyte chemoattractant protein-1 and macrophage infiltration in hypertensive kidney injury. *Kidney Int,* 2000;58:2408–2419.

[303] Hernandez-Presa, M; Bustos, C; Ortego, M; Tunon, J; Renedo, G; Ruiz-Ortega, M; Egido, J. Angiotensin-converting enzyme inhibition prevents arterial nuclear factor-kappa B activation, monocyte chemoattractant protein-1 expression, and macrophage infiltration in a rabbit model of early accelerated atherosclerosis. *Circulation, 1*997;95:1532–1541.

[304] *Ruiz*-Ortega, M; Ruperez, M; Lorenzo, O; Esteban, V; Blanco, J; Mezzano, S. Angiotensin II regulates the synthesis of proinflammatory cytokines and chemokines in the kidney. *Kidney Int,* 2002;62(suppl 82):12–22.

[305] Tham, DM; Martin-McNulty, B; Wang, YX; Wilson, DW; Vergona, R; Sullivan, ME. Angiotensin II is associated with activation of NF-kappa B-mediated genes and downregulation of PPARs. *Physiol Genom,* 2002;11:21–31.

[306] Yoshimura, T; Leonard, EJ. Identification of high affinity receptors for human monocyte chemoattractant protein-1 on human monocytes. *J Immunol,* 1990;145:292–297.

[307] Charo, IF; Myers, SJ; Herman, A; Franci, C; Connolly, AJ; Coughlin, SR. Molecular cloning and functional expression of two monocyte chemoattractant protein-1 receptors reveals alternative splicing of the carboxyl-terminal trails. *Proc Natl Acad Sci USA,* 1994;91:2752–2756.

[308] Uetama, T; Ohno-Matsui, K; Nakahama, K; Morita, I; Mochizuki, M. Phenotypic change regulates monocyte chemoattractant protein-1 (MCP-1) gene expression in human retinal pigment epithelial cells. *J Cell Physiol,* 2003; 197: 77-85.

[309] Higgins, GT; Wang, JH; Dockery, P; Cleary, PE; Redmond, HP. Induction of angiogenic cytokine expression in cultured RPE by ingestion of oxidized photoreceptor outer segments. *Invest Ophthalmol Vis Sci*, 2003; 44: 1775-1782.

[310] Ambati, J; Anand, A; Fernandez, S; Sakurai, E; Lynn, BC. An animal model of age-related macular degeneration in senescent Ccl-2- or Ccr-2-deficient mice. *Nat Med,* 2003; 9: 1390-1397.

[311] Tuo, J; Bojanowski, CM; Zhou, M; Shen, D; Ross, RJ. Murine ccl2/cx3cr1 deficiency results in retinal lesions mimicking human age-related macular degeneration. *Invest Ophthalmol Vis Sci*, 2007; 48: 3827-3836.

[312] Basso, N; Paglia N, Stella I, de Cavanagh, EM; Ferder, L; Arnaiz, M; Inserra, F. Protective effect of the inhibition of the renin-angiotensis system on aging. *Regul Pept,* 2005;128:247-252.

[313] Diz, D; Lewis, K. Dahl memorial lecture: the renin-angiotensisn system and aging. *Hypertension*, 2008;52:37-43.

[314] Cushman, WC. Are there benefits to specific antihypertensive drug therapy? *Am J Hypertens,* 2003;16:31–35.

[315] Timmermans, PB; Wong, PC; Chiu, AT; Herblin, WF; Benfield, P; Carini, DJ. Angiotensin II receptors and angiotensin II receptor antagonists. *Pharmacol Rev,*1993;45:205–251.

[316] Heart Outcomes Prevention Evaluation Study Investigators. Effects of an angiotensin-converting enzyme inhibitor, ramipril, on cardiovascular events in high-risk patients. *N Engl J Med.* 2000;342:145–153.

[317] Dahlof, B; Devereux, RB; Kjeldsen, SE; Julius, S; Beevers, G; Faire, U. for the LIFE Study Group. Cardiovascular morbidity and mortality in the Losartan Intervention For Endpoint reduction in hypertension study (LIFE): a randomised trial against atenolol. *Lancet,* 2002;359:995–1003.

[318] Hisada, Y; Sygaya, T; Yamanouchi, M; Uchida, H; Fujimura, H; Sakurai, H. Angiotensin II plays a pathologic role in immune-mediated renal injury in mice. *J Clin Invest,*1999;103:627–635.

[319] Behr, TM; Willette, RN; Coatney, RW; Berova, M; Angermann, CE; Anderson, K. Eprosartan improves cardiac performance, reduces cardiac hypertrophy and mortality and downregulates myocardial MCP-1 and inflammation in hypertensive heart disease. *J Hypertens,* 2004;22:583–592

[320] Funakoshi, Y; Ichiki, T; Shimokawa, H; Egashira, K; Takeda, K; Kaibuchi, K. Rho-kinase mediates angiotensin II-induced monocyte chemoattractant protein-1 expression in rat vascular smooth muscle cells. *Hypertension,* 2001;38:100–104.

[321] Wu, L; Iwai, M; Nakagami, H; Li, Z; Chen, R; Suzuki, J. Roles of angiotensin II type 2 receptor stimulation associated with selective angiotensin II type 1 receptor blockade

with valsartan in the improvement of inflammation-induced vascular injury. *Circulation,* 2001;104:2716–2721.

[322] Sozzani, S; Luini, W; Molino, M; Jilek, P; Bottazzi, B; Cerletti, C. The signaling transduction pathway involved in the migration induced by a monocyte chemotactic cytokine. *J Immunol,* 1991;147:2215–2221.

[323] Chen, XL; Tummala, PE; Olbrych, MT; Alexander, RW; Medford, RM. Angiotensin II induces monocyte chemoattractant protein-1 gene expression in rat vascular smooth muscle cells. *Circ Res,* 1998;83:952–959.

[324] Locati, M; Zhou, D; Luini, W; Evangelista, V; Mantovani, A; Sozzani, S. Rapid induction of arachidonic acid release by monocyte chemotactic protein-1 and related chemokines: role of Ca^{2+} influx, synergism with platelet-activating factor and significance for chemotaxis. *J Biol Chem,* 1994;269:4746–4753

[325] Yu, BP; Chung, HY. Adaptive mechanisms to oxidative stress during aging. *Mech Ageing Dev*, 2006; 127:436–443.

[326] Kim, HJ; Jung, KJ; Yu, BP; Cho, CG; Choi, JS; Chung, HY. Modulation of redox-sensitive transcription factors by calorie restriction during aging. *Mech Ageing Dev*, 2002; 123:1589–1595.

[327] Chung, HY; Kim, HJ; Kim, KW; Choi, JS; Yu, BP. Molecular inflammation hypothesis of aging based on the anti-aging mechanism of calorie restriction. *Microsc Res Tech*, 2002; 59:264–272.

[328] Chung, HY; Cesari, M; Anton, S; Marzetti, E; Giovannini, S; Seo, AY; Carter, C; Yu, BP; Leeuwenburgh, C. Molecular inflammation: underpinnings of aging and age-related diseases. *Ageing Res Rev*, 2009; 8:18–30.

[329] Miyata, N; Yamakoshi, Y; Nakanishi, I. Reactive species responsible for biological actions of photo excited fullerenes. *Yakugaku Zasshi*, 2002; 120:1007–1016.

[330] Murkies, A. Phytoestrogens what is the current knowledge? *Aust Fam Physician*, 1998; 27:S47–S51.

[331] Praddaude, F; Cousins, SW; Pêcher, C; Marin-Castaño, ME. Angiotensin II-induced hypertension regulates AT1 receptor subtypes and extracellular matrix turnover in mouse retinal pigment epithelium. *Exp Eye Res*, 2009;15;89(1):109-118.

[332] Espinosa-Heidmann, DG; Sall, J; Hernandez, EP; Cousins, SW. Basal laminar deposit formation in APO B100 transgenic mice: complex interactions between dietary fat, blue light, and vitamin E. *Invest Ophthalmol Vis Sci*, 2004;45(1):260-266.

[333] Cousins, SW; Marin-Castano, ME; Espinosa-Heidmann, DG; Alexandridou, A; Striker, L; Elliot, S. Female gender, estrogen loss, and Sub-RPE deposit formation in aged mice. *Invest Ophthalmol Vis Sci*, 2003;44(3):1221-1229.

In: Angiotensin: New Research
Editors: S. Harada, I. Moi, pp. 273-302

ISBN: 978-1-62100-773-9

Chapter 12

DO ANGIOTENSIN II RECEPTORS PLAY A ROLE IN CEREBELLAR DEVELOPMENT AND NEURONAL MIGRATION?

Susana I. Sánchez, Maria E. Arce, Leonardo R. Seguin, and Gladys M. Ciuffo

IMIBIO-SL CONICET, Facultad de Química, Bioquímica y Farmacia,
Universidad Nacional de San Luis,
Ejército de los Andes 950, San Luis, Argentina.

ABSTRACT

Angiotensin II (Ang II), the active peptide of the renin–angiotensin system, binds and activates two major receptor subtypes, namely AT_1 and AT_2. The classical effects of Ang II in the control of blood pressure and fluid homeostasis are mediated by AT_1 receptors. The AT_2 receptor is involved in vasodilatation, inhibition of the cell proliferation, induction of programmed cell death and cellular differentiation. Ang II AT_2 receptor expression is highly modulated during development. In the fetus, AT_2 receptors predominate in all tissues and decline shortly after birth, being restricted to a few organs including brain.

Interpretation of the function of Ang II in cerebellum necessitates a thorough understanding about the localization and signal transduction of Ang II receptors. A clear complementary pattern of AT_1 and AT_2 binding labeled by $[^{125}I]$ Ang II was observed on adjacent layers in young rats within the cerebellar cortex. By using specific markers of the Purkinje cells (PCs) (Zebrin II and calbindin28K), we demonstrated that Ang II AT_2 receptors co-localized with the PCs as a monolayer, in correspondence with the well-defined layer observed by binding autoradiography at differential developmental stages (P0 to P60). Blockade of AT_2 receptors with PD123319 during late pregnancy caused a lost of AT_2 binding in the external granular layer (EGL) in P0 pups. A detailed histological analysis evidenced an enlarged EGL in the cerebellar cortex. It is well known that PCs migrate early during fetal stage (E14) toward the cerebellar cortex. Aiming to elucidate the non-classical signaling pathway of Ang II AT_2 receptors in rat hindbrain we selected P15, a critical developmental stage. Following Ang II stimulation, SHP-1 associates to AT_2 receptors but not to AT_1 subtype. Immunocomplexes obtained with anti-AT_2 or anti-SHP-1 exhibited PTPase activity, blocked by PD123319 (AT_2 antagonist) or PP2. SHP-1 activation was correlated with tyr-phosphorylation level of SHP-1 in immunocomplexes. Both immunocomplexes contained c-Src and PP2 blocked SHP-1 tyr-phosphorylation as well as activation and association SHP-1 to c-Src.

Taken together, the localization of AT_2 receptors in the Purkinje cells, the effect of blockade during late pregnancy on the development of the cerebellar cortex and the signal transduction mechanisms, a potential role for AT_2 receptors can be assigned on neuronal migration and cerebellar cortex organization.

1. Introduction

1.1. The Renin-Angiotensin System, History and Perspective

The renin-angiotensin system (RAS) is a major regulatory system of blood pressure and electrolyte homeostasis, among multiple actions. The RAS has been and still is an active field of intensive research as reflected by the number of publications produced. The discovery of a pressor principle named "renin", extracted from the kidney, in 1898 by Tigerstedt and Bergman [1], constituted an initial step in understanding the regulation of blood pressure. However, it was not until 1940 [2] that a vasoconstrictor substance was isolated from renal venous blood from the ischemic kidney of a Goldblatt hypertensive dog. At the same time, Page and Helmer [3] identified a similar factor, after the injection of renin into an intact animal. The pressor substance, named "hypertensin" in Argentina and "angiotonin" in the United States was later identified as an octapeptide (Asp-Arg-Val-Tyr-Ile-His-Pro-Phe) [4-6]. In 1958, both groups agreed on the hybrid term Angiotensin for this highly potent pressor octapeptide. Although the active principle, Ang II was discovered seventy years ago, many of the functions of the RAS remain elusive.

Angiotensin II (Ang II) considered the main effector peptide of the RAS, has been related to the control of blood pressure either peripherally, by acting on the cardiovascular system and key organs such as kidney, lung, adrenal, or centrally, acting on brain nucleus related to blood pressure control [7-9]. Recently, a potential role for Ang II in development as a growth modulating factor was proposed [10-14] The trophic effects of Ang II have been studied *in vitro* in primary cultures or in established cell lines [7,8,14,15].

The classical RAS is systemic in nature and it is a cascade of enzymatic and sequential reactions, starting from a precursor molecule, Angiotensinogen (Aogen), released from the liver [16-18]. Aogen is cleaved in the circulation by rennin, an enzyme secreted from the juxtaglomerular apparatus of the kidney [7] to form the decapeptide Ang I. The angiotensin converting enzyme (ACE), a membrane-bound metalloproteinase, predominantly expressed at high concentrations on the surface of endothelial cells in the pulmonary circulation, cleaves the decapeptide Ang I to produce Ang II.

The classical RAS, described above, had to be expanded significantly by more recent findings that increased the complexity of the system. At present, receptors have been identified for the renin and pro-renin peptides [19]. Besides, the system generates several active peptides: Ang II, Ang III, Ang (1-7) and Ang IV. Ang II can be metabolized by aminopeptidases producing small peptides, Ang III and Ang IV (Figure 1).

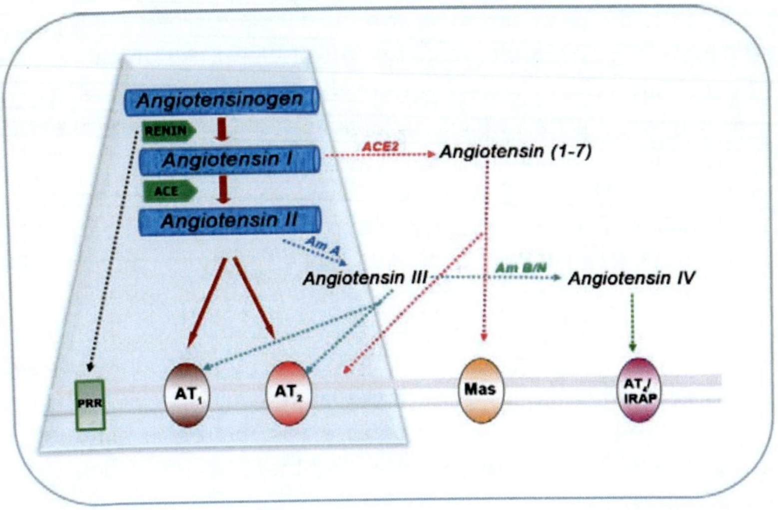

Figure 1. The present RAS components. Biosynthesis of neuroactive angiotensins from the precursor angiotensinogen. The "classical" biosynthesis pathway that leads to the formation of Angiotensin II is in light blue. ACE: angiotensin-converting enzyme, Am: aminopeptidase, PRR: renin-prorenin receptor.

While Ang II and Ang III recognize the same receptors, Ang IV exhibited specific receptors (AT_4) which differ at their location and functions with those for Ang II and Ang III. Recently, a new active peptide of the RAS has been recognized, Ang (1-7), showing opposite effects to those of Ang II, as vasodilator and cardioprotective peptide [20.21]. Ang (1-7) is a cleavage product of Ang I or Ang II caused by the action of a new carboxipeptidase named ACE2. Ang (1-7) acts on specific receptors, described earlier as Mas receptors (Figure 1) [22,23].

A number of studies demonstrated the presence and the importance of a local RAS in different tissues, such as the kidney, brain, heart, peripheral vasculature and adrenal glands [24-34]. The existence of a brain local RAS was proposed by the discovery of a renin-like activity in the brain [35], in combination with the finding of most components of the RAS, including angiotensinogen, angiotensins, and converting enzymes [36]. An essential requirement for a tissue RAS is that the different components necessary for biosynthesis of the active peptide, Ang II, has to be expressed *in situ* [31].

Local RAS systems have been identified in most organs and tissues investigated as recently reviewed by Paul [34].

Thus, Ang II is not just a circulating hormone, but also is synthesized *in situ* in different tissues. The discovery of Ang II in brain areas located within the blood-brain barrier was a clear evidence of the existence of a local RAS. Renin and Ang II are unable to cross the blood-brain barrier [37,38].

2. Angiotensin II

In the present chapter we will refer mainly to the classical active principle Ang II and its receptors. Ang II is one of the major hypertensive peptides present in all organisms and its effects are mediated by the interaction with two membrane receptor subtypes, AT_1 and AT_2, described on the basis of pharmacological properties [39,40]. AT_1 receptors are specifically blocked by Losartan and AT_2 receptors, selectively displaced by CGP42112 or PD123319 [7,8,39,40]. Losartan and PD123319 are non-peptidic antagonists, while CGP42112 is a peptide agonist derived from the Ang II sequence.

Besides their pharmacological differences, Ang II receptors have been cloned and their derived structure indicates that both receptor subtypes belong to the superfamily of G-protein coupled receptors (GPCRs) [41-44]. However, both receptor subtypes induce opposite biological effects, such as vasoconstriction/vasodilatation and cell growth/anti-growth [45,46] by acting via different intracellular signaling pathways. Another clear difference between AT_1 and AT_2 receptors refers to the time during development when they are expressed. AT_1 receptors predominate in adult tissues: cardiovascular system, kidneys, lungs, adrenals, liver, brain nucleus related to blood pressure and homeostasis control. In contrast, AT_2 receptors predominate in fetal tissues and decline shortly after birth, being restricted to a few organs including brain [8,38].

Autoradiography as well as *in situ* hybridization studies provide evidence suggesting that Ang II AT_1 and AT_2 receptors are developmentally regulated, being Ang II AT_2 receptors more abundant at early stages of development, while AT_1 receptors predominate in adult tissues [7,10,26,47-57]. The high expression of Ang II AT_2 receptors during fetal and early postnatal life implies an important role in organ development, the regulation of growth, cell proliferation and apoptosis [7]. Different tissues, such as kidneys, aorta, cerebral nuclei, cerebellum exhibit a developmentally regulated pattern of expression [10,47,54-57].

2.1. AT_1 Receptors

Ang II controls blood pressure and homeostasis acting both at the central level and on peripheral organs. Most of the known central effects of Ang II are mediated by AT_1 receptors [7,13,58,59], including blood pressure regulation, electrolyte balance and the central control of thirst and salt ingest. The principal organs involved in homeostasis control, kidneys and adrenal, also expressed AT_1 receptor subtype in adult tissues. AT_1 receptors exhibit high and selective affinity for biphenylimidazoles, the ´sartan´ family, including losartan, candesartan and ibersartan, while have none or low affinity for tetrahydroimidazo-pyridine, such as PD123177 and PD123319 and the peptide analogue CGP42112.

AT_1 receptors were first cloned in 1991, allowing the identification of a peptide of 359 amino acids, belonging to the seven transmembrane domain family (7-TMR) [41,42]. Two isoforms were recognized in rodents, designated as AT_{1A} and AT_{1B} which share a 94% homology [60,61]. Both isoforms show similar pharmacological behavior but different tissue distribution. Gene AT_{1A} localized at chromosome 17 while AT_{1B} gene localized at chromosome 2 [62]. The human genome present a single gene for AT_1 receptor, localized in chromosome 3 [63].

AT_1 receptors behave as classical GPCRs and activate several signaling pathways interacting with $G_{q/11}$, G_i, G_{12} and G_{13}, thus producing second messengers such as IP3, DAG and ROS [13,14]. It has been well establish its participation in growth promoting mechanisms and remodeling ([64]. AT_1 receptors activate various intracellular protein kinases, including the MAPK family [65].

2.2. AT_2 Receptors

Ang II AT_2 receptors exhibit high affinity for PD123319, PD123177 and the peptide Ang II-derived analogue CGP42112 and low affinity for the ´sartan´ family [7,58]. Ang II binds with similar affinity to AT_2 receptors as well as to AT_1 receptors. AT_2 receptors, first cloned from cDNA libraries, belong to the seven-transmembrane-type G protein-coupled receptor containing 363 amino acids with an estimated mass of 41 kDa [43,44].

AT_2 receptor genes were cloned from different species including humans, rat and mouse as a single copy on the X chromosome [66-68] and knock-out mice were obtained [69,70]. In spite of the similar affinity for Ang II, low amino acid sequence homology (34%) is shared for AT_2 and AT_1 receptors, resident mainly in the transmembrane domains [43,44]. Residues considered important in the AT_1 receptor for binding of Ang II are preserved in AT_2 receptors.

AT_2 receptors do not behave as classical GPCRs and its signaling mechanism is much less well characterized, and its physiological role is not completely understood [72,73]. Earlier studies proposed a role of AT_2 receptors to induced programmed cell death mediated by a PTPase [74] and dephosphorylation of Bcl-2 [75]. Activation of the PTPase SHP-1 by AT_2 receptors was associated to cellular apoptosis in different cell lines [76-78]. Increasing evidence supports a role of AT_2 receptors mediated by protein tyrosine dephosphorylation [8,72,78,79].We will devote a special section to AT_2 signaling transduction mechanism in this chapter.

2.3. Tissue Distribution of Ang II Receptors

AT_1 and AT_2 receptors show differential tissue distribution in adult tissues with a clear predominance of AT_1 receptors. In adult organisms, AT_1 receptors show a wide expression [7,58]. AT_1 receptors are expressed in circumventricular nuclei related to central control of blood pressure and homeostasis and peripherally in the lungs, liver, heart, vascular system, adrenal gland, kidneys. In contrast, in adult tissues AT_2 receptor expression is restricted to a few central nucleus, like Superior Collicullus (SC), Locus Coeruleus (LC), Geniculate nucleus, cerebellum (cb), Inferior olive complex (IOC) in the brainstem, adrenals, ovary [7,36,47]. Besides, AT_2 receptors are present at a very low level in the adult heart, vascular endothelium, kidney, miometrium [7,50,58] where the expression increases under pathological conditions such as cardiac infarct, renal damage, ischemia and vascular lesions [8].

A number of ontogenic studies demonstrated that both the localization pattern and mRNA expression of Ang II receptors varies with development. The $AT_2 : AT_1$ ratio changes during development, with maximum AT_2 receptor level at the end of fetal development, followed by a rapid decrease after birth. However, in rodents this pattern varies in different tissues, particularly in those which exhibit an important postnatal development, like kidneys, aorta and cerebellum [10,54,57,80]. In contrast, AT_1 receptor expression during embrionary development is low and reflects the localization observed in adult tissues.

2.4. Ang II in the Central Nervous System (CNS)

Ang II is recognized as an important neuropeptide with multiple roles in the CNS. The classical and well defined actions of Ang II in the brain include the central control of blood pressure, the regulation of hormone synthesis and release, the central regulation of water and salt intake and the modulation the sympathetic activity. It is well known that Ang II acts via the AT_1 to increase neuron excitability in the cardiovascular regulatory centers of the hypothalamus and brainstem. The different components of the RAS have been identified in the brain. Pharmacological evidences and those from genetic manipulation support a role of the RAS in central control of blood pressure and hypertension [81]. Besides, not only Ang II receptors are present in the CNS, yet receptors have been identified for Ang IV and Ang (1-7) in brain areas. Table 1 summarizes the major actions attributed to the different Angiotensins in the brain.

Most of the Ang II actions in the CNS are induced by circulating Ang II while a few other actions are controlled by locally produced Ang II. Thus, the circumventricular nuclei, including the Subfornical organ (SFO), vascular organ of the lamina terminal (OVLT), median eminence (ME), anterior pituitary and area postrema exhibit high levels of Ang II AT_1 receptors [7,36,58,82]. These areas, exposed to circulating Ang II, are related to the central vasopressor Ang II actions, which stimulate water and salt intake and hormone release from the pituitary. AT_1 receptors are also expressed in the nucleus of the solitary tract (sol) and the rostral ventrolateral medulla (RVLM) of the brainstem [81].

AT_2 receptor´s localization in adult brain is limited to a few selected areas, the limbic system (septum and amygdala), various thalamic and subthalamic nuclei, IOC, LC and hipoglosal motor nucleus [83,84]. Although the role of AT_2 receptors is still under revision, the expression pattern of AT_2 receptors points to a number of central actions involving the sensory and motor control nuclei and a possible role in behavior [55,69,70]. AT_2 receptors may also antagonize the central effects of Ang II in blood pressure and homeostasis regulation mediated via AT_1 receptors [85].

It was suggested that AT_4 receptors might influence learning and memory, suggesting an important role for the brain RAS in normal cognitive processing [86]. However, the anatomical and physiological ontogeny and functions of Ang IV and AT_4 receptors in the fetal brain remain unclear.

Table 1. Angiostesin peptides and major responce in the brain

RECEPTORS	ACTIVE ANGIOTENSIN PEPTIDES	LIGAND	STRUCTURAL FEATURES	CHROMOSOME	MAYOR RESPONSE IN BRAIN	Ref.
AT1	Ang II	Losartan	GPCRs- 7TM 41 kDa	3 (human), 17and 2 (rat)	Increased sympathetic tone Blood pressure Water intake Salt appetite Vasopressin release Impaired cardiac baroreflex sensitivity	36
AT_2		PD123319, PD123177, CGP42112	GPCRs- 7TM 41 kDa	X (human and rat)	Vasodilatation Anti-proliferation Cerebral ischemia Nitric oxide release	7, 46, 71
Mas	Ang (1-7)		GPCRs- 7TM 41 kDa	6(human)	Increased cardiac baroreflex sensitivity Prostaglandin synthesis Vasopressin release Nitric oxide release Substance P release	21-23
AT_4/IRAP	Ang IV	LVV-hemorphin7	M1 family Aminopeptidase	N/D	Learning and memory Increased cerebral blood flow	86

N/D.: not determined.

3. RAS in Development

All the components of the RAS show early expression during development, including Aogen, renin, ACE, Ang II and both Ang II receptors subtypes [48,84]. Recently, a potential role for Ang II in development as a growth modulating factor was proposed [11-14]. Ang II AT_1 and AT_2 receptors are developmentally regulated, being Ang II AT_2 receptors more abundant at early stages of development, while AT_1 receptors appear later in development and remain in adulthood. The high expression of Ang II AT_2 receptors during fetal and early postnatal life suggest an important role in cellular differentiation, the regulation of growth, cell proliferation and apoptosis [7], all processes participating of organogenesis. In the rat, several organs complete their differentiation postnatally, such as the kidney, aorta, lung, cerebellum and brainstem. While in a few organs (i.e., lung, liver), the receptor subtype expressed during embryonic life remains in the adult, in other tissues, the expression of Ang II receptor subtypes encompasses differentiation, like in the aorta, kidney, cerebellum, among others, where a spatial and temporal pattern of expression was observed [10,32,47-49,54,56, 80,87].

Studies over the last decades have shown that the central RAS plays an important role in the control of fetal cardiovascular responses, body fluid balance, and neuroendocrine regulation. Since these initial discoveries, most intrinsic components of the RAS, including Angiotensiogen, angiotensins, and converting enzymes, have been well documented in the early developing brain.

Angiotensinogen: Rat brain angiotensinogen mRNA was shown on embrionic day 15 (E15) and its levels increased about ten times during gestation [88-90] reaching higher levels after birth [89]. In the fetal brain, Aogen protein was also evidenced by immunoreactivity, present from E19 in rats [91,92] being more abundant in rat brain than in liver from fetuses. The timing of Aogen appearance during brain development supports the hypothesis about the establishment of a central RAS by late gestation. Aogen predominance in fetal hypothalamic nuclei and in thalamic, cerebellar, and cortical neurons suggests a potential role in brain maturation, in prenatal fluid and electrolyte balance, and in sensor motor development [93].

Renin: Renin was first detected in rat at E15 in the gonadic arteries, and at E17 in the aorta and branches of the renal, adrenal, and gonadic arteries [94]. Although information about renin in the fetal brain is limited, the presence of major components of the RAS such as Aogen in the rat fetal brain before E19, supports an early onset of fetal brain renin. Renin activity as well as Aogen, ACE, and Ang II immunoreactivity was identified in fetal rat brain at E19 [91,92,95,96].

Angiotensin converting enzyme (ACE): ACE is widely distributed in the adult brain and particularly high concentrations of ACE were found in the circumventricular nuclei [97]. ACE immunoreactivity and mRNA have been detected on fetal brain from different species [98-103]. Functional brain ACE was demonstrated by exogenous administration of Ang I applied into the lateral ventricle in late gestation, causing Ang II-like physiological actions, such as increased blood pressure and release of the neuropeptide vasopressin [84]. In rat fetal brain, ACE was detected at E19 in the SFO and posterior pituitary [99,104].

Ang II: Immunohistochemical identification of Ang II in rat brain was first described by Changaris et al. [105], revealing a wide distribution of Ang II in brain areas. Neuronal cell bodies exhibiting Ang II immunoreactivity were described in brain regions such as the sol, cb,

PVN and SFO. Ang II was also detected in the central nucleus of the amygdala (Ce), bed nucleus of the stria terminalis (BST), amygdalo-hippocampal zone, lateral parabrachial nucleus (LPB) and ME [106,107]. In rat fetuses, Ang II was detected as early as E20, formed and released from primary neuron cultures in brain cells [108,109].

Ang II receptors: The distribution of AT_1 receptors has been mapped in the nervous system of a number of species by *in vitro* autoradiography [7,36,38,47,58,82,83,87,100, 104,110] and *in situ* hybridization [56,83]. Studies from binding autoradiography showed that both AT_1 and AT_2 receptors were located in the brain at E18 in fetal rats [47,84,104]. In E19 rat brain, AT_1 receptors are located in SFO, PVN, sol, choroid plexus and anterior pituitary [47]. AT_2 receptors are also expressed during fetal development [34,36,104].

Nuyt et al. detected mRNA for *in situ* hybridization to determine the expression during development of the two AT_1 isoforms (AT_{1a} and AT_{1b}) and AT_2 receptors mRNA [55,56]. The first appearance of AT_{1a} receptors mRNA was at E19 in many brain regions, and AT_2 receptors mRNA appeared at E13 in the differentiating lateral hypothalamus [55,56]. At E17, AT_2 mRNA was detected in the pedunculopontine nucleus, cb, motor facial nucleus and the IOC; at E19 at the supragenual nucleus (SGe) and at E21 in the SC. AT_2 mRNA persists until brain maturity, in nuclei involved in motor functions and sensory integration. In young rats, AT_2 binding was observed in the developing cerebellum and brainstem [111,112]. In this chapter, we will describe in detail receptor localization in the rat hindbrain.

4. Hindbrain: Development and RAS Expression

4.1. Cerebellar Development

The cerebellum consists of a highly organized set of folia that, in rodents, are largely generated postnatally, providing a convenient model to study ongoing developmental processes [113,114]. Cerebellar neurons are generated from two anatomically and molecularly distinct progenitor zones within the primordia or cerebellar anlage: the rooth of the fourth ventricule, named as ventricular zone (VZ), and the dorsally located rhombic lip (RL) [115]. The ventricular zone (VZ) generates neurons of the cerebellar nuclei, Purkinje cells (PCs), and cerebellar interneurons. On the other hand, the anterior rhombic lip (aRL) gives rise to precursors of granule neurons of the cerebellum, the most abundant neuron in the brain, neurons of the precerebellar nuclei and the olivary complex [116].

Neurons of the cerebellar cortex do not grow simultaneously and a complex mechanism is required in order to establish the adult pattern of the cerebellar cortex. While PCs precursors are formed during the embryonic stage, most granule cells are generated postnatally. PCs migration in small rodents starts during the second half of gestation (E12 in mice and E14 in rats) and lasts until postnatal days 4-6. In the rat, the dendritic arbors of PCs reach their maximal length by postnatal day 30 (P30) [117].

The cerebellum plays crucial roles in sensory integration, motor planning and cognitive processing [117]. The cerebellum is also a major anatomical site of cardiovascular regulation [118]. Early studies pointed out that destruction of the fastigial nucleus leads to hypertension [119,120]. This observation suggests that either neurons within the nucleus or pathways connecting through the fastigial nucleus may be critical in maintaining blood pressure [118].

Recent studies, confirmed the participation of the cerebellar fastigial nuclei in regulating large blood pressure changes [121].

From the hundred neuropeptides that are expressed in the CNS, 22 neuropeptides have been identified in the cerebellum [122], being Ang II, one of them. By using *in situ* hybridization and immunocytochemistry Aogen mRNA, Aogen, Ang II and Ang (1-7) were demonstrated in the rat cerebellum [118,123,124].

Both Ang II AT_1 and AT_2 receptors have been described in cerebellum of young rats [57,111]. In 2-week-old animals, AT_2 receptors and its mRNA are discretely localized in neurons of the inferior olive [47,125]. Chemical lesion of the inferior olive (IO) in 2-week-old rats decreased binding to AT_2 receptors and its mRNA levels in the IO and AT_2 receptor binding in the molecular layer of the cerebellar cortex [112]. At present, data suggesting the subtype receptor localization at the cerebellar neuronal layers are controversial [57,111,126]. The AT_2 mRNA expression during fetal and neonatal brain development was studied from 11 days of gestation (E11) to postnatal day 28 (P28) [55]. Table 2 summarizes the finding of Ang II receptors mRNA or protein in the hindbran during development.

Studies from knock-out mice reinforce the hypothesis that AT_2 receptors play a role in neuronal development. AT_2 knock-out mice suffer from perturbations in exploratory behavior and locomotor's activity [69,70], as well as anxiety-like behavior [127]. Genetic deletion of AT_2 receptors lead to increased cell number in different brain structures in mice [128,129].

Table 2. Receptor localization and mRNA expression of Ang II receptors in hindbrain development

Areas	Embrionic day								Postnatal day							
	E15		E17		E19		E21		P2		P7		P15		P28	
	AT1	AT2	AT1	AT2	AT1	AT2	AT1	AT2	AT1	AT2	AT1	AT2	AT1	AT2	AT1	AT2
Cerebellum, areas 1–10				√		√		√		√		√	+	+		√
Inferior colicullus complex													-	+		
Inferior cerebellar peduncle													-	+		
Superior cerebellar peduncle													-	+		
Inferior olive				√ +		√		√		√		√	√ +	√ +		√
Supragenual nucleus		√				√		√				√	-	+		√
Locus coeruleus						√		√		√		√				√
Sensory root trigeminal nerve nucleus													-	+		
Genu facial nucleus													-	+		
Spinal trigeminal nucleus, oral													+	-		
Subcoeruleus													-	+		
Principal sensory root													-	+		
Dorso tegmental nucleus													-	+		
Principal sensory root trigeminal nucleus													+	+		
Vestibular nucleus												√	-	+		√
Lateral nucleus													-	+		
Facial nucleus				√	√	√	√	√	√	√	√	√	-	+	√	√
Simple lobule													+	-		
Raphe magnus											√		+	-		
Raphe pallidus					√		√				√		+	-	√	

√: Expression of Ang II receptor mRNA; +: Angiotensin II binding site(47,55,57).

4.2. Ang II Receptors During Cerebellar Development

Despite the multiple functions of the cerebellum and a clear presence of the RAS in the cerebellum, very little effort has been dedicated to study the localization and potential role of Ang II receptors in the cerebellum during development. Besides, a possibly important role of AT_2 receptors in neuronal differentiation and organogenesis has been previously suggested. In the rat, the cerebellar development is mainly postnatal. In the following sections we will focus on the localization of Ang II receptors during hindbrain development, studying receptor localization, the effect of pharmacological blockade of Ang II receptors during neuronal migration and cerebellar organogenesis and the transduction mechanism of Ang II AT_2 receptors at a critical development stage.

4.2.1. Ang II AT_2 Receptors in Purkinje Cells

A detailed study by binding autoradiography of the Ang II receptor localization in the 2-week-old (P15) rat hindbrain showed a localization of both receptor subtypes in different structures [57] (Table 2). Cerebellar cortex at all the antero-posterior levels showed the presence of both receptor subtypes of Ang II in the cerebellar cortex of 2-week old animals. Ang II receptor subtypes AT_1 and AT_2 localized at adjacent layers of the cerebellar cortex at different Bregma levels, in all lobes. A similar pattern was observed in the cerebellar cortex of rat hindbrain from P8 animals [130].

At P8 and P15, the neuronal layers of the cerebellar cortex exhibited differential AT_1 (arrowhead) or AT_2 (arrows) labeling in a complementary pattern (Figure 2) when compared to the total binding, in opposition to the overlapping binding observed at P30 and P60, where AT_2 binding appears superimposed with AT_1 binding (see Figure 2). AT_2 binding was higher at early stages being maximal at P15, but low levels remain in adult animals, while AT_1 binding increase with age [87].

Figure 3 shows that the total binding within the cerebellar cortex comprises both, the molecular and PC layers, with a clear correspondence of AT_1 binding with the molecular layer. The thin layer showing AT_2 binding seems localized at the Purkinje cell layer while no binding was observed at the granular layer (intensively stained nuclei, Figure 3). By immunohistochemistry and immunofluorescence staining of the cerebellar cortex form P8, P15, P30 and P60 rats, AT_2 binding was demonstrated at the PCs bodies.

At P8 the Purkinje cells have already migrated to their final localization and constitute a monolayer. At this developmental stage the pyramidal somata appeared very well defined and the efferent processes were weakly immunostained [87].

Consecutive coronal sections of P8, P15, P30 and P60 cerebellum were incubated with $[^{125}I]$ Ang II (0.2 nM) in the absence (Total) or in the presence of PD123319 (AT_1 receptors, AT_1-R 10^{-6} M) or Losartan (AT_2 receptors, AT_2-R 10^{-6} M). The differential localization of Ang II receptors is indicated at the cerebellar cortex: AT_1 (arrowhead) and AT_2 (arrow). 2: area 2 of the cerebellar cortex. Representative image from n= 5-6 animals. (Adapted from Ref. 87)

The presence of Ang II AT_2 receptors in cerebellum of older animals has not been extensively studied and only recently, it was recognized the presence of Ang II AT_2 receptors in adult cerebellum [131]. Similarly to the localization observed in young animals (P8, P15), in P30 and P60 animals, AT_2 receptors localized to PCs, as shown by immunostaining with anti-AT_2 and calbindin antibodies [87]. In P60 animals, a weak AT_2 immunolabeling was observed in glial processes which enter into the molecular layer. The pattern seems to correspond to Bergmann glial processes, which are fully developed around P60 [132].

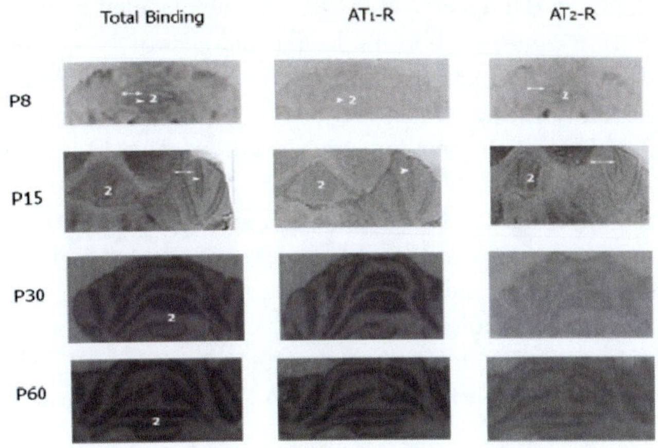

Figure 2. Autoradiographic localization of the Ang II receptors in rat cerebellum at different postnatal ages.

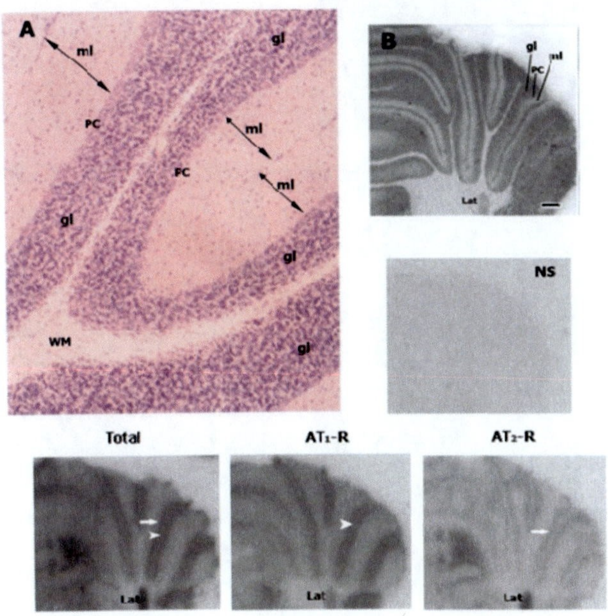

Figure 3. Binding autoradiography at the cerebellar cortex (level Bregma -10.52 mm) of P15 rats. **A–B**: hematoxylin-eosin staining at high (A) and low (B) resolution. Consecutive coronal sections of P15 cerebellum were incubated with [^{125}I] Ang II (0.2 nM) in the absence (Total) or in the presence of PD123319 (AT_1 receptors, AT_1-R 10^{-6} M) or Losartan (AT_2 receptors, AT_2-R 10^{-6} M). AT_2 (arrow) and AT_1 (arrowhead) binding localized on adjacent neuronal layers, in correspondence with the Purkinje cell layer (PC) and the molecular layer (ml), respectively. No Ang II binding was observed at the granular (gl) layer. NS, non-specific binding; Lat, lateral nucleus; WM, white matter. (Adapted from Ref. 87).

These observations might account for the low Ang II AT_2 binding at this stage and apparent co-localization of AT_1 and AT_2 binding observed by autoradiography (Figure 2).

The cellular layer of the cerebellar cortex expressing Ang II receptors was further characterized in P15 rats by confocal immunofluorescence using specific antibodies that recognize either glial or Purkinje cells. PCs were immunolabeled by AT_2 antibodies, as well as calbindin and zebrin (Figure 4), both molecular markers of PCs. The glial marker GFAP did not co-localize with AT_2 labeling [87]. PC migration in small rodents starts during the second half of gestation (E12 in mice and E14 in rats) and lasts until postnatal days 4-6, but the dendrite arbors of PCs reach their maximal length by P30 [117]. Thus, the well-defined pattern of binding observed in P8 and P15 cerebellum is in clear coincidence with the formation of the monolayer of PCs and previous to the complete differentiation of these cells.

Previous studies have suggested that AT_2 binding in the cerebellar cortex of young rats localized to the molecular layer and it was attributed to the climbing fibers from the inferior olivary complex [112]. Other studies reported the presence AT_2 receptor-immunoreactivity in granule cells in culture [71]. The double immunolabeling with specific molecular markers for PCs and AT_2 immunolabeling clearly show that AT_2 binding observed by autoradiography corresponds to PCs [87].

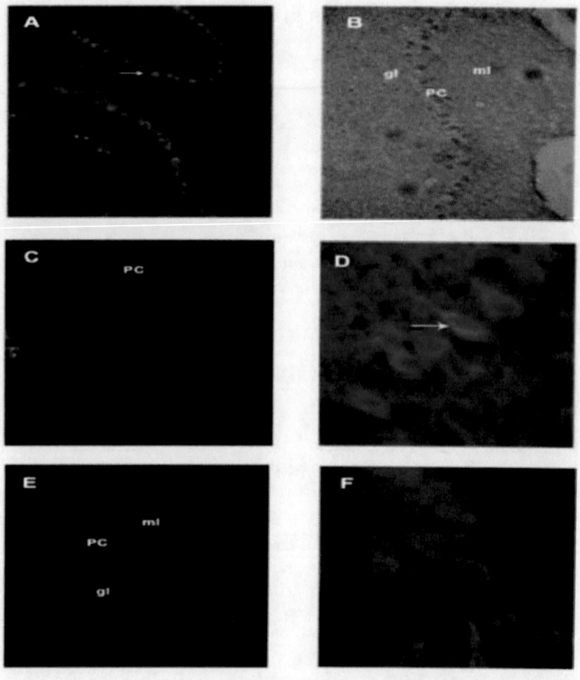

Figure 4. Inmunolabeling of PC layer in P15 rats with AT_2 receptor and PC molecular markers. **A.** Immunofluorescence localization of AT_2 receptor in parasagittal sections of rat P15 cerebellum. Arrow points to a representative AT_2-immunoreactive PC. **B.** Peroxidase-DAB immunoreactivity of AT_2 showing the same pattern. **C.** Immunofluorescence staining of PC bodies with Calbindin, a specific Purkinje cell marker in cerebellum (arrow points to an immunostained PC). **D.** Immunofluorescence staining of calbindin at higher magnification (400x) of cell bodies and processes in the PC layer of P15 rat cerebellum. **E-F.** Immunofluorescence staining of Zebrin II marker at lower (100x, E) and higher (400x, F) magnification showing PCs and their processes intensely stained. Abbreviations: ml, molecular layer; gl, granular layer; PC, Purkinje cells.

4 2.2. *Ang II Receptors at Cerebellar Structures and Brainstem*

In P15 rat hindbrain AT_2 binding to the cerebellar peduncles was surprisingly high. A strong AT_2 binding was observed in the inferior, medium and superior cerebellar peduncles (icp, mcp, scp). Also cerebellar nuclei, the vestibular (Ve) and lateral (Lat) nuclei, expressed AT_2 subtype. Similar observations were made in P8 rat hindbrain [130].

In P15 brainstem, nuclei which selectively express AT_2 receptors were: dorso tegmental nucleus (DTg), central tegmental nucleus (DTgC), subcoeruleus (SubC), subcoeruleus nucleus alpha (SubCA), sensory root of the trigeminal nerve (s5), primary sensory trigeminal nucleus (Pr5), principal sensory trigeminal nucleus ventrolateral (Pr5VL) and the classical areas such as the (IOC) and (LC). Areas which contain predominantly AT_2 labeling, but also AT_1 receptors were the SGe, genu facial nerve (g7), facial nucleus (7). We also identified structures expressing mainly or only AT_1 receptor subtype: raphe pallidus nucleus (RPa), raphe magnus nucleus (RMg), spinal trigeminal nucleus oral (Sp5O) (see Table 2) [57]. Similar finding were observed in P8 animals [130].

5. Effect of the Pharmacological Blockade of RAS on Hindbrain Development

As pointed out before, Ang II receptor expression seems to be regulated during fetal and early postnatal life [7]. Both clinical as well as experimental evidence have shown the importance and potential role of the RAS during development [133]. The cloning of genes for the different components of the RAS allowed the development of knock-out mice for Aogen, ACE, renin and Ang II receptors, AT_{1A}, AT_{1B} or double knock-out for AT_{1A} plus AT_{1B} [134].

Studies from knock-out mice reinforce the hypothesis that AT_2 receptor plays a role in neuronal development [69,70]. Although a first evaluation of the phenotype revealed only subtle differences, like changes in the exploratory behavior and water intake, posterior analysis showed an anxiety-like behavior in knock-out mice [127] and hypersensitivity to Ang II of blood pressure and sodium secretion [135]. The increased cell number in different brain structures, like the hippocampus, supports a role for AT_2 receptors in the control of cellular proliferation [128]. In human, X-linked mental retardation has been linked to AT_2 receptor mutations [136]. Recently, impaired spatial memory and altered dendrite morphology was described in AT_2 knock-out mice [129]. These evidences, plus the temporal coincidence of the maximal expression of AT_2 receptors with movement acquisition by the rat (P15), suggest a potential important role of Ang II AT_2 receptors in hindbrain development.

Pharmacological studies, performed by blockade of the RAS allowed to evaluate a potential role of RAS components on growth and development. In adult animals, blockade of AT_2 receptors with a low dose up-regulates AT_1 receptor expression in PV, SFO and ME [137]. Several studies have been performed with blockade of the AT_1 or AT_2 receptors [80,137-141] however, no study has so far examined receptor localization or expression in the hindbrain after receptor blockade in developing rats.

We performed a study where Ang II inhibitors were administered to pregnant rats during late gestation E13-E21. The period of drug administration (E13 to E21) and the doses employed (1.0 mg/kg/day) were selected in order to study the potential role of Ang II receptors during hindbrain organogenesis (see Figure 5). In rodents, cerebellar development begins at E10–E11 and lasts until the third postnatal week [115]. Thus, treatment was performed during a crucial stage in the establishment of cell progenitors of the cerebellar structures [116]. Although treatments were performed with either over-stimulation of Ang II receptors or blockade of both receptor subtypes, in this chapter we will refer mainly to blockade of AT_2 receptors with the specific competitor PD123319.

Low doses of PD123319 (1.0 mg/kg/day) did not cause changes in the blood pressure of the mother or changes in the weight, survival and number of pups [80]. The effect of treatment with PD123319 on hindbrain development was evaluated at the histomorphological level and receptor localization by binding autoradiography at different antero-posterior levels in P0 and P8 animals.

In the cerebellar nuclei, binding was present in animals from different treatment groups. However, for those treated with PD123319, AT_2 binding was higher in the cerebellar nuclei, where the nucleus appeared with higher cellular density (Figure 6). Quantification of binding at the cerebellar cortex evidenced that AT_1 as well as AT_2 binding were significantly reduced in animals treated with Losartan o PD123319.

On the contrary, treatment with PD123319 induced an increased binding to AT_2 receptors in cerebellar nuclei and the IO [130].

In the cerebellar cortex, control animals showed binding in the incipient cerebellar cortex in P0, corresponding mainly to the AT_2 subtype. Blockade of AT_2 receptors during late pregnancy caused a lost of Ang II AT_2 binding in the external granular layer (EGL) of the cerebellar cortex in P0 pups (see Figure 6).

A detailed histological analysis evidenced a gross alteration at the histological level in the cerebellar layers, where the EGL appeared over-developed is well known that PCs migrate early during fetal stage (E14) toward the cerebellar cortex. The differential effect on the cerebellar cortex and nuclei needs further attention.

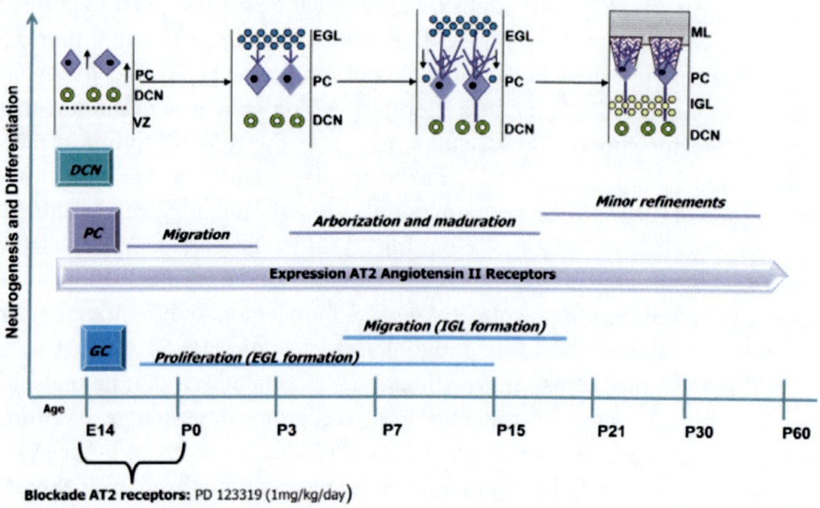

Figure 5. Pattern of histogenesis and migration of the cerebellar neurons and period of treatment. Abbreviations: DCN, deep cerebellar nuclei; EGL, external granule layer; GC, granule cells; IGL, internal granule layer; ML, molecular layer; PC, Purkinje cells; VZ, ventricular zone.

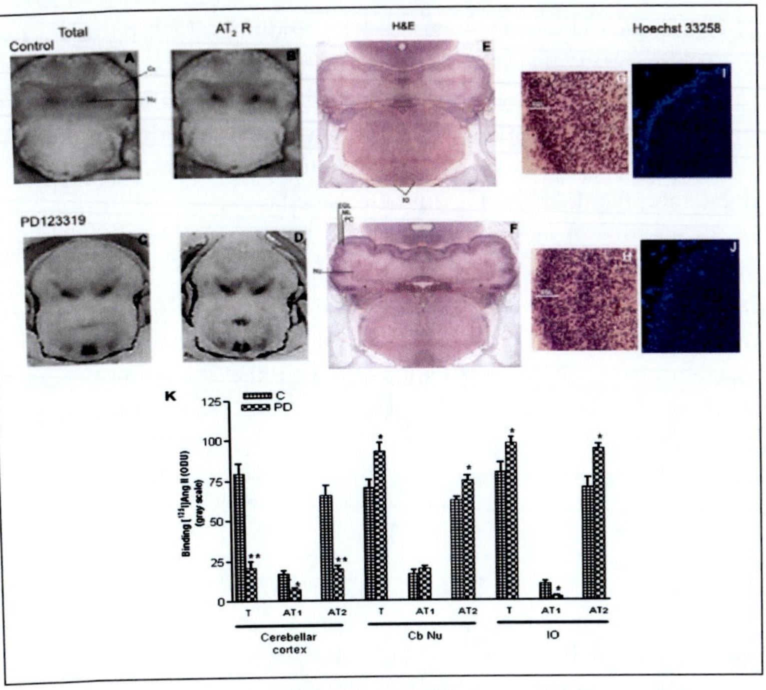

Figure 6. Comparative analysis of new-born hindbrains from control and PD123319 treated animals. **A-D:** Autoradiographic localization of Ang II receptors in P0 rat hindbrain, level P0-69. Consecutive coronal sections were incubated with [125I]Ang II (0.2 nM) in the absence (Total) or in the presence of the selective AT_1 blocker (Losartan) which reveal the localization of AT_2 receptors. Rows correspond to Control or PD123319 treated animals. **E-H:** H&E: hematoxylin–eosin staining at lower (20x) or higher magnification (100X). I, J: Hoechst staining of nuclei in parallel sections. **K:** Effects of treatment with PD123319 on binding densities in P0 animals. ** $p< 0.01$, * $p< 0.05$ vs. control. Abbreviations: PC: Purkinje cell layer (cerebellum); Ml: molecular layer of cerebellum; EGL: external germinal layer of Cb; IO: inferior olive; nu: cerebellar nuclei. (Adapted from Ref. 130).

Why if increased number of cells was observed in both, the cerebellar cortex and the nuclei, in one case we observed a lost of binding while an increased binding was present in cerebellar nuclei? As pointed out before, the precursors of PCs originate from the ventricular zone and postmitotic PCs migrate toward the cerebellar cortex at an early stage (E14), while granule cells generate mainly postnatally [116] (Figure 5). Considering that treatment with PD123319 was performed during a prenatal period critical for PCs migration, this might cause an altered cerebellar cortex in P0 animals. The lack of binding at the enlarged EGL in P0 animals treated with PD123319, not only agrees with our data that AT_2 receptors localized at the PCs (Figure 4) but also suggest a potential role for Ang II AT_2 receptors during PCs migration. Besides, it was reported that PCs regulate proliferation of the granulose cells [142]. Previous studies conducted in cell lines support the role of AT_2 receptor in neurite elongation, neuron migration, neuronal death/ survival balance, and in the establishment and maintenance of synaptic connections [71, 143-146].

Since a pro-apoptotic role has been attributed to AT_2 receptors [73,74], blockade of these receptors could inhibit apoptosis, a normal process in organogenesis, leading to an increased number of cells, as shown by Hoechst staining (Figure 6). This observation is in agreement with previous ones, showing that AT_2 knock-out animals exhibited a larger number of neurons in several brain areas [128]. In PD123319-treated animals, the cerebellar nuclei and the inferior olive complex showed increased AT_2 binding, which parallels an increased cell number [130]. While blockade of AT_2 receptors with PD123319 during late pregnancy significantly increased AT_2 binding in cerebellar nuclei and IO, it produced a loss of binding in the EGL in P0 animals. Morales and Hatten [116] provided evidence that different progenitor cells give raise to the EGL, Purkinje cell progenitors and those for the cerebellar nuclei. Taken together, the thicker EGL in the cerebellar cortex and the lack of binding at the EGL, suggest either that a certain type of cells overproliferate or that cells do not differentiate/migrate when AT_2 receptors were blocked.

Although treatments lasted for 1 week before birth, we observed important effects on hindbrain development both at the histological and receptor localization level in P8 animals born from treated-mothers. These observations indicate that the damage persisted even when there was no longer exposure to drugs, suggesting that treatment during late pregnancy seriously disrupts the organogenesis pattern. These data, together with previous studies, strongly support a potential role for both Ang II receptors during cerebellar development.

6. AT_2 Receptors and Neuronal Differentiation

Recently, a potential role for Ang II in development as a growth modulating factor was proposed [11-14]. Studies from knock-out mice reinforce the hypothesis that AT_2 receptors play a role in neuronal development [69,70,127]. Our studies from pharmacological blockade and receptor localization during hindbrain development also support this hypothesis. A number of studies on AT_2-receptor signaling have been performed in cells of neuronal origin (PC12W, N1E-115 and NG 108-15 cell lines), where activation of the AT_2 receptor was shown to induce neurite outgrowth and elongation [71,146], neuronal differentiation [145], promote cellular migration and, in particular conditions, induce neuronal cell death [147].

Although the predicted structure of the AT_2 receptor indicates that it belongs to the G-protein coupled receptors, the signaling pathway for this receptor is still controversial since it does not stimulate classical second messengers [71,72,148]. AT_2 receptors share some features with the somatostatin receptor, both activate the PTPase SHP-1, associated to cellular apoptosis in different cell lines [75-79]. The first evidence of this association was described by Nahmias et al. [78].

Four major signaling mechanisms can be attributed to Ang II AT_2 receptors, involving phosphatase activation, NO/cGMP synthesis, phospholipase A2 stimulation and arachidonic acid release, ceramide synthesis [71,72,79,148,149] (Figure 7). A brief description of these mechanisms follows:

1. Phosphatase activation: AT_2 receptor stimulation induces protein dephosphorylation of regulatory proteins that participate in anti-proliferation, apoptosis, differentiation and vasodilatation. Three phosphatases have been identified: the Protein Tyrosine Phosphatase (PTPase) SHP-1, Mitogen Activated Protein Kinases (MAPK) phosphatase-1 (MKP-1) and the Ser/Thr phosphatase PP2A. AT_2 receptors inhibited MAPK by activation of several phosphatases such as MKP-1 [73,74], SHP-1 [75-77,148,150] and PP2A [151] and in this way inhibited cellular proliferation. SHP-1 (also named as SH-

PTP-1, HCP, PTP-1C) is a non transmembrane PTPase that contains two Src homology 2 domains (SH2), allowing its association with multiple adaptor molecules [152,153]. MKP-1 activation in PC12W cells led to dephosphorylation of Bcl-2, an anti-apoptotic protein, and a positive regulation of the pro-apoptotic protein Bax, inducing apoptosis [74]. Besides, in neural cells from rat hippocampus, AT_2 receptor induced the activation (mediated by G_i) of K channels via PP2A [71,154].

2. Activation of the NO/GMPc: NO release with an increase in intracellular cGMP during neuronal differentiation was described in NG108-15 cells [155]. NO, when produced at low levels, is known to induce neuronal differentiation. In NG108–15 cells, Côté et al. [146] demonstrated that AT_2 induced differentiation with participation of the neuronal NO synthase (nNOS) and cGMP production (Gi-dependent) [71,149,155]. Different tissues from spontaneously hypertensive rats (SHR) evidenced an activation of the NO/GMPc pathway, mediated by AT_2 receptors [156].
3. Phospholipase A2 stimulation: it was proposed that release of arachidonic acid and PP2A activation would be mediated by AT_2 receptor activation (G_i-dependent). Arachidonic acid might contribute to the activation of a unidirectional transport of Na^+/HCO^{3-} which regulate pH [148,149].
4. Ceramide synthesis: long-term stimulation of AT_2 receptor with Ang II increases ceramide synthesis, which can activate stress kinases and caspases involved in apoptosis induction [157,158]. Ceramide is an intracellular messengers generated by *de novo* synthesis following AT_2 receptor stimulation in neuronal cells, thus inducing caspase activation and then apoptosis. Ceramide can also induce activation of the stress-activated protein kinase family (SAPK) and the c-Jun N-terminal kinase (JNK) which is known to be involved in various types of apoptosis [148,149].

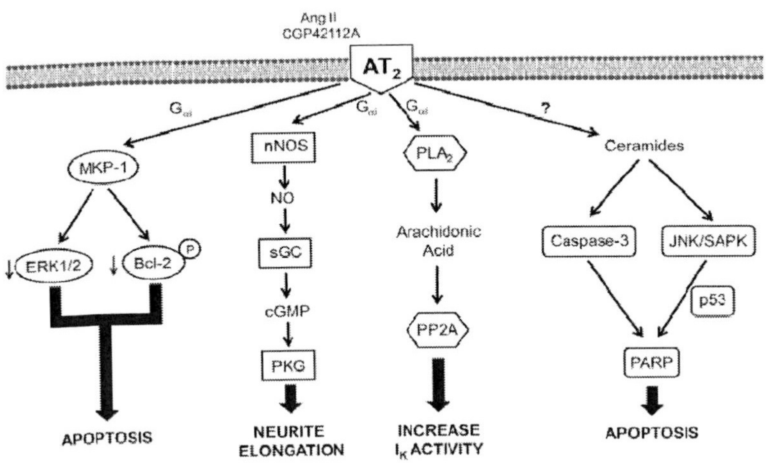

Figure 7. Signal transduction mechanisms and physiological effects of the AT_2 receptor. ERK, extracellular signal-regulated kinase; $G_{\alpha i}$, αi-subunit of GPCR; JNK, c-Jun kinase; MKP-1, mitogen-activated protein kinase phosphatase 1; nNOS, neuronal nitric oxide synthase; NO, nitric oxide; PARP, poly (ADP-ribose) polymerase; PKG, cGMP-dependent protein kinase; PLA2, phospholipase A2; PP2A, protein phosphatase 2A; sGC, soluble guanylyl cyclase; SAPK, stress-activated protein kinase; SHP-1, SH2 domain-containing Phosphatase 1.

7. Signal Transduction for Ang II AT_2 Receptors in RAT Hindbrain

As stated in the previous section, AT_2 receptors activate unconventional signaling pathways which in general do not involve a classical activation of a G-protein [72,149]. Besides, the physiological role of AT_2 receptors is still under discussion. Receptor localization during development evidenced maximal expression of Ang II AT_2 receptors in the cerebellum and brainstem from P15 rats [57,87]. In the search of a potential role for Ang II AT_2 receptors, we selected P15 rat hindbrain, which represent a physiological developmental condition, to investigate the transduction mechanism for AT_2 receptors in an *ex vivo* preparation. In a previous study in fetal tissues we demonstrated the formation of a SHP-1/c-Src complex by activation of AT_2 receptors [79].

By using P15 rat hindbrain membrane preparations, which represent a physiological condition, we showed association and activation of the PTPase SHP-1 to AT_2 receptor in immunocomplexes obtained either with anti-AT_2 antibodies or with anti-SHP-1 antibody. Complex formation as well as tyr-phosphorylation and activation of SHP-1 were inducible but not constitutive [159]. Activation of SHP-1 requires a tyr-phosphorylation that triggers tyrosine phosphatase activity [160]. Ang II induced SHP-1 activation in P15 rat hindbrain, which was blocked by AT_2 antagonist PD123319, measured in immunocomplexes obtained either with anti-SHP-1 or anti-AT_2 antibodies.

Considering that AT_2 receptors belong to the superfamily of GPCR, we wonder for the mechanism involved in SHP-1 tyr-phosphorylation. Thus, we searched for the presence of c-Src in the immunocomplexes obtained with anti-AT_2 antibodies. Ang II induced a marked increase of the association, selectively blocked by the AT_2 antagonist PD123319. Participation of members of SFK in the transduction mechanism of AT_2 receptors has been recently proposed in rat cerebellum [161] and neuronal cell lines [162]. Recently, Guimond et al. [162] observed neurite outgrowth mediated by Ang II AT_2 receptors in NG108-15 cells, with participation of Fyn, member of the SFK. In our model, we demonstrated the formation of a tertiary complex, containing AT_2/SHP-1/c-Src, following stimulation with Ang II. Previous reports suggest a constitutive activation of AT_2 receptors [163,164]. Our data clearly show AT_2 receptors recruit c-Src and SHP-1 in response to Ang II stimulation, being c-Src responsible for SHP-1 tyr-phosphorylation and its activation. Thus, a member of SFK was required in order to produce SHP-1 activation. MALDI-TOF analysis confirmed the presence of the components in immunocomplexes [159].

Focal Adhesion Kinase (FAK) is a substrate of c-Src which participates in extracellular signaling mediated by integrins in growth process, differentiation and cell migration [165-168]. It has been shown recently that FAK knock-out mice suffer from a serious damage on cerebellar foliation, Bergmann glia positioning and climbing fiber territory on Purkinje cells [166]. Cleavage of FAK by caspase 3 and 6 results in an 85 kDa fragment, which has been related to apoptosis [169]. Thus, we explored the presence of FAK in AT_2-immunocomplexes obtained in P15 rat hindbrain. To our surprise, we found the p85FAK fragment (85 kDa) but not paxillin in immunocomplexes. The absence of the full-length FAK and the presence of the p85 fragment in AT_2 immunocomplexes explain the absence of paxillin in those immunocomplexes [165]. The serious cerebellar damage observed in the FAK knock-out mice reinforces the interest in this model of study.

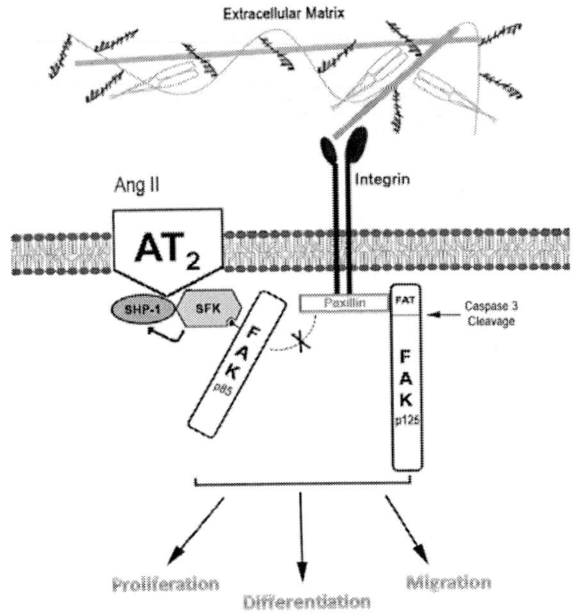

Figure 8. Proposed model for AT_2 receptor signal transduction in rat hindbrain. (Adapted from Ref. 159).

In this *ex vivo* model in P15 rat hindbrain we provide evidences for an inducible signal transduction mechanism for Ang II AT_2 receptors and demonstrated that Ang II stimulation induces the formation of a complex containing AT_2/SHP-1/c-Src/p85FAK (Figure 8). The demonstrated participation of FAK might have a possible implication in either cell migration or apoptosis induction, two mechanisms critical in cerebellar development.

8. Conclusions

In spite that a number of studies report the role of the AT_2 receptors in neurite elongation, neuronal excitability and axonal regeneration, the role of the Ang II AT_2 receptor in neuronal differentiation and brain development is a matter of discussion. Receptor localization has been extensively explored in the CNS, while very little information is available on cerebellar and brainstem development. Studies from autoradiography in normal development allowed us to identify Ang II receptor expression at different levels in the hindbrain. AT_2 receptor expression was maximal in P15 rat cerebellar cortex and limited to a thin layer. Immunohistochemistry and confocal analysis confirmed that Ang II AT_2 receptors co-localize with molecular markers of PCs during cerebellar development, from P8 to P60. Studies from knock-out mice reinforce the hypothesis that AT_2 receptors play a role in neuronal development. Pharmacological blockade of Ang II AT_2 receptor with PD123319 caused a serious morphological and receptor expression alteration in P15 rat hindbrain.

Most of the AT_2 signal transduction studies have been performed in cell lines. We selected an *ex vivo* model, which represents a physiological condition. In this model, formation of a complex containing AT_2/SHP-1/c-Src/p85FAK was demonstrated. Taken together, studies from receptor localization, the particular characteristics of cerebellar development, the effect of pharmacological blockade of Ang II AT_2 receptor and the role of FAK in cerebellar development, we propose a possible implication of Ang II AT_2 receptor signaling in cell migration or apoptosis induction, two mechanisms critical in cerebellar development.

ACKNOWLEDGEMENTS

G.M. Ciuffo is a member of the researcher's career of CONICET (Consejo Nacional de Investigaciones Científicas y Tecnológicas, Argentina). LR Seguin has a fellowship from CONICET, Argentina. This work was supported by grants from CONICET, PICT 15-32350 (ANPCYT) and Universidad Nacional de San Luis, Argentina.

REFERENCES

[1] Tigerstedt R, Bergman PG. Niere und Kreislauf. Skand *Arch Physiol.* 1898;8:223–71.

[2] Braun-Menendez E, Fasciolo JC, Leloir LF, Muñoz JM. The substance causing renal hypertension. *J Physiol* (Lond.). 1944;98:283–98.

[3] Page IH, Helmer OM. A crystaline pressor substance (angiotonin) resulting from the action between renin and renin-activator. *J Exp Med.* 1940;71:29–42.

[4] Skeggs LT, Kahn JR, Shumway NP. The purification of hypertensin II. *J Exp Med.* 1956;103(3):301-7.

[5] Bumpus FM, Schwarz H, Page IH. Synthesis and pharmacology of the octapeptide angiotonin. *Science.* 1957;125(3253):886-7.

[6] Elliott DF, Peart WS. The amino acid sequence in a hypertensin. *Biochem J.* 1957;65(2):246-54.

[7] de Gasparo M, Catt KJ, Inagami T, Wright JW, Unger TH. International Union of Pharmacology. XXIII. The Angiotensin II *Receptors. Pharmacol Rev.* 2000;52:415-472.

[8] Gallinat S, Busche S, Raizada MK, Summers C. The Angiotensin II type 2 receptor: an enigma with multiple variations. *Am J Physiol Endocrinol Metab.* 2000;278:E357-E374.

[9] Saavedra JM. Emerging features of brain angiotensin receptors. *Regul Pept.* 1999;85:31–45.

[10] Ciuffo GM, Viswanathan M, Seltzer AM, Tsutsumi K, Saavedra JM. Glomerular Angiotensin II receptor subtypes during development of rat kidney. *Am J Physiol.* 1993;265:F264-71.

[11] Landon EJ, Inagami T. Beyond the G protein: the saga of the type 2 angiotensin II receptor. *Arterioscler Thromb Vasc Biol.* 2005;25(1):15-6.

[12] Deshayes F, Nahmias C. Angiotensin receptors: a new role in cancer? *Trends Endocrinol Metab.* 2005;16(7):293-9.

[13] Hunyady L, Catt KJ. Pleiotropic AT1 receptor signaling pathways mediating physiological and pathogenic actions of angiotensin II. *Mol Endocrinol.* 2006 ;20(5):953-70.

[14] Godeny MD, Sayeski PP. ANG II-induced cell proliferation is dually mediated by c-Src/Yes/Fyn-regulated ERK1/2 activation in the cytoplasm and PKCzeta-controlled ERK1/2 activity within the nucleus. *Am J Physiol Cell Physiol.* 2006;291(6):C1297-307.

[15] Wu L, Iwai M, Li Z, Shiuchi T, Min LJ, Cui TX, et al. Regulation of inhibitory protein-kappa B and monocyte chemoattractant protein-1 by angiotensin II type 2 receptor-activated Src homology protein tyrosine phosphatase-1 in fetal vascular smooth muscle cells. *Mol Endocrinol.* 2004;18(3):666-78.

[16] Menard J, Bouhnik J, Clauser E, Richoux JP, Corvol P. Biochemistry and regulation of angiotensinogen. *Clin Exp Hypertens.* 1983;5:1005–1019.

[17] Deschepper CF. Angiotensinogen: hormonal regulation and relative importance in the generation of angiotensin II. *Kidney Int.* 1994;46:1561–1563.

[18] Hall JE. Historical perspective of the renin-angiotensin system. *Mol Biotechnol.* 2003;24:27–39.

[19] Nguyen G, Delarue F, Burckle C, Bouzhir L, Giller T, Sraer JD. Pivotal role of the renin/prorenin receptor in angiotensin II production and cellular responses to renin. *J Clin Invest.* 2002;109:1417–1427.

[20] Ferrario CM, Brosnihan KB, Diz DI, Jaiswal N, Khosla MC, Milsted A, et al. Angiotensin-(1-7): a new hormone of the angiotensin system. *Hypertension.*1991;18 (SIII):III-126 –III-133.

[21] Ferrario CM, Chappell MC, Tallant EA, Brosnihan KB, Diz DI. Counterregulatory actions of angiotensin-(1-7). *Hypertension.*1997;30:535-541.

[22] Santos RA, Simoes e Silva AC, Maric C, Silva DM, Machado RP, de Buhr I, et al. Angiotensin-(1-7) is an endogenous ligand for the G protein coupled receptor Mas. *Proc Natl Acad Sci USA.* 2003;100: 8258–8263.

[23] Santos RA, Ferreira AJ. Angiotensin(1–7) and the renin-angiotensin system. *Curr Opin Nephrol Hypertens.* 2007;16:122– 128.

[24] Kifor I, Dzau VJ. Endothelial renin-angiotensin pathway: evidence for intracellular synthesis and secretion of angiotensins. *Circ Res.* 1987;60:422–428.

[25] Pieruzzi F, Abassi ZA, Keiser HR. Expression of renin-angiotensin system components in the heart, kidneys, and lungs of rats with experimental heart failure. *Circulation.* 1995;92:3105–3112.

[26] Harris RC, Cheng HF. The intrarenal renin-angiotensin system: a paracrine system for the local control of renal function separate from the systemic axis. *Exp Nephrol.* 1996; Suppl 1:2–7

[27] Mulrow PJ, Franco-Saenz R. The adrenal renin-angiotensin system: a local hormonal regulator of aldosterone production. *J Hypertens* 1996;4:173–176.

[28] Dell'Italia LJ, Meng QC, Balcells E, Wei CC, Palmer R, Hageman GR, et al. Compartmentalization of angiotensin II generation in the dog heart. Evidence for independent mechanisms in intravascular and interstitial spaces. *J Clin Invest.*1997;100:253–258.

[29] Dostal DE, Baker KM. The cardiac renin-angiotensin system: conceptual, or a regulator of cardiac function? *Circ Res.*1999;85:643–650.

[30] Baltatu O, Bader M. Brain renin-angiotensin system. Lessons from functional genomics. *Neuroendocrinology*. 2003;78: 253–259.

[31] Carey R, Siragy HM. Newly Recognized Components of the Renin-Angiotensin System: Potential Roles in Cardiovascular and Renal Regulation. *Endocrine Revs.* 2003;24(3):261–271.

[32] Jensen BL, Stubbe J, Madsen K, Nielsen FT, Skott O. The renin-angiotensin system in kidney development: role of COX-2 and adrenal steroids. *Acta Physiol Scand.* 2004;181:549–559.

[33] Sakai K, Sigmund CD. Molecular evidence of tissue renin angiotensin systems: a focus on the brain. *Curr Hypertens Rep.* 2005;7:135–140.

[34] Paul M, Poyan Mehr A, Kreutz R. Physiology of Local Renin-Angiotensin Systems. *Physiol Rev*. 2006; 86:747–803.

[35] Ganten D, Minnich JL, Granger P, Hayduk K, Brecht HM, Barbeau A, et al. Angiotensin-forming enzyme in brain tissue. *Science*. 1971;173:64–65.

[36] Saavedra JM. Brain and pituitary angiotensin. *Endocrinol Rev*. 1992;13:329–380.

[37] McKinley MJ, Albiston AL, Allen AM, Mathai ML, May CN, McAllen RM, et al. The brain renin–angiotensin system: location and physiological roles. *Int J Biochem Cell Biol*. 2003;35: 901–918.

[38] Saavedra JM. Brain angiotensin II: new developments, unanswered questions and therapeutic opportunities. *Cell Mol Neurobiol*. 2005;(3-4):485-512.

[39] Chiu AT, Herbin WF, Mc Call DE, Ardecky RJ, Carini DJ, Duncia JV, et al. Identification of angiotensin II receptor subtypes. *Biochem Biophys Res Commun.* 1989;165:196-203.

[40] Whitebread S, Mele M, Kamber B, de Gasparo M. Preliminary biochemical characterization of two angiotensin II receptor subtypes. *Biochem Biophys Res Commun.* 1989;163:284–291.

[41] Murphy TJ, Alexander RW, Griendling KK, Runge ME, Bernstein KE. Isolation of a cDNA encoding the vascular type-I angiotensin II receptor. *Nature*. 1991;351: 233-236.

[42] Sasaki K, Yamano Y, Bardhan S, Iwai N, Murray JJ, Hasegawa M,et al. Cloning and expression of a complementary DNA encoding a bovine adrenal angiotensin II type-I receptor. *Nature*. 1991;351:230-233.

[43] Kambayashi Y, Bardhan S, Takahashi K, Tsuzuki S, Inui H, Hamakubo T, et al. Molecular Cloning of a novel angiotensin II receptor isoform involved in phosphotyrosine phosphatase inhibition. *J Biol Chem*. 1993;268:24543-24546.

[44] Mukoyama M, Nakajima M, Horiuchi M, Sasamura H, Pratt RE, Dzau VJ.. Expression Cloning of type 2 angiotensin II receptor reveals unique class of seven-transmembrane receptors. *J Biol Chem*. 1993;268:24539-24542.

[45] Horiuchi M, Lehtonen J, Daviet L.. Signaling Mechanism of the AT_2 Angiotensin II Receptor: Crosstalk between AT_1 and AT_2 Receptors in Cell Growth. *Trends Endocrinol Metab.* 1999;10:391-396.

[46] Steckelings UM, Kaschina E, Unger T. The AT_2 receptor: A matter of love and hate. *Peptides*. 2005;26:1401-1409.

[47] Tsutsumi K, Viswanathan M, Strömberg C, Saavedra JM.. Type-1and type-2 angiotensin II receptors in fetal rat brain. *European J Pharmacol*. 1991;198: 89-92.

[48] Tufro-McReddie A, Gomez RA.. Ontogeny of the renin-angiotensin system. *Semin Nephrol.* 1993;13:519-530.

[49] Aguilera G, Kapur S, Feuillan P, Sunar-Akbasak B, Bathia AJ Developmental changes in angiotensin II receptor subtypes and AT_1 receptor mRNA in rat kidney. *Kidney Int.* 1994;46: 973–979.

[50] Hunt RA, Ciuffo GM, Saavedra JM, Tucker DC. Quantification and Localization of Angiotensin II receptors and Angiotensin Converting Enzyme in the developing rat heart. *Cardiovas Res.* 1995;29:834-840.

[51] Bastien NR, Ciuffo GM, Saavedra JM, Lambert C. Angiotensin II receptor expression in the conduction system and arterial duct of neonatal and adult rat hearts. *Regul Pep.* 1996;163:19-16.

[52] Wolf G. Angiotensin II and tubular development. *Nephrol Dial Transplant.* 2002;17:48–51.

[53] Garcia-Villalba P, Denkers ND, Wittwer CT, Hoff C, Nelson RD, Mauch TJ. Real-time PCR quantification of AT_1 and AT_2 angiotensin receptor mRNA expression in the developing rat kidney. *Nephron Exp Nephrol.* 2003;94:154-159.

[54] Viswanathan M, Tsutsumi K, Correa FM, Saavedra JM. Changes in expression of angiotensin receptor subtypes in the rat aorta during development. *Biochem Biophys Res Commun.* 1991;179:1361–1367.

[55] Nuyt AM, Lenkei Z, Palkovits M, Corvol P, LLorens-Cortes C. Ontogeny of angiotensin II type-2 receptor mRNA expression in fetal and neonatal rat brain. *J Comp Neurol.* 1999; 407:193-206.

[56] Nuyt AM, Lenkei Z, Corvol P, Palkovits M, Llorens-Cortes C. Ontogeny of angiotensin II type 1 receptor mRNAs in fetal and neonatal rat brain. *J Comp Neurol.* 2001;440(2):192-203.

[57] Arce ME, Sanchez S, Seltzer A, Ciuffo GM. Autorradiographic localization of Angiotensin II receptors in developing rat cerebellum and brainstem. *Regul Pept.* 2001; 99: 53-60.

[58] Timmerman PBMWM, Wong PC, Chiu AT, Herblin WF, Carini DJ, Lee RJ. Angiotensin II receptor and angiotensin II receptor antagonist. *Pharmacol Rev.*1993;45: 205-51.

[59] Higuchi S, Ohtsu H, Suzuki H, Shirai H, Frank GD, Eguchi S. Angiotensin II signal transduction through the AT_1 receptor: novel insights into mechanisms and pathophysiology. *Clin Sci.* 2007;112:417-428.

[60] Iwai N, Inagami T. Identification of two subtypes in the rat type I angiotensin II receptor. *FEBS Lett.* 1992;289:257-260.

[61] Sasamura H, Hein L, Krieger JE. Pratt RE, Kobilka BK, DzauVJ. Cloning, characterization, and expression of two angiotensin receptor (AT_1) isoforms from the mouse genome. *Biochem Biophys Res Commun.* 1992;185:253-259.

[62] Lewis JL, Serikawa T, Warnock DG. Chomosomal localization of angiotensin II type receptor isoforms in the rat. *Biochem Biophys Res Commun.* 1993;194.677-682.

[63] Guo DF, Furuta H, Mizukoshi M, Inagami, T. The genomic organization of human angiotensin II type 1 receptor. *Biochem Res Commun.* 1994;200:313-319.

[64] Hernandez Schulman Zhou MS, Raij L. Cross-talk between angiotensin II receptor types 1 and 2: potential role in vascular remodeling in humans. *Hypertension.* 2007;49(2):270-1.

[65] Saito M, Shinohara Y, Sasaki H, Netsu Y, Yoshida M, Nakahata N. Type 1 angiotensin receptor (AT1-R)-mediated decrease in type 2 angiotensin receptor mRNA level is

dependent on Gq and extracellular signal-regulated kinase 1//2 in AT1-R-transfected PC12 cells. *J Neuroendocrinol.* 2008;20(3):299-308.

[66] Koike G, Horiuchi M, Yamada T, Szpirer C, Jacob HJ, Dzau VJ. Human type 2 angiotensin II receptor gene: cloned, mapped to the X chromosome, and its mRNA is expressed in the human lung. *Biochem Biophys Res Commun.* 1994;203: 1842–1850.

[67] Koike G, Winer ES, Horiuchi M, Brown DM, Szpirer C, Dzau VJ, Jacob, HJ. Cloning, characterization, and genetic mapping of the rat type 2 angiotensin II receptor gene. *Hypertension.*1995; 26: 998–1002.

[68] Lazard D, Briend-Sutren MM, Villageois P, Mattei MG, Strosberg AD, Nahmias C. Molecular characterization and chromosome localization of a human angiotensin II AT_2 receptor gene highly expressed in fetal tissues. *Receptors Channels* 1994;2:271–280.

[69] Hein L, Barsh GS, Pratt RE, Dzau VJ, Kobilka BK. Behavioral and cardiovascular effects of disrupting the angiotensin II type-2 receptor gene in mice. *Nature.* 1995; 377:744-747.

[70] Ichiki T, Labosky PA, Shiota C, Shigeru O, Imagawa I, Fogo A, et al. Effects on blood pressure and reduced exploratory behavior in mice lacking angiotensin II type 2 receptor. *Nature.* 1995;377:748-750.

[71] Gendron L, Payet MD, Gallo-Payet N. The Angiotensin type 2 receptor of angiotensin II and neuronal differentiation: from observations to mechanisms. *J Mol Endocrinol.* 2003;31:359-372.

[72] Porrello ER, Delbridge LM, Thomas WG. The angiotensin II type 2 (AT_2) receptor: an enigmatic seven transmembrane receptor. *Front Biosci.* 2009;1(14):958-972.

[73] Yamada T, Horiuchi M, Dzau VJ Angiotensin II type 2 receptor mediates programmed cell death. *Proc Natl Acad USA.* 1996;93:156–160.

[74] Horiuchi M, Hayashida W, Kambe T, Yamada T, Dzau VJ. Angiotensin Type 2 Receptor Dephosphorylates Bcl-2 by Activating Mitogen-activated Protein Kinase Phosphatase-1 and Induces Apoptosis. *J Biol Chem.* 1997; 272(30):19022-19026.

[75] Bedecs K, Elbaz N, Sutren M, Masson M, Susini C, Strosberg AD, et al. Angiotensin II type 2 receptors mediate inhibition of mitogen-activated protein kinase cascade and functional activation of SHP-1 tyrosine phosphatase. *Biochem J.* 1997;325:449-454.

[76] Shibasaki Y, Matsubara H, Nozawa Y, Mori Y, Masaki H, Kosaki A, et al. Angiotensin II type 2 receptor inhibits epidermal growth factor receptor transactivation by increasing association of SHP-1 tyrosine phosphatase. *Hypertension.* 2001;38:367–372.

[77] Cui T, Nakagami H, Nahmias C, Shiuchi T, Takeda-Matsubara Y, Li JM, et al. Angiotensin II subtype2 receptor activation inhibits insulin-induced phosphoinositide3-kinase and Akt and induces apoptosis in PC12W cells. *Mol Endocrinol.* 2002;16:2113–2123.

[78] Nahmias C, Strosberg AD. The angiotensin AT_2 receptor: searching for signal-transduction pathways and physiological function. *Trends Pharmacol Sci.* 1995;7:223-235

[79] Alvarez SE, Seguin LR, Villarreal RS, Nahmias C, Ciuffo GM. Involvement of c-Src tyrosine kinase in SHP-1 phosphatase activation by Ang II AT_2 receptors in rat fetal tissues. *J Cell Biochem.* 2008;105(3):703-711.

[80] Sanchez SI, Seltzer AM, Fuentes LB, Forneris ML, Ciuffo GM. Inhibition of Angiotensin II receptors during pregnancy induces malformations in developing rat kidney. *Eur J Pharmacol.* 2008;588:114–123.

[81] Cuadra AE, Shan Z, Sumners C, Raizada MK. A current view of brain renin–angiotensin system: Is the (pro)renin receptor the missing link?. *Pharmacol Ther.* 2010;125(1):27-38.

[82] Song K, Allen AM, Paxinos G, Mendelsohn FA. Mapping of angiotensin II receptor subtype heterogeneity in rat brain. *J Comp Neurol.*1992, 316(4):467-84.

[83] Lenkei Z, Palkovits M, Corvol P, Llorens-Cortes C. Expression of angiotensin type-1 (AT_1) and type-2 (AT_2) receptor mRNAs in the adult rat brain: a functional neuroanatomical review. *Front. Neuroendocrinol.* 1997;18:383–439.

[84] Mao C, Shi L, Xu F, Zhang L, Xu Z. Development of fetal brain renin–angiotensin system and hypertension programmed in fetal origins. *Progress in Neurobiol.* 2009;87:252–263.

[85] Höhle S, Culman J, Boser M, Qadri F, Unger T. Effect of angiotensin AT_2 and muscarinic receptor blockade on osmotically induced vasopressin release. *Eur J Pharmacol.* 1996;300(1-2):119-23.

[86] Wright JW, Harding J. The Brain angiotensin system and the extracellular matrix molecules in neural plasticity, learning and memory. *Progress in Neurobiol.* 2004;72:263-293.

[87] Arce ME, Sánchez SI, López Aguilera F, Seguin LR, Seltzer AM, Ciuffo GM. Purkinje cells express Angiotensin II AT_2 receptors at different developmental stages. *Neuropeptides.* 2011;45 69–76.

[88] Lee HU, Campbell DJ, Habener JF. Development expression of the angiotesinogen gene in rat embryos. *Endocrinology.* 1987;121:1335–1342.

[89] Kalinyak JE, Hoffman AR, Perlman AJ. Ontogeny of angiotensinogen mRNA and angiotensin II receptors in rat brain and liver. *J Endocr Invest.* 1991;14:647–653.

[90] Yang G, Sigmund CD. Developmental expression of human angiotensinogen in transgenic mice. *Am J Physiol.* 1998;274:F932–F939.

[91] Sood PP, Panigel M, Wegmann R. The existence of renin–angiotensinogen system in the rat fetal brain: I. Immunocytochemical localization of renin-like activity at the 19th day of gestation. *Cell Mol Biol.* 1987;33:675–680.

[92] Sood PP, Richoux JP, Panigel M, Bouhnik J, Wegman R. The existence of renin–angiotensinogen system in the rat fetal brain. II. Immunocytochemical localization of angiotensinogen in the telencephalon and the diencephalons. *Cell Mol Neurobiol.* 1987;33:681–689.

[93] Mungall BA, Shinkel TA., Sernia C. Immunocytochemical localization of angiotensinogen in the fetal and neonatal rat brain. *Neuroscience* 1995;67:505–524.

[94] Richoux JP, Amsaguine S, Grignon G, Bouhnik J, Menard J, Corvol P. Earliest renin containing cell differentiation during ontogenesis in the rat. An immunocytochemical study. *Histochemistry.* 1987;88(1):41-6

[95] Sood PP, Panige Ml, Wegmann R. Co-existance of renin-like immunoreactivity in the rat maternal and fetal neocortex. *Neurochem Res.* 1989;14:499–502.

[96] Sood PP, Richoux JP, Panigel M, Bouhnik J, Wegmann R. Angiotensinogen in the developing rat fetal hindbrain and spinal cord from 18th to 20th day of gestation: an immunocytochemical study. *Neuroscience.* 1990;37:517–522.

[97] Saavedra JM, Chevillard C. Angiotensin-converting enzyme is present in the subfornical organ and other circumventricular organs of the rat. *Neuroscience Lett.* 1982;29:123-127.

[98] Strittmatter SM, Lo MMS, Javitch JA, Snyder SH. Autoradiographic visualization of angiotensin-converting enzyme in rat brain with [3H]captopril: localization to a striatonigral pathway. *Proc Natl Acad Sci USA*. 1984;81:1599–1603.

[99] Strittmatter SM, Lynch DR, Synder SH. Differential ontogeny of rat brain peptidases: prenatal expression of enkephalin converytase and postnatal development of angiotensin-converting enzyme. *Brain Res*. 1986;394:207–215.

[100] Mendelsohn FAO, Chai SY, Dunbar M. In vitro autoradiographic localization of angiotensin-converting enzyme in rat brain using 125I-labelled MK351A. *J Hypertens Suppl*. 1984;2:S41–S44.

[101] Chai SY, Mendelsohn FAO, Paxinos G. Angiotensin converting enzyme in rat brain visualized by quantitative in vitro autoradiography. *Neuroscience*. 1987;20:615–627.

[102] Whiting P, Nava S, Mozley L, Eastham H, Poat J. Expression of angiotensin converting enzyme mRNA in rat brain. *Mol Brain Res*. 1991;11:93–96.

[103] Baltatu O, Lippoldt A, Hansson A, Ganten D, Bader M.. Local renin– angiotensin system in the pineal gland. *Brain Res*. 1998;54:237–242.

[104] Tsutsumi, K, Seltzer A, Saavedra JM, Angiotensin II receptor subtypes and angiotensin-converting enzyme in the fetal rat brain. *Brain Res*. 1993;631:12–220.

[105] Changaris DG, Severs WB, Keil LC. Localization of Angiotensin II in rat brain. *J Histochem and Cytochem*. 1978;26(7):593-607.

[106] Chappell MC, Brosnihan KB, Welches WR, Ferrario CM. Characterization by high performance liquid chromatography of angiotensin peptides in the plasma and cerebrospinal fluid of the dog. *Peptides*. 1987;8:939–942.

[107] Chappell MC, Brosnihan KB, Diz DI, Ferrario CM. (. Identification of angiotensin-(1–7) in rat brain. Evidence for differential processing of angiotensin peptides. *J Biol Chem*. 1989;264:16518–16523.

[108] Weyhenmeyer JA, Raizada MK, Phillips MI, Fellows RE. Presence of angiotensin II in neurons cultured from fetal rat brain. *Neurosci Lett*. 1980;16(1):41-6.

[109] Gadbut AP, Cash SA, Noble JA, Radice TR, Weyhenmeyer JA. The effect of Ca^{2+} channel antagonists (cadmium, omega-conotoxin GIVA, and nitrendipine) on the release of angiotensin II from fetal rat brain in vitro. *Neurosci Lett*. 1991;123(1):91-4.

[110] Allen A M, Moeller I, Jenkins TA, Zhuo J,. Aldred GP, et al. Angiotensin receptors in the nervous system. *Brain Research Bull*.1998, 47(1):17–28.

[111] Jöhren O, Saavedra JM. Gene expression of angiotensin II receptor subtypes in the cerebellar cortex of young rats. *Neuroreport* 1996;7(8):1349-52.

[112] Jöhren O, Hauser W, Saavedra JM. Chemical lesion of the inferior olive reduces [125I] Sarcosine1–Angiotensin II binding to AT_2 receptors in the cerebellar cortex of young rats. *Brain Res*. 1998;793:176–186.

[113] Altman J. Postnatal development of the cerebellar cortex in the rat. II. Phases in the maturation of Purkinje cells and of the molecular layer. *J Comp Neurol* 1972;145:399–463.

[114] Swinny JD, van der Want JJL, Gramsbergen A. Cerebellar Development and Plasticity: Perspectives for Motor coordination Strategies, Motor Skills, and Therapy. *Neural Plasticity*. 2005;12:153-160.

[115] Millen KJ, Gleeson JG. Cerebellar development and disease. Curr Op Neurobiol. 2008;18:12–19.

[116] Morales D, Hatten ME.. Molecular Markers of Neuronal Progenitors in the Embryonic Cerebellar Anlage. *J Neurosci*. 2006;26:12226–12236.
[117] Sotelo C, Dusart I. Intrinsic versus extrinsic determinants during the development of Purkinje cell dendrites. *Neurosci* 2009;162(3):589-600.
[118] Phillips MI, Sumners C. Angiotensin II in central nervous system physiology. *Regul Pept*. 1998;78:1-11.
[119] Doba N, Reis DJ. Changes in regional blood flow and cardio- dynamics evoked by electrical stimulation of the fastigial nucleus in the cat and their similarity to orthostatic reflexes. *J Physiol London*. 1972;227:729–47
[120] Bradley DJ, Paton JFR, Spyer KM. Cardiovascular responses evoked from the fastigial region of the cerebellum in anesthetized and decerebrate rabbits. *J Physiol London*. 1987;392:475–92.
[121] Rector DM, Richard CA, Harper RM. Cerebellar fastigial nuclei activity during blood pressure challenges. *J Appl Physiol*. 2006;101:549–555.
[122] Ito M. Cerebellar circuitry as a neuronal machine. *Prog Neurobiology*. 2009;162;666-672.
[123] Lippoldt A, Bunnemann B, Ueki A, Rosén L, Cintra A, Hasselrot U, Metzger R, Hilgenfeldt U, Brosnihan B, Ganten D, et al. On the plasticity of the cerebellar renin-angiotensin system: localization of components and effects of mechanical perturbation. *Brain Res*. 1994;668(1-2):144-59.
[124] Erdmann Bettina; K Fuxe; D Ganten. Subcellular Localization of Angiotensin II Immunoreactivity in the Rat Cerebellar Cortex. *Hypertension*. 1996;28:818-824.
[125] Häuser W, Jöhren O, Saavedra JM. Characterization and distribution of Angiotensin II receptor subtypes in the mouse brain. *Eur J Pharmacol*. 1998;348(1):101-14.
[126] Reagan LP, Flanagan-Cato LM, Yee DK, Ma LY, Sakai R, Fluharty SJ. Immunohistochemical mapping of angiotensin type 2 (AT2) receptors in rat. *Brain Res*. 1994.662:45-59.
[127] Okuyama S, Sakagawa T, Chaki S, Imagawa T, Ichiki T, Inagami T.. Anxiety-like behavior in mice lacking the angiotensin II type-2 receptor. *Brain Res*. 1999;821:150–159.
[128] von Bohlen und Halbach O, Walther T, Bader M, Albrecht D.. Genetic deletion of angiotensin AT_2 receptor leads to increased cell numbers in different brain structures of mice. *Regul Pept*. 2001; 99:209–216.
[129] Maul B, von Bohlen und Halbach O, Becker A, Sterner-Kock A, Voigt J, Siems W, Grecksch et al. Impaired spatial memory and altered dendritic spine morphology in angiotensin II type 2 receptor-deficient mice. *J Mol Med*. 2008;86:563–571.
[130] Sánchez SI, Arce ME, Fuentes LB, Ciuffo GM. Prenatal blockade of Ang II receptors affects neonatal rat hindbrain structure and receptor localization. *Exp Neurol*. 2009;220:246-254.
[131] Fogarty DJ, Matute C. Angiotensin receptor-like immunoreactivity in adult brain white matter astrocytes and oligodendrocytes. *Glia*. 2001;35:131–146.
[132] Bellamy, T.C. Interactions between Purkinje neurons and Bergmann glia. *Cerebellum*. 2006;5:116-126.
[133] Alwan S, Polifka JE, Friedman JM. Angiotensin II receptor antagonist treatment during pregnancy. Birth Defects Res. A. *Clin. Mol. Teratol*. 2005;73:123-130.

[134] Lake-Bruse, S. Transgenic and knockout mice to study the rennin-angiotensin system and other interacting vasoactive pathways. *Curr Hypertens Rep*. 2000; 2:211-6

[135] Siragy HM, , Inagami T, Ichiki T, Carey RM. Sustained hypersensitivity to Angiotensin II and its mechanism mice lacking the subtype-2 (AT_2) angiotensin receptor. *Proc Natl Acad Sci USA*.1999;96: 6506-10

[136] Vervoot VS, Beachem MA, Edwards PS, Ladd S, Miller KE, De Mollrat X, et al. AGTR2 mutations in X-linked mental retardation. *Science*. 2002;296:2401-2403.

[137] Macova M, Pavel J, Saavedra JM. A Peripherally administered, centrally acting angiotensin II AT_2 antagonist selectively increases brain AT_1 receptors and decreases brain tyrosine hydroxylase transcription, pituitary vasopressin and ACTH. *Brain Res*. 2009;1250:130-40

[138] Lakó-Futó Z, Szokodi I, Sármán B, Földes G, Tokola H, Ilves M, et al. Evidence for a Functional Role of Angiotensin II Type 2 Receptor in the Cardiac Hypertrophic Process In Vivo in the Rat Heart. *Circulation*. 2003;108:2414-2422.

[139] Chen J, Lasaitiene D. Gabrielsson BG, Carlsson LMS, Billig H, Carlsson B, et al. Neonatal Losartan tratment suppresses renal expression of molecules involved in cee-cell and cell-matrix interactions. *J Am Soc Nephrol*. 2004; 15: 1232-1243.

[140] Lasaitiene D. Friberg P, Sundelin B, Chen J. Neonatal RAS inhibition changes the phenotype of the developing think ascending limb of Henle. *Am J Physiol Renal Physiol*. 2004.286:1144-1153.

[141] Izu Y, Mizoguchi F, Kawamata A, Hayata T Nakamoto T, Nakshima K et al. Angiotensin II type 2 receptor blockade increases bone mass. *J Biol Chem*. 2009; 284: 4857-64.

[142] Carletti B, Rossi F. Neurogenesis in the cerebellum. *Neurocientist*. 2008; 14 (1):91-100.

[143] Gallinat S, Csikos T, Meffert S, Herdegen T, Stoll M, Unger T. The angiotensin AT_2 receptor down-regulates neurofilament M in PC12W cells. *Neurosci Lett*. 1997; 227(1):29-32.

[144] Kilian P, Campbell S, Bilodeau L, Guimond MO, Roberge C, Gallo-Payet N, Payet MD. Angiotensin II type 2 receptor stimulation increases the rate of NG108-15 cell migration via actin depolymerization. *Endocrinology*. 2008;149(6):2923-2933.

[145] Laflamme L, Gasparo M, Gallo JM, Payet MD, Gallo-Payet N Angiotensin II induction of neurite outgrowth by AT_2 receptors in NG108-15 cells. Effect counteracted by the AT_1 receptors. *J Biol Chem*. 1996 ;271(37):22729-35. 2005;8:1401-1409

[146] Côté F, Do TH, Laflamme L, Gallo JM, Gallo-Payet N. Activation of the AT(2) receptor of angiotensin II induces neurite outgrowth and cell migration in microexplant cultures of the cerebellum. *J Biol Chem*. 1999;27 (44):31686-31692.

[147] Chamoux E, Breault L, Lehoux JG, Gallo-Payet N. Involvement of the angiotensin II type 2 receptor in apoptosis during human fetal adrenal gland development. *J Clin Endocrinol Metab*. 1999;84(12):4722-30.

[148] Nouet S, Amzallag N, Li JM, Louis S, Seitz I, Cui TX, et al. Trans-inactivation of receptor tyrosine kinases by novel angiotensin II AT_2 receptor-interacting protein, ATIP. *J Biol Chem*. 2004;279(28):28989-28997.

[149] Li JM, Mogi M, Tsukuda K, Tomochika H, Iwanami J, Min LJ, et al. Angiotensin II-induced neural differentiation via angiotensin II type 2 (AT_2) receptor-MMS2 cascade involving interaction between AT_2 receptor-interacting protein and Src homology 2 domain-containing protein-tyrosine phosphatase 1. *Mol Endocrinol*. 2007;21:499-511.

[150] Shenoy UV, Richards EM, Huang XC, Sumners C. Angiotensin II type 2 receptor-mediated apoptosis of cultured neurons from newborn rat brain. *Endocrinology*. 1999;140:500-509.

[151] Wu C, Sun M, Liu L, Zhou GW. The function of the protein tyrosine phosphatase SHP-1 in cancer. *Gene*. 2003;306:1–12

[152] Chong ZZ, Maiese K. The Src homology 2 domain tyrosine phosphatases SHP-1 and SHP-2: diversified control of cell growth, inflammation, and injury. *Histol Histopathol*. 2007; 22:1251–1267.

[153] Buisson B, Laflamme L, Bottari SP, de Gasparo M, Gallo-Payet N, Payet MD. A G protein is involved in the angiotensin AT_2 receptor inhibition of the T-type calcium current in non-differentiated NG108-15 cells. *J Biol Chem*. 1995;270(4):1670-1674.

[154] Gendron L, Oliny JF, Payet MD, Gallo-Payet N. Cyclic AMP-independent involvement of Rap1/B-Raf in the Angiotensin II AT_2 receptor signalling pathway in NG108-15 cells. *J Biol Chem*. 2003; 278:3606-3614.

[155] Liu H, Terrell ML, Bui V, Summy-Long JY, Kadekaro M. NO and angiotensin II effects on blood pressure and fluid homeostasis. *J Neuroendocrinol*. 1997;(7):545-552.

[156] Lehtonen JYA, Daviet L, Nahmias C, Horiuchi M, Dzau VJ. Analysis of Functional Domains of Angiotensin II Type 2 Receptor Involved in Apoptosis. *Mol Endocrinol*. 1999;13(7)1051-1060.

[157] Gallinat S, Busche S, Schütze S, Krönke M, Unger T. AT_2 receptor stimulation induces generation of ceramides in PC12W cells. *FEBS Lett*1999; 443(1):75-79.

[159] Seguin LR, Ciuffo GM. AT_2 receptors recruit c-Src, SHP-1and FAK upon activation by Ang II in PND15 rat. *Neurochem Int*. (in press).

[160] Frank C, Burkhardt C, Imhof D, Ringel J, Zschörnig O, Wieligmann K, et al. Effective dephosphorylation of Src substrates by SHP-1. *J Biol Chem*. 2004;279:11375-11383.

[161] Clark MA, Gonzalez N. Src and Pyk2 mediate angiotensin II effects in cultured rat astrocytes. *Regul Pept*. 2007;143(1-3):47-55.

[162] Guimond MO, Roberge C, Gallo-Payet N. Fyn is involved in angiotensin II type 2 receptor-induced neurite outgrowth, but not in p42/p44mapk in NG108-15 cells. *Mol Cell Neurosci*. 2010;45:201-212.

[163] Feng Y-H, Sun Y, Douglas JG. $G_{\beta\gamma}$-independent constitutive association of $G_{\alpha s}$ with SHP-1 and angiotensin II receptor AT_2 is essential in AT_2-mediated ITIM-independent activation of SHP-1. *Proc Natl Acad Sci.USA*. 2002;99:12049–12054.

[164] Miura S, Karnik SS, Saku K. Constitutively active homo-oligomeric angiotensin II type 2 receptor induces cell signaling independent of receptor conformation and ligand stimulation. *J Biol Chem*. 2005;280:18237-44.

[165] Wen LP, Fahrni JA, Troie S, Guan JL, Orth K, Rosen GD. Cleavage of focal adhesion kinase by caspases during apoptosis. *J Biol Chem*. 1997;272:26056-61.

[166] Watanabe F, Miyazaki T, Takeuchi T, Fukaya M, Nomura T, Noguchi S, et al. Effects of FAK ablation on cerebellar foliation, Bergmann glia positioning and climbing fiber territory on Purkinje cells. *Eur J Neurosci*. 2008;4:836-854.

[167] Otis M, Campbell S, Payet MD, Gallo-Payet N. In adrenal glomerulosa cells, angiotensin II inhibits proliferation by interfering with fibronectin-integrin signaling. *Endocrinology*. 2008; 149:3435-45.

[168] Lal H, Verma SK, Foster DM, Golden HB, Reneau JC, Watson LE, et al. Integrins and proximal signaling mechanisms in cardiovascular disease. *Front Biosci.* 2009;14:2307-2334.

[169] Shani V, Bromberg Y, Sperling O, Zoref-Shani E. Involvement of Src tyrosine kinases (SFKs) and of focal adhesion kinase (FAK) in the injurious mechanism in rat primary neuronal cultures exposed to chemical ischemia. *J Mol Neurosci.* 2009;37:50-59.

In: Angiotensin: New Research
Editors: S. Harada, I. Moi, pp. 303-318

ISBN: 978-1-62100-773-9

Chapter 13

ADVANCES IN NON-INVASIVE IMAGING OF RENIN ANGIOTENSIN SYSTEM

Kumiko C. Mackasey, Rob S. Beanlands and Jean N. DaSilva

[1] Molecular Function and Imaging, National Cardiac PET Centre, Division of Cardiology, University of Ottawa Heart Institute, Ottawa, Ontario, Canada K1Y 4W7.

[2] Department of Cellular and Molecular Medicine, Faculty of Medicine, University of Ottawa, Roger Guindon Hall, Ottawa, Ontario, Canada K1H 8MS.

1. ABSTRACT

The Renin Angiotensin System (RAS) has been shown to be involved in the progression of several diseases. The association of RAS and disease is the mechanistic basis behind medications that block its components, such as Angiotensin II (ANGII) Type 1 Receptor (AT_1R) blockers (ARBs) or Angiotensin Converting Enzyme (ACE) inhibitors (ACEi). Disorders such as hypertension, heart disease, chronic renal disease and diabetic nephropathy are treated with these medications; however, blocking the RAS is not effective in all patients. The exact role the RAS plays in the progression of disease is not completely understood. *In vivo* imaging techniques to investigate RAS alterations would be of great value to further understand RAS contribution to disease states. Characterization experiments and initial testing in animal disease models of AT_1R and ACE specific radiotracers are ongoing, with several potential candidate tracers having been identified which would allow for non-invasive *in vivo* imaging modalities such as Single Photon Emission Tomography (SPECT) and Positron Emission Tomography (PET). This chapter will summarize RAS alterations in diseased tissue, the relevance of *in vivo* imaging, and novel tracer development and evaluation.

2. Introduction

2.1. Renin Angiotensin System

Angiotensinogen is cleaved by renin, which is produced primarily in the kidney, to produce Angiotensin I (ANGI) which is then converted to ANGII by ACE or to a lesser extent, by chymase. ANGII is further cleaved by ACE2 to produce ANG(1-7). The RAS is an endocrine system; however, tissues such as the heart, brain and kidneys produce components of the system which suggests a role of locally produced ANGII in the function of these tissues [1-3].

ANGII binds to at least 3 different receptors, AT_1R, AT_2R and AT_4R [4]. The most physiologically important of these receptors is the AT_1R which will be the focus of this chapter. This receptor is a G-protein coupled receptor (GPCR) which upon agonist binding is internalized similarly to other GPCRs. The AT_1R acts through secondary messengers to promote downstream effects such as vasoconstriction, inflammation, atherogenicity, cellular proliferation and matrix production. AT_1Rs are expressed in heart, brain, kidney, gut, adrenal and vascular tissue [1-3, 5-11]. While AT_1R is dominant in adult tissues, AT_2R is the main ANGII receptor in fetus however; AT_2R may reappear in response to disease [12, 13]. AT_2R is documented as having the opposite downstream effects to AT_1R. The AT_2R promotes apoptosis, inhibits growth, lowers blood pressure and reduces inflammation [13, 14]. Although less is known of the AT_4R, it is present in endothelial cells and its possible role is to control expression of procoagulant species.

While most mammalian species have only one form of the AT_1R, mice and rats have two forms of the receptor, $AT_{1A}R$ and $AT_{1B}R$. The amino acid sequences of these two forms of the receptor are 95% identical [15]. The subtypes are similar in terms of ligand binding and activation properties, but differ in tissue distribution, chromosomal location and transcriptional regulation. A suggested explanation as to the presence of two subtypes in rodents is that AT_1R duplicated during evolution after the branching of rodents [16].

$AT_{1A}R$ mRNA is most prominent in all tissues with the exception of adrenal and pituitary glands [7]. $AT_{1A}R$ is expressed in the kidney, heart, liver, adrenal gland, brain, lung, fat and gonads. $AT_{1B}R$ expression is limited to adrenal gland, brain and testis [17]. From here on, subtypes of AT_1R will not be differentiated.

2.2. RAS in Disease States

Local and circulating RAS are thought to play a role in the progression of diabetes, cardiac, renal, neurodegenerative and pulmonary diseases. ANGII promotes oxidative stress, hypertrophy, inflammation, and vasoconstriction. The negative effects of ANGII in disease have led to the treatment of patients with therapies which inhibit either the production of ANGII by blocking ACE, or blocking the AT_1R.

2.2.1. Heart Failure

Heart failure is a common end point for many cardiac diseases. Despite advances in therapy, the mortality associated with heart failure remains high [18-23]. Blocking the RAS with either ACEi or ARBs has shown to improve heart failure symptoms as seen by several clinical trials [18, 19, 24-27]. According to studies in animal models of heart failure induced by myocardial infarct (MI), cardiac AT_1R levels are reported to increase shortly after MI[28-33]. The changes in human cardiac AT_1R levels are not completely understood during progression of heart disease and remain to be elucidated.

2.2.2. Hypertension

RAS blockers are the most widely prescribed treatment for hypertension [34]. In addition to ARB and ACEi therapies, renin blockers have also been found to lower blood pressure [35]. Despite the effectiveness of RAS blockade, RAS antagonists are not equally effective in all patients [36]. For example, it has been reported that ARBs and ACEi's are not as effective in lowering blood pressure in certain ethnic groups unless coadministered with other medication [37,38]. The ability to personalize treatment of hypertension to each patient will be possible using non invasive methods to monitor activity of AT_1R and determine if certain therapies are more effective than others.

2.2.3. Nephropathy

RAS blockade has renoprotective properties in diabetic and non diabetic renal disease. In animal models of experimental diabetes and renal mass ablation, glomerulosclerosis and glomerular pressure were reduced after RAS blockade [39, 40]. Locally produced ANGII triggers pathways that promote proteinuria and increased activity of profibrotic factors [41-46]. Renoprotection resulting from RAS blockade is independent of the anti-hypertensive effect of ARBs or ACEi [39-45, 47-49]. While amelioration of kidney function is seen *in vitro, in vivo* and in patients, RAS blockade is not a cure for renal disease [50-55]. The complexity of the RAS and its apparent involvement in the progression of disease makes it an intriguing target to study more thoroughly *in vivo*. A more complete mechanistic understanding of temporal changes in AT_1R and ACE expression in these disease states will lead to more effective treatment.

2.3. Imaging

Both SPECT and PET imaging use the concept of labeling pharmaceuticals with radioisotopes. These radioligands may be specific for structures of interest. By quantifying tracer accumulation in regions of the body, it is possible to extrapolate the amount of these structures. Using the small animal SPECT or PET systems in experimental research minimizes the number of animals needed for the experiment because an animal need not be sacrificed before examination allowing the animal to serve as its own control.

Radiotracers used for SPECT and PET scans with higher specific activity (low amount of radioactivity/amount of tracer mass) will allow one to detect low concentrations of receptors. The tracer is used in small doses and according to Jagoda et al receptor saturation should be below 5% for accurate extrapolation [56].

SPECT and PET are the most sensitive of the non-invasive imaging techniques available today, however, the spatial resolution is low [57]. Therefore, it is common to combine SPECT and PET with Computed Tomography (CT) or Magnetic Resonance Imaging (MRI).

CT and MRI are less sensitive but have smaller spatial resolution which will enhance the anatomical detail of the scan. SPECT and PET are used clinically to noninvasively diagnose and study cancer, cardiac, neurodegenerative and psychiatric diseases.

3. SPECT AT_1R TRACER

SPECT imaging uses radiotracers that are labeled with gamma ray emitting isotopes. As the radiotracer decays, the gamma rays are detected externally by a gamma camera. The angle and direction of the gamma rays emitted are determined by a collimator which is placed in front of the gamma camera. The advantages of SPECT over PET lie in the longer half lives of the radionuclides and lower cost of the gamma camera which make SPECT imaging more widely available in research and clinic.

3.1. ^{99m}Tc Losartan

3.1.1. Synthesis

Losartan, an ARB, is retained on a resin via its tetrazole group. The hydroxyl group of losartan is replaced with a leucine and further attached to tetraethylene glycol and diglycolic acid which serves as a linker between losartan and tetraamine [58].

3.1.2. In Vivo

Verjans et al used male Swiss Webster mice in their *in vivo* micro-SPECT and micro-CT studies to image the AT_1R. The mice were scanned 3 weeks post-MI caused by left coronary artery ligation. ^{99m}Tc Losartan injected uptake per gram of cardiac tissue was significantly higher in infarcted hearts, 0.52±0.21%, when compared to control hearts, 0.21±0.13% [58]. Within the MI hearts, uptake in the infarct zone was 2.4 times higher compared to remote regions [58]. To our knowledge, no other reports using this tracer or SPECT to measure AT_1R changes have been published.

4. PET AT_1R TRACERS

When a PET radiotracer is injected into the subject, it decays releasing a positron. After travelling a short distance, this positron will interact with an electron in the surrounding area. The positron and electron will annihilate each other, releasing two gamma rays of 511keV that travel in opposite directions. The two gamma rays emitted are captured by PET detectors at 180° from each other.

PET imaging is more sensitive than SPECT which leads to higher resolution in the images. However, the half lives of the isotopes are usually shorter than those of SPECT tracers and an onsite cyclotron and complex radiochemistry may be required.

4.1.[^{11}C] MK-996

4.1.1. Synthesis

The synthesis of [^{11}C]MK-996 is described by Mathews et al, this tracer is the first AT_1R PET radioligand reported in the literature [59]. First, α-[^{11}C] benzyl chloride is produced by reacting [^{11}C]CO_2 and phenylmagnesium chloride in tetrahydrafuran (THF). α-[^{11}C]Benzyl chloride in hexane is then added to the precursor, L-159,221 dissolved in THF, to produce [^{11}C]MK-996. Average synthesis time is 38minutes. The tracer is produced with non-decay corrected radiochemical yield of 3%, >95% radiochemical purity and an average specific activity of 1162 mCi/μmol [59]. Due to difficulty of tracer synthesis, further reports were not published and [^{11}C]L-159,884 was developed by the same group [60].

4.2.[^{11}C]L-159, 884

4.2.1.Synthesis

The phenolic precursor of [^{11}C]L-159,884 is prepared through coupling of activated benzoic acids to the sulphonamide nitrogen of L-159,221. To prepare the precursor, L-162,914, for methylation it must undergo reductive debenzylation. Synthesis of [^{11}C]L-159,884 involves the *O*-methylation of its phenolic precursor in dimethylformamide (DMF) and tetrabutylammonium hydroxide. The average synthesis time is 18minutes, average non-decay corrected radiochemical yield is 5% and radiochemical purity over 95%. The average specific activity measured is 2979mCi/μmol [61].

4.2.2. Ex Vivo

Biodistribution studies were performed on CD-1 mice by Kim et al using [^{11}C]L-159,884 [62]. Animals were injected with tracer and sacrificed at 5, 15, 30, 60 and 90minute time points after injection to measure radioactivity in various tissues using a gamma counter. Peak values of tracer uptake were noted in the kidney, lungs and heart at 15minutes post-injection and remained until 90minutes post-injection. Radioactivity accumulated in the intestine throughout the observation while only 8% was measured in the urine, suggesting that [^{11}C]L-159,884 is likely excreted through the hepatobiliary system. To examine specificity of the tracer, animals were pre-treated with known AT_1R, AT_2R, α-adrenergic receptor, and β-adrenergic receptor blockers. It was found that only AT_1R specific blockade reduced tracer uptake in kidney, heart and lungs while uptake was unaffected by other drugs used in the study. With the evidence supporting the appropriate regional distribution, pharmacology and selectivity, [^{11}C]L-159,884 was a promising candidate for further PET imaging.

4.2.3. In Vivo

PET imaging using [^{11}C]L-159,884 was first reported by Szabo et al in Beagle dogs [63]. Dogs were chosen for the similar homology of amino acid sequence to human AT_1R and because dogs, like humans, have only one subtype of AT_1R. Animals were scanned under control conditions and also after pre-treatment with MK-996, a potent AT_1R antagonist. In control scans, accumulation of [^{11}C]L-159,884 was observed in the renal cortex. When scanned after MK-996 treatment, influx rate of tracer into the cortex was reduced by 66%

[63]. Similarities between arterial input function suggest that the lower tracer influx in the treated animals was not caused by a reduced tracer delivery but was in fact caused by the reduced tracer accumulation.

[^{11}C]L-159,884 was injected into a baboon and binding characteristics were compared to [^{11}C]KR31173, another AT_1R PET tracer that is described below. The tracers were injected into the same animal two months apart. After pre-treating the animal with SK-1080, an ARB, the renal cortical uptake of AT_1R tracer was decreased by 81% and 34% using [^{11}C]KR31173 and [^{11}C]L-159,884, respectively when compared to baseline scan [64]. Specific binding of the tracers was found to be higher in [^{11}C]KR31173 (92% vs 12%) [64]. With the development of [^{11}C]KR31173, [^{11}C]L-159,884 was no longer used in further published studies.

4.3. [^{11}C]KR31173

4.3.1. Synthesis

The tetrazole moiety of the phenolic precursor of [^{11}C]KR31173 is protected prior to the radiolabeling. The precursor is then methylated with [^{11}C]methyl iodide in presence of NaH in DMF or THF. The protecting group is finally removed by acid hydrolysis. The average synthesis time is reported at 25minutes, non-decay radiochemical yield 5% and the average specific activity was 6981.08mCi/μmol [60].

4.3.2. Ex Vivo

Biodistribution studies of [^{11}C]KR31173 were performed in CD-1 mice at 5, 15, 30, 60 and 90minutes post-tail vein injection [60]. Highest uptake of the tracer was measured at 30minutes after injection in the kidneys and adrenal glands. Blocking studies using MK-996 and KR31173 (AT_1R antagonists) treatment 10minutes prior to tracer injection displayed decreased retention in adrenal glands (91%), kidneys (90%), lungs (88%), and heart (92%) [60]. Pre-treatment with AT_2R antagonist, PD123,319, did not affect uptake of [^{11}C]KR31173 [64].

Another report studied AT_1R in male Wistar rats after undergoing transient left anterior descending (LAD) coronary artery ligation surgery [32]. The LAD was occluded for 20-25minutes then released. Autoradiography binding studies using [^{125}I]-[Sar^{1}Ile^8]ANGII were performed on left ventricles (LV) of animals sacrificed at 1hour, 1day, 1week, 3weeks post-surgery. ^{201}Tl-chloride injected for delineation of nonperfused scar area and ^{99m}Tc-tetrofosmin injected during occlusion to delineate area at risk. ^{125}I-labeled ANGII binding increased in LAD territory of the LV 1week and 3weeks post-surgery while non infarcted control rats and rats 1hour post-surgery expressed no change in labeled ANGII binding. Ratio of uptake in infarct/remote increased approximately 4 fold after 1 and 3weeks when compared to control [32]. The specificity of ^{125}I signal was demonstrated by strong blocking effect of SK-1080. Immunohistochemistry with AT_1R antibody confirmed increased expression in histological area of infarct. Autoradiography studies following *in vivo* injection of [^{11}C]KR31173 1-3 weeks post-surgery expressed a 2-3 fold increase in infarct uptake to remote uptake ratio [32].

The effect of [^{11}C]KR31173 binding in response to valsartan (ARB) and enalapril (ACEi) suggests that only the ARB can reduce tracer binding. While the reduction in AT_1R binding may seem positive, the authors state that the medication doses used in this investigation were much higher than relative clinical dose.

4.3.3. In Vivo

First PET imaging with this tracer was done in mice, dogs and baboons to determine the *in vivo* binding characteristics. PET scans were done in control animals and also after pre-treatment with SK-1080. In all three species, renal and adrenal tissues had highest uptake. In pre-treated animals, renal uptake was reduced by 49%, 48% and 81% in mice, dogs and a baboon respectively [64]. From these experiments, it was determined that [^{11}C]KR31173 would be most appropriate to use in future human PET studies.

Xia et al used this tracer to study a porcine model of renovascular hypertension (RVH) [65]. A tissue irritating coil was placed inside the renal artery of the domestic pig which leads to approximately 70% occlusion of the renal artery within 2 to 3weeks. Animals were scanned using [^{11}C]KR31173 to investigate changes in renal AT_1R levels in response to renal artery stenosis. Time activity curves exhibited a lower activity peak in stenotic kidneys compared to contralateral control kidneys. While uptake was decreased because of reduced blood flow to the kidney, binding was increased by 40% in the stenotic kidney [65]. The reduced uptake in stenotic kidneys was directly related to reduced perfusion as measured by [^{15}O]H_20 [65]. The increased [^{11}C]KR31173 binding observed in *in vivo* PET studies was corroborated with [^{125}I]-[Sar^{1}Ile^8]ANGII autoradiography, with significant correlation between *in vivo* and *in vitro* binding of AT_1R in renal cortex [65]. Specific binding in the porcine renal cortex, determined by scans completed after SK-1080 treatment, was estimated to be between 70-80% [65] .

Small animal *in vivo* PET scans were done by Higuchi et al in male Wistar rats following 20-25 minute LAD ligation surgery. The animals were scanned one week post-surgery and the uptake ratio of infarct to remote areas, as defined by [^{13}N]NH_3 myocardial blood flow PET scans, was 2.2 ±0.9, similar to that of the autoradiography results (see in section 4.3.2.) [32]. The number of animals used in this study was small (n=3) and the authors describe the successful cardiac PET scans as a proof of concept and a launching point for further cardiac studies.

4.3.4. Human Studies

A preliminary study (published in abstract form) was completed in four healthy human subjects who were scanned with [^{11}C]KR31173 [66]. Twenty four hours later, two subjects were pre-treated with olmesartan, an ARB, and then scanned again. Pre-treatment with olmesartan lead to a 51% decrease in myocardial [^{11}C]KR31173 retention index [66]. Retention in the human heart was significantly higher in the inferior wall of the left ventricle than the anterior wall; this heterogeneity is thought to be caused by spillover from the liver. This report is the first AT_1R radiotracer study involving human subjects.

4.4. [^{11}C]Methyl-Candesartan

4.4.1. Synthesis

The production of ^{11}C-labeled derivative of the clinically used candesartan is described by Hadizad et. al [67]. The tetrazole group of unlabeled candesartan is protected with trityl chloride. The precursor is then methylated with the [^{11}C]methyl iodide trapped in the reaction vessel. Finally the radiolabeled tetrazole-protected methyl-candesartan is deprotected using 1N hydrochloric acid hydrolysis for 2min at 65-70°C. Total synthesis time is approximately 30minutes. The radiochemical purity is reported at >99%, yield at 50-70%, and specific activity ranges from 300-1500 mCi/μmol [67].

4.4.2. Ex Vivo

Ex vivo time course and biodistribution studies were performed on male Sprague-Dawley rats. Animals were injected with [^{11}C]methyl-candesartan and sacrificed at 5, 15, 30, 45 or 60minutes post-tracer injection. Ratio of tissue to blood activity was highest at 15minutes after injection and this time point was used for further competition studies. In the competition experiments, rats were coadministered or pre-injected with AT_1R blockers (candesartan and losartan), AT_2R blocker (PD123,319), ANG(1-7) Mas receptor blocker (A-779), β-adrenergic receptor blocker (propranolol), or α_2-adrenergic receptor blocker (yohimbine). Animals were sacrificed 15minutes post-radioligand injection and tracer retention was expressed as injected dose normalized to tissue weight. Rats treated with ARBs showed dose dependent decrease in tracer uptake in renal cortex and renal outer medulla while the other treatments did not affect tracer uptake. This initial report of [^{11}C]methyl-candesartan did not include *in vivo* experiments but the ex vivo experiments show high binding selectivity for AT_1R and potential for further studies.

4.5. [^{11}C]TH4

4.5.1. Synthesis

[^{11}C]TH4 is the desethyl derivative of [^{11}C]methyl-candesartan and was also synthesized by Hadizad et al. The synthesis procedure is similar for the two tracers however, the methylation and deprotection steps for [^{11}C]TH4 were completed at a higher temperature (90°C). Radiochemical purity, chemical purity, yield and specific activities were similar to those of [^{11}C]methyl-candesartan (see 4.4.1) [67].

4.5.2. Ex Vivo

[^{11}C]TH4 has similar time course characteristics as [^{11}C]methyl-candesartan. Peak tissue tracer accumulation was measured at 15minutes post-injection [67]. Male Sprague Dawley rats were used in competition studies using the ARBs, AT_2R blocker, Mas receptor blocker, β-adrenergic receptor blocker, and α_2-adrenergic receptor blocker as in the [^{11}C]methyl-candesartan competition studies. It was observed that AT_1R blockade reduced [^{11}C]TH4 uptake but not to the extent of [^{11}C]methyl-candesartan uptake. [^{11}C]TH4 uptake was also reduced by the ANG(1-7) Mas receptor blockade, suggesting that the radiotracer was not selective of AT_1R over ANG(1-7) Mas receptor. Because of the reduced selectivity of

[^{11}C]TH4, it was suggested that [^{11}C]methyl-candesartan would be a more appropriate renal AT_1R imaging agent.

4.6 [^{11}C]Methyl-Losartan

4.6.1. Synthesis

[^{11}C]Methyl-losartan is the ^{11}C-methyl derivative of the ARB, losartan. The tetrazole group of the losartan molecule was protected with trityl chloride. The protected precursor was then methylated with [^{11}C]methyl iodide. Finally the methylated protected precursor is deprotected using hydrochloric acid for 3min at 80°C. The radiotracer was produced in 30-60% (decay-corrected) radiochemical yield, radiochemical purity of >99%, and total synthesis time is approximately 35minutes. Specific activity ranged from 700-3600mCi/µmol [68].

4.6.2. Ex Vivo

Biodistribution studies were used to investigate binding properties of [^{11}C]methyl-losartan in male Sprague Dawley rats. Animals were treated with AT_1R antagonist (losartan and candesartan), AT_2R antagonist (PD-123,319) or ANG(1-7) Mas receptor antagonist (A-779) prior to injection of [^{11}C]methyl-losartan. Rats were sacrificed at 10minutes post-injection. Highest uptake was observed in kidney cortex, kidney medulla and liver. AT_1R blocker treatment reduced tracer uptake in renal cortex and medulla by 74-86% [69]. This decrease was not seen in animals treated with AT_2R or ANG(1-7) Mas receptor blockade. This data was presented as an abstract and further evaluation and optimization studies are ongoing [68,69].

5. PET ACE TRACERS

5.1. [^{18}F]Fluorocaptopril

5.1.1. Synthesis

The first step of [^{18}F]fluorocaptopril ([^{18}F]FCAP) is the production of the triflate analogue of the ACEi, captopril. Diisopropylethyl amine was added to 4-trans-hydroxyl-L-proline methyl ester hydrochloride which was suspended in methyl chloride. (R)-3-(acetylthio)-2-methylpropanyl chloride was added to the resulting mixture. Crude product was recrystallized and added to pyridine with triflic anhydride. The mixture was transferred to a silica gel column to purify the triflate analogue. To create the cold *cis*-fluorocaptopril (FCAP), the triflate analogue was reacted with tetra-*n*-butylammonium fluoride. This mixture was reacted with [^{18}F]potassium fluoride and purified. Pure [^{18}F]FCAP was synthesized in a 12% radiochemical yield and a specific activity of >300mCi/µmol [70]

5.1.2. Ex Vivo

Biodistribution studies were performed in female Sprague Dawley rats sacrificed at 0.5, 1, 2, or 4hours after [^{18}F]FCAP injection into a femoral vein. Multiple tissues were removed and counted in a gamma counter. High uptake was measured in organs known to have high levels of ACE: kidneys, lungs and aorta. Washout from these organs was slow with maintained activity until the 4hour post-injection time point [70].

Titration studies found that co-injecting animals with varying doses of cold FCAP reduces tissue uptake as amount of cold tracer increases. This shows the saturability of the tracer as larger amounts of cold compound will compete and saturate ACE binding sites. Uptake was also decreased in blood (78%), lung (96%), kidney (95%), heart (92%) and aorta (90%) in animals pre-treated with captopril [70]. These ex vivo results displayed promising specificity and desirable kinetics of [^{18}F]FCAP as an ACE PET tracer.

5.1.3. In Vivo

The first *in vivo* application of [^{18}F]FCAP was in mongrel dogs [71, 72]. The tracer was used to study healthy animals and those with induced left pulmonary caudal lobe hypoxia. Animals were scanned with [^{18}F]FCAP to assess pulmonary ACE levels and [^{15}O]H_2O to measure pulmonary blood flow. The study found that the ACE expression (B_{max}) was decreased hypoxic lungs compared to controls. This result could have been caused by the limited access of tracer to hypoxic lung tissue or the effect of hypoxia on ACE levels. Ideally, because ACE is an endothelium bound enzyme that is distributed evenly on vessels, B_{max} should be given per unit of endothelial surface. However, the endothelial surface value is not available. To account for the diminished blood flow in the hypoxic lung, the investigators normalized B_{max} to lung volume, blood volume (BV) and extravascular lung water (EVLW). Lung volume normalization would only work if all regions of the lungs were inflated evenly (due to hypoxic gas ventilation). Blood volume would account for different lung volumes; however, blood volume is not linearly related to vessel surface area. Finally, EVLW should be constant in normal tissues, but this is not the case for hypoxic lungs. This study did not conclude which was the most appropriate way to normalize B_{max}. Regardless, B_{max} normalized to lung volume, BV and EVLW were consistently lower in a ratio comparing left lung (hypoxic)/right lung (normoxic) values. This study also found no relationship between flow and B_{max} suggesting that lowered B_{max} observed in hypoxic lungs was not due to reduced tracer access but rather to diminished vascular ACE recruitment [72].

5.1.4. Humans

[^{18}F]FCAP has been studied in healthy human subjects and patients with primary pulmonary hypertension (PPH) [70, 73]. The subjects were separated into the following groups: healthy subjects were scanned twice to test for reproducibility, healthy subjects scanned before and after treatment with enalapril (ACEi), and PPH patients before and after enalapril treatment. All subjects were also scanned with [^{15}O]H_20 to assess regional pulmonary blood flow. Pulmonary blood flow normalized to body weight was 45% lower in PPH patients than healthy subjects [73]. Enalapril reduced binding by 83% and 76% in healthy and PPH patients respectively [73]. Finally, ACE binding was found to be 60% lower in PPH patients compared to control suggesting ACE inhibition as a treatment and [^{18}F]FCAP PET imaging as a monitoring tool [73].

5.2. [^{18}F]Fluorobenzoyl-Lisonopril

5.2.1. Synthesis

The production of [^{18}F]fluorobenzoyl-lisonopril ([^{18}F]FBL) involves synthesis of N-succininidyl-4-^{18}F fluorobenzoate and then coupling this active ester to lisonopril, an ACEi. The radiochemical yield of the tracer is 15% and average synthesis time is 130minutes [74]. The advantages of [^{18}F]FBL over [^{18}F]FCAP are that [^{18}F]FBL is more specific to tissue ACE, which is thought to play a more pivotal role in disease progression than circulating ACE and simpler synthesis. [^{18}F]FCAP has an unstable sulfhydryl moiety that leads to *in vitro* conversion into other isomers [71, 72]. [^{18}F]FBL is a non sulfhydryl and is therefore more stable.

5.2.2. In vitro

[^{18}F]FBL has been investigated in *in vitro* studies using explanted human heart tissue [74]. The subjects of this study were patients with ischemic cardiomyopathy with severe heart failure and angina awaiting heart transplants. The *in vitro* human tissue study investigated the distribution of collagen, ACE and chymase mast cells in the LV of the diseased heart. Firstly, it was found that [^{18}F]FBL is specific to ACE through competition studies with lisonopril. Once the tracer was determined specific for ACE, ACE binding was found to be 1.3 fold higher in the peri-infarct areas compared to infarct and non-infarct LV tissue [74]. The peri-infarct of the LV is associated with areas of replacement fibrosis. The areas with the lowest increase in ACE binding were found to have the highest amount of chymase, a mast cell enzyme that produces ANGII in an ACE independent mechanism. At the time of this publication, no PET studies have been published using this tracer.

6. CONCLUSION

Imaging the RAS remains a target in the understanding of several diseases which are associated with altered RAS. *In vivo* imaging in humans of RAS components such as AT_1R and ACE will allow for a deeper understanding of disease progression and guide therapy. While ARB and ACEi therapies are a main component of cardiovascular treatment, variability in response among patients remains significant. Non-invasive imaging may offer clinicians a reliable way to predict patient response. There is great potential in investigating different RAS radiotracers. The development of molecular nuclear imaging will lead to a further understanding of temporal changes of RAS components through disease progression and insight into effective treatment pathways for patients on an individual basis. Further human studies are required to integrate nuclear imaging technology into clinical intervention of cardiovascular and pulmonary diseases. The studies presented in this chapter are an encouraging and promising start to implementing RAS imaging in humans.

REFERENCES

[1] Dostal DE., Baker KM. (1999).The cardiac renin-angiotensin system:conceptual, or a regulator of cardiac function? *Circ. Res.*85,643-650.

[2] Wagenaar LJ.;Voors AA.;Buikema H., van Gilst WH. (2002).Angiotensin receptors in the cardiovascular system. *Can. J. Cardiol.*18,1331-1339.

[3] Goodfriend TL.;Elliott ME., Catt KJ. (1996).Angiotensin receptors and their antagonists. *N Engl. J. Med.*334,1649-1654.

[4] Berk BC. (2003).Angiotensin type 2 receptor (AT2R): a challenging twin. *ScI STKE.*2003,PE16.

[5] Li Z.; Iwai M.;Wu L.;Shiuchi T.;Jinno T.;Cui TX., Horiuchi M. (2003).Role of AT2 receptor in the brain in regulation of blood pressure and water intake. *Am. J. Physiol. Heart Circ. Physiol.*284,H116-121.

[6] Gard PR. (2002).The role of angiotensin II in cognition and behaviour. *EUR. J. Pharmacol.*438,1-14.

[7] De Gasparo M.;Catt KJ.;Inagami T.;Wright JW., Unger T.(2000).International union of pharmacology, XXIII. The angiotensin II receptors. *Pharmacol. Rev.*52,415-472.

[8] Opie LH., Sack MN. (2001).Enhanced angiotensin II activity in heart failure: reevaluation of the counterregulatory hypothesis of receptor subtypes. *Circ. Res.*88,654-658.

[9] Timmermans PB.;Chiu AT.;Herblin WF.;Wong PC., Smith RD. (1992).Angiotensin II receptor subtypes. *Am. J. Hypertens.*5,406-410.

[10] Allen AM.;Zhuo J., Mendelsohn FA. (2000).Localization and function of angiotensin AT1 receptors. *Am. J. Hypertens.*13,31S-38S.

[11] Allen AM.;Zhuo J., Mendelsohn FA. (1999).Localization of angiotensin AT1 and AT2 receptors. *J. Am. Soc. Nephrol.*10 Suppl. 11,S23-29.

[12] Akishita M.;Horiuchi M.;Yamada H.;Zhang L.;Shirakami G.;Tamura K.;Ouchi Y., Dzau VJ. (2000).Inflammation influences vascular remodeling through AT2 receptor expression and signaling. *Physiol. Genomics.*2,13-20.

[13] Masaki H.;Kurihara T.;Yamaki A.;Inomata N.;Nozawa Y.;Mori Y.;Murasawa S.;Kizima K.;Maruyama K.;Horiuchi M.;Dzau VJ.;Takahashi H.;Iwasaka T.;Inada M., Matsubara H. (1998).Cardiac-specific overexpression of angiotensin II AT2 receptor causes attenuated response to AT1 receptor-mediated pressor and chronotropic effects. *J. Clin. Invest.*101,527-535.

[14] Nakajima M.;Hutchinson HG.;Fujinaga M.;Hayashida W.;Morishita R.;Zhang L.;Horiuchi M.;Pratt RE., Dzau VJ. (1995).The angiotensin II type 2 (AT2) receptor antagonizes the growth effects of the AT1 receptor: gain-of-function study using gene transfer. *Proc. Natl. Acad. Sci. U S A.*92,10663-10667.

[15] Kakar SS.;Sellers JC.;Devor DC.;Musgrove LC., Neill JD. (1992).Angiotensin II type-1 receptor subtype cDNAs: differential tissue expression and hormonal regulation. Biochem. *Biophys. Res. Commun.*183,1090-1096.

[16] Aiyar N.;Baker E.;Wu HL.;Nambi P.;Edwards RM.;Trill JJ.;Ellis C., Bergsma DJ. (1994).Human AT1 receptor is a single copy gene:characterization in a stable cell line. *Mol. Cell Biochem.*131,75-86.

[17] Burson JM.;Aguilera G.;Gross KW., Sigmund CD. (1994).Differential expression of angiotensin receptor 1A and 1B in mouse. *Am J Physiol.*267,E260-267.

[18] Effects of enalapril on mortality in severe congestive heart failure. Results of the Cooperative North Scandinavian Enalapril Survival Study (CONSENSUS). Thc CONSENSUS Trial Study Group. (1987). *N Engl. J. Med.*316,1429-1435.

[19] Cowie MR.;Mosterd A.;Wood DA.;Deckers JW.;Poole-Wilson PA.;Sutton GC., Grobbee DE. (1997).The epidemiology of heart failure. Eur. Heart J.18,208-225.

[20] Massie BM., Packer M. (1990).Congestive heart failure: current controversies and future prospects. *Am. J. Cardiol.*66,429-430.

[21] Ghali JK.;Cooper R., Ford E. (1990).Trends in hospitalization rates for heart failure in the United States, 1973-1986. Evidence for increasing population prevalence. *Arch. Intern. Med.*150,769-773.

[22] Yousef ZR.;Redwood SR., Marber MS. (2000).Postinfarction left ventricular remodelling: where are the theories and trials leading us? *Heart.*83,76-80.

[23] Zannad F.;Briancon S.;Juilliere Y.;Mertes PM.;Villemot JP.;Alla F., Virion JM. (1999).Incidence, clinical and etiologic features, and outcomes of advanced chronic heart failure: the EPICAL Study. Epidemiologie de l'Insuffisance Cardiaque Avancee en Lorraine. *J. Am. Coll.* Cardiol.33,734-742.

[24] GISSI-3: effects of lisinopril and transdermal glyceryl trinitrate singly and together on 6-week mortality and ventricular function after acute myocardial infarction. Gruppo Italiano per lo Studio della Sopravvivenza nell'infarto Miocardico. (1994). *Lancet.*343,1115-1122.

[25] Pfeffer MA.;Braunwald E.;Moye LA.;Basta L.;Brown EJ. Jr.;Cuddy TE.;Davis BR.;Geltman EM.;Goldman S.;Flaker GC.; klein m.;lamas ge.;packer m.;rouleau j.;rouleau jl.;rutherford j.;werheimer jh., hawkins cm. (1992).Effect of captopril on mortality and morbidity in patients with left ventricular dysfunction after myocardial infarction. Results of the survival and ventricular enlargement trial. The SAVE Investigators. *N Engl. J. Med.*327,669-677.

[26] Hall AS.;Murray GD., Ball SG. (1997).Follow-up study of patients randomly allocated ramipril or placebo for heart failure after acute myocardial infarction: AIRE Extension (AIREX) Study. Acute Infarction Ramipril Efficacy. *Lancet.*349,1493-1497.

[27] A randomized trial of beta-blockade in heart failure. The Cardiac Insufficiency Bisoprolol Study (CIBIS). CIBIS Investigators and Committees. (1994). *Circulation.* 90,1765-1773.

[28] Leenen FH.;Skarda V.;Yuan B., White R. (1999).Changes in cardiac ANG II postmyocardial infarction in rats: effects of nephrectomy and ACE inhibitors. *Am. J. Physiol.*276,H317-325.

[29] Silvestre JS.;Heymes C.;Oubenaissa A.;Robert V.;Aupetit-Faisant B.;Carayon A.;Swynghedauw B., Delcayre C. (1999).Activation of cardiac aldosterone production in rat myocardial infarction: effect of angiotensin II receptor blockade and role in cardiac fibrosis. *Circulation.*99,2694-2701.

[30] Van Kats JP.;DUNCKER DJ.;Haitsma DB.; SCHUJIT MP.;NIEBUUR R.;STUBENITSKY R.; BOOMSMA F.; SCHALEKAMP MA.; VERDOUW PD., DANSER AH. (2000).Angiotensin-converting Enzyme inhibition and angiotensin II type 1 receptor blockade prevent cardiac remodelinG in pigs after myocardial infarction:ROLE OF TISSUE ANGIOTENSIN II.*Circulation.*102.1556-1563.

[31] Tan J.;Wang H.; Leenen FH. (2004).Increases in brain and cardiac AT1 receptor and ACE densities after myocardial infarct in rats. *Am. J. Physiol. Heart Circ. Physiol.*286,H1665-1671.

[32] Higuchi T.;Fukushima K.;Xia J.;Mathews WB.;Lautamaki R.;Bravo PE.;Javadi MS.;Dannals RF.;Szabo Z., Bengel FM. (2010) Radionuclide imaging of angiotensin II type 1 receptor upregulation after myocardial ischemia-reperfusion injury. *J. Nucl. Med.*51,1956-1961.

[33] Meggs LG.;Coupet J.;Huang H.;Cheng W.;Li P.;Capasso JM.;Homcy CJ., Anversa P. (1993).Regulation of angiotensin II receptors on ventricular myocytes after myocardial infarction in rats. *Circ. Res.*72,1149-1162.

[34] Laight DW. (2009).Therapeutic inhibition of the renin angiotensin aldosterone system. *Expert. Opin. Ther. Pat.*19,753-759.

[35] Branch K. AliSkiren (Tekturna®) for Hypertension. Pharmacotherapy udate. Vol X: Cleveland Clinic; May/June 2007.

[36] Catanzaro DF., Frishman WH. (2010). Angiotensin receptor blockers for management of hypertension. *South Med. J.*103,669-673.

[37] Burnier M. (2001).Angiotensin II type 1 receptor blockers. *Circulation.*103,904-912.

[38] Plosker GL., Robinson DM. (2008).Amlodipine/Valsartan: fixed-dose combination in hypertension. *Drugs.*68,373-381.

[39] Anderson S.;Meyer TW.;Rennke HG., Brenner BM. (1985).Control of glomerular hypertension limits glomerular injury in rats with reduced renal mass. *J. Clin. Invest.*76,612-619.

[40] Neuringer JR., Brenner BM. (1993).Hemodynamic theory of progressive renal disease: a 10-year update in brief review. *Am. J. Kidney Dis.*22,98-104.

[41] Wolf G., Neilson EG. (1993).Angiotensin II as a renal growth factor. *J. Am. Soc. Nephrol.*3,1531-1540.

[42] Ketteler M.;Noble NA., Border WA. (1995).Transforming growth factor-beta and angiotensin II: the missing link from glomerular hyperfiltration to glomerulosclerosis? *Annu. Rev. Physiol.*57,279-295.

[43] Fogo AB. (2000).Glomerular hypertension, abnormal glomerular growth, and progression of renal diseases. *Kidney Int. Suppl.*75,S15-21.

[44] Long DA.;Price KL.;Herrera-Acosta J., Johnson RJ. (2004).How does angiotensin II cause renal injury? *Hypertension.*43,722-723.

[45] Ma LJ.;Nakamura S.;Aldigier JC.;Rossini M.;Yang H.;Liang X.;Nakamura I.;Marcantoni C., Fogo AB. (2005).Regression of glomerulosclerosis with high-dose angiotensin inhibition is linked to decreased plasminogen activator inhibitor-1. *J. Am. Soc. Nephrol.*16,966-976.

[46] Fogo A., Ichikawa I. (1989).Evidence of central role of glomerular growth promoters in the development of sclerosis. *Semin. Nephrol.*9,329-342.

[47] Kakinuma Y.;Kawamura T.;Bills T.;Yoshioka T.;Ichikawa I., Fogo A. (1992).Blood pressure-independent effect of angiotensin inhibition on vascular lesions of chronic renal failure. *Kidney Int.*42,46-55.

[48] Lafayette RA.;Mayer G.;Park SK., Meyer TW. (1992).Angiotensin II receptor blockade limits glomerular injury in rats with reduced renal mass. *J. Clin. Invest.*90,766-771.

[49] Taal MW.; Brenner BM. (2000).Renoprotective benefits of RAS inhibition: from ACEI to angiotensin II antagonists. *Kidney Int.*57,1803-1817.

[50] Ruster C.; Wolf G. (2006).Renin-angiotensin-aldosterone system and progression of renal disease. *J. Am. Soc. Nephrol.*17,2985-2991.

[51] Kanno Y.;Takenaka T.;Nakamura T., Suzuki H. (2006).Add-on angiotensin receptor blocker in patients who have proteinuric chronic kidney diseases and are treated with angiotensin-converting enzyme inhibitors. *Clin. J. Am. Soc. Nephrol.*1,730-737.

[52] Kunz R.;Friedrich C.;Wolbers M.; Mann JF. (2008).Meta-analysis: effect of monotherapy and combination therapy with inhibitors of the rennin angiotensin system on proteinuria in renal disease. *Ann. Intern. Med.*148,30-48.

[53] Lewis EJ.;Hunsicker LG.;Clarke WR.;Berl T.;Pohl MA.;Lewis JB.;Ritz E.;Atkins RC.;Rohde R., Raz I. (2001).Renoprotective effect of the angiotensin-receptor antagonist irbesartan in patients with nephropathy due to type 2 diabetes. *N Engl. J. Med.*345,851-860.

[54] Li PK.;Leung CB.;Chow KM.;Cheng YL.;Fung SK.;Mak SK.;Tang AW.;Wong TY.;Yung CY.;Yung JC.;Yu AW., Szeto CC. (2006).Hong Kong study using valsartan in IgA nephropathy (HKVIN): a double-blind, randomized, placebo-controlled study. *Am. J. Kidney Dis.*47,751-760.

[55] Wolf G. (2008).Novel aspects of the renin-angiotensin-aldosteronesystem. *Front Biosci.*13,4993-5005.

[56] Jagoda EM.;Vaquero JJ.;Seidel J.;Green MV., Eckelman WC. (2004).Experiment assessment of mass effects in the rat: implications for small animal PET imaging. *Nucl. Med. Biol.*31,771-779.

[57] Pimlott SL., Sutherland A. (2011) Molecular tracers for the PET and SPECT imaging of disease. *Chem. Soc. Rev.*40,149-162.

[58] Verjans JW.;Lovhaug D.;Narula N.;Petrov AD.;Indrevoll B.;Bjurgert E.;Krasieva TB.;Petersen LB.;Kindberg GM.;Solbakken M.;Cuthbertson A.;Vannan MA.;Reutelingsperger CP.;Tromberg B. J.;Hofstra L.; Narula J. (2008).Noninvasive imaging of angiotensin receptors after myocardial infarction. *JACC Cardiovasc. Imaging.*1,354-362.

[59] Mathews W. B.;Burns HD.;Dannals RF.;Ravert HT., Naylor EM. (1995).Carbon-11 Labeling of a Potent, Nonpeptide, AT1-Selective Angiotensin-II Receptor Antagonist: MK-996. Journal of Labelled Compounds and Radiopharmaceuticals.XXXVI,729-737.

[60] Mathews WB.;Yoo SE.;Lee SH.;Scheffel U.;Rauseo PA.;Zober TG.;Gocco G.;Sandberg K.;Ravert HT.;Dannals RF., Szabo Z. (2004).A novel radioligand for imaging the AT1 angiotensin receptor with PET. *Nucl. Med. Biol.*31,571-574.

[61] Hamill TG.;Burns HD.;Dannals RF.;Mathews WB.;Musachio JL.;Ravert HT., Naylor EM. (1996).Development of [11C]L-159,884: a radiolabelled, nonpeptide angiotensin II antagonist that is useful for angiotensin II, AT1 receptor imaging. *Appl. Radiat. Isot.*47,211-218.

[62] Kim SE.;Scheffel U.;Szabo Z.;Burns HD.;Gibson RE.;Ravert HT.;Mathews WB.;Hamill TG., Dannals RF. (1996).In vivo labeling of angiotensin II receptors with a carbon-11-labeled selective nonpeptide antagonist. *J. Nucl. Med.*37,307-311.

[63] Szabo Z.;Kao PF.;Burns HD.;Gibson RE.;Hamill TG.;Ravert HT.;Kim SE.;Mathews WB.;Musachio JL.;Scheffel U., Dannals RF. (1998).Investigation of angiotensin II/AT1 receptors with carbon-11-L-159,884: a selective AT1 antagonist. *J. Nucl. Med.*39,1209-1213.

[64] Zober TG.;Mathews WB.;Seckin E.;Yoo SE.;Hilton J.;Xia J.;Sandberg K.;Ravert HT.;Dannals RF., Szabo Z. (2006).PET Imaging of the AT1 receptor with [11C]KR31173. *Nucl. Med. Biol.*33,5-13.

[65] Xia J.;Seckin E.;Xiang Y.;Vranesic M.;Mathews WB.;Hong K.;Bluemke DA.;Lerman LO., Szabo Z. (2008).Positron-emission tomography imaging of the angiotensin II subtype 1 receptor in swine renal artery stenosis. *Hypertension.*51,466-473.

[66] Bravo P.;Fukushima K.;Higuchi T.;Voicu C.;Lodge M.;Mathews WB.;Dannals RF.;Szabo Z., Bengel F. M. (2011).Translational imaging of the myocardial angiotensin II type 1 receptor using C-11 KR31173 PET: From animal model to human application. *J. Nucl. Med.*52(Supplement 1).

[67] Hadizad T.;Kirkpatrick SA.;Mason S.;Burns K.;Beanlands RS., Dasilva JN. (2009).Novel O-[(11)C]methylated derivatives of candesartan as angiotensin II AT(1) receptor imaging ligands: radiosynthesis and ex vivo evaluation in rats. *Bioorg. Med. Chem.*17,7971-7977.

[68] Hadizad T.;Collins J.;Antoun R.;Beanlands RS., Dasilva JN.[11C]Methyl-losartan as a potential ligand for PET imaging angiotensin II AT1receptors. *J. Label Compd. Radiopharm.* In Press.

[69] Antoun R.;Hadizad T.;Thorn S.;Lortie M.;deKemp R.;Beanlands RS., Dasilva JN. (2010).In vivo evaluation of [11C]methyl-Losartan as a selective AT1R radioligands in rats. *J. Nucl. Med.*51(Supplement 2),1490.

[70] Hwang DR.;Eckelman WC.;Mathias CJ.;Petrillo EW. Jr.;Lloyd J., Welch MJ. (1991).Positron-labeled angiotensin-converting enzyme (ACE) inhibitor: fluorine-18-fluorocaptopril. Probing the ACE activity in vivo by positron emission tomography. *J. Nucl. Med.*32,1730-1737.

[71] Markham J.;McCarthy TJ.;Welch MJ., Schuster DP. (1995).In vivo measurements of pulmonary angiotensin-converting enzyme kinetics. I. Theory and error analysis. *J. Appl. Physiol.*78,1158-1168.

[72] Schuster DP.;McCarthy TJ.;Welch MJ.;Holmberg S.;Sandiford P., Markham J. (1995).In vivo measurements of pulmonary angiotensinconverting enzyme kinetics. II. Implementation and application. *J .Appl. Physiol.*78,1169-1178.

[73] Qing F.;McCarthy TJ.;Markham J., Schuster DP. (2000).Pulmonary angiotensin-converting enzyme (ACE) binding and inhibition in humans. A positron emission tomography study. *Am. J. Respir. Crit. Care Med.*161,2019-2025.

[74] Dilsizian V.;Eckelman WC.;Loredo ML.;Jagoda EM., Shirani J. (2007).Evidence for tissue angiotensin-converting enzyme in explanted hearts of ischemic cardiomyopathy using targeted radiotracer technique. *J. Nucl. Med.*48,182-187.

INDEX

A

B

C

D

E

F

G

H

I

J

K

L

M

N

O

P

Q

R

T

U

V

W

X

Y

Z